Gynecological Oncology

Kavita Singh • Bindiya Gupta
Editors

Gynecological Oncology

Basic Principles and Clinical Practice

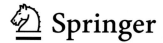

Editors
Kavita Singh
Pan Birmingham Gynaecology Cancer
Centre, City Hospital
Birmingham, UK

Bindiya Gupta
Department of Obstetrics & Gynecology
University College of Medical
Sciences & Guru Teg Bahadur Hospital
Delhi, India

ISBN 978-3-030-94109-3   ISBN 978-3-030-94110-9   (eBook)
https://doi.org/10.1007/978-3-030-94110-9

© The Editor(s) (if applicable) and The Author(s), under exclusive license to Springer Nature Switzerland AG 2022
This work is subject to copyright. All rights are solely and exclusively licensed by the Publisher, whether the whole or part of the material is concerned, specifically the rights of translation, reprinting, reuse of illustrations, recitation, broadcasting, reproduction on microfilms or in any other physical way, and transmission or information storage and retrieval, electronic adaptation, computer software, or by similar or dissimilar methodology now known or hereafter developed.
The use of general descriptive names, registered names, trademarks, service marks, etc. in this publication does not imply, even in the absence of a specific statement, that such names are exempt from the relevant protective laws and regulations and therefore free for general use.
The publisher, the authors and the editors are safe to assume that the advice and information in this book are believed to be true and accurate at the date of publication. Neither the publisher nor the authors or the editors give a warranty, expressed or implied, with respect to the material contained herein or for any errors or omissions that may have been made. The publisher remains neutral with regard to jurisdictional claims in published maps and institutional affiliations.

This Springer imprint is published by the registered company Springer Nature Switzerland AG
The registered company address is: Gewerbestrasse 11, 6330 Cham, Switzerland

Preface

Decision-making in gynaeoncology is critical for achieving best outcome of different treatment modalities in Gynaeoncology. This book is an attempt to develop easier and practical understanding for day-to-day management of clinical cases in gynaeoncology and at the same time incorporate scientific evidence in daily clinical practice in a simplistic manner. The concept of this book was conceived during Covid pandemic when direct exposure to patients was rationed and therefore more accurate understanding of assessment and management was critical.

The main motivation behind it was a quest for perfection and desire to do the best for our patients; a principle we both are passionate about. This book has been conceived in two volumes—the first volume focusses on basic principles and practices in Gynaecological oncology and the second volume shall discuss practical clinical management of real-time anonymised clinical case scenarios.

For an effective decision in a clinical case, one has to have a sound understanding of basics in gynaecological oncology relating to case assessment and examination, radiological and pathology investigations, knowledge of different treatment modalities and their impact on patient outcome, management of complications, optimisation and improvement of perioperative outcome and palliative care. We have included various chapters covering in detail the above-mentioned aspects, and, in addition, have incorporated chapters to facilitate obtaining information for practice of evidence-based care, consenting, effective communication, multidisciplinary approach to decision-making, hereditary cancers, and holistic treatment therapies.

It is humbling to see this book materialise from what started off as management discussions and scientific reading between both of us and then various experts and specialists joined us to get it into print. We are extremely thankful to the eminent authors who have kindly contributed in the book, sharing their vast clinical experience and expertise.

This book is a starter book for individuals wishing to pursue a subspeciality career in Gynaeoncology and is also a quick and easy reference guide for practicing clinicians.

Our book is dedicated to our patients who are our constant source of inspiration and learning…

Birmingham, UK Kavita Singh
New Delhi, India Bindiya Gupta

Contents

1. **Approach to a Case of Gynae Oncology** 1
   Bindiya Gupta and Kavita Singh

2. **Multidisciplinary Decision Making in Gynaeoncology: Guidance, Conduct and Legalities** 11
   Andrew Phillips and Benjamin Burrows

3. **Consent and Communication Skills in Management of Gynaeoncology** 19
   Aarti Lakhiani and Sudha Sundar

4. **Holistic Approach Towards Managing Patients in Case Management in Gynaeoncology** 27
   Audrey Fong Lien Kwong, Catherine Spencer, and Sudha Sundar

5. **Clinical Evidence in Gynaeoncology: Sources and Application** 35
   Elaine Leung and Sudha Sundar

6. **Surgical Principles and Practices in Gynaecological Oncology: Achieving the Best Outcome** 51
   Janos Balega and Desmond Barton

7. **Techniques of Enhanced Recovery in Post Operative Care** 61
   Shweta Sharma and Bindiya Gupta

8. **Surgical Complications in Gynaecological Oncology** 73
   Kavita Singh and Bindiya Gupta

9. **Minor Procedures in Gynaecological Oncology** 87
   Felicia Elena Buruiana, Rajendra Gujar, and Bindiya Gupta

10. **Management of Complications: Chemotherapy Related Complications, Acute Bowel Obstruction, Symptomatic Ascites and Pleural Effusion, Pulmonary Embolism, Deep Vein Thrombosis, Severe Pain, Chylous Ascites** 107
    Anastasios Tranoulis, Howard Joy, and Bindiya Gupta

11	**Chemotherapy in Gynaecological Cancers and Newer Developments** 123
	Michael Tilby, Sarah Williams, and Jennifer Pascoe
12	**Hormonal Treatment in Gynaecological Malignancies** 139
	Anastasios Tranoulis and Indrajit N. Fernando
13	**Radiation Protocols Relevant for Gynaecological Oncology and Management of Complications** 147
	Beshar Allos, Indrajit N. Fernando, and Nawaz Walji
14	**Palliative Care in Gynaecologic Oncology** 161
	Seema Singhal, Milind Arolker, and Rakesh Garg
15	**Clinical Interpretation of Immunohistochemistry in Gynaecological Cancers** 173
	William Boyle, Matthew Evans, and Josefa Vella
16	**Genomics in Gynaecological Cancer: What the Clinician Needs to Know** 193
	Anca Oniscu, Ayoma Attygalle, and Anthony Williams
17	**Role of Genetics in Gynaecological Cancers** 207
	Ashwin Kalra, Monika Sobocan, Dan Reisel, and Ranjit Manchanda
18	**Radiology Investigations and Interventions in Gynaeoncology** 221
	Lohith Ambadipudi
19	**Post-operative Care in Gynaecological Oncology** 235
	Christine Ang

Annexure: Staging of Gynaecological Cancers 253

Index 259

Editors and Contributors

About the Editors

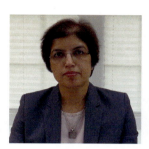

Kavita Singh is an experienced clinician working in a reputed busy cancer centre in the UK based at Pan Birmingham Gynaecology Cancer Centre. She is the clinical lead for surgical delivery of care for all types of gynaecological cancers and is also the Programme Director for subspeciality training in Gynaeoncology. She is well known in the UK for her surgical performance and surgical training skills and attracts trainees to come and train under her from the UK and abroad. She is a keen teacher with immense clinical experience and has achieved the best survival outcomes in Gynaecological oncology care in the UK for her centre.She has innovated several surgical techniques in her clinical practice and her complex surgical expertise attracts referrals from the UK and abroad. She communicates well and has presented in several professional meetings.She has contributed several book chapters and has been the subeditor for Gynaecological oncology sections in books and published several papers in peer reviewed journals. She is a reviewer for several journals and holds regular training courses in anatomy and surgical techniques. Her training experience extends from having worked in India, UK, France, Africa, and the USA. She is well recognised in her NHS performance by obtaining several clinical excellence awards.

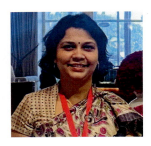

Bindiya Gupta works as an Associate Professor in Obstetrics and Gynaecology at UCMS & GTB Hospital, Delhi, India. She completed her fellowship in gynaecologic oncology from Pan Birmingham Gynaecology Cancer Centre, Birmingham, UK under the Commonwealth Exchange Programme. She is an editor of five books, has more than 75 indexed publications in national and international journals of repute, and has contributed several chapters in books. She is also a reviewer of several international journals and has received several awards including the FIGO award for best paper from a developing country. She is an active member of various organisations like ISCCP, AOGIN-India, etc., and has delivered lectures in various national and international conferences.

Contributors

Beshar Allos Cancer Centre, University Hospitals Birmingham NHS Foundation Trust, Birmingham, UK

Lohith Ambadipudi Department of Radiology, University Hospital of North Durham, County Durham and Darlington NHS Foundation Trust, Durham, UK

Christine Ang Northern Gynaecological Oncology Centre, Queen Elizabeth Hospital, Gateshead, UK

Milind Arolker University of Birmingham, Birmingham, UK

Ayoma Attygalle The Royal Marsden NHS Foundation Trust, London, UK

Janos Balega Pan-Birmingham Gynaecological Cancer Centre, City Hospital, Birmingham, UK

Desmond Barton The Royal Marsden Hospital, London, UK

William Boyle Birmingham Women's and Children's NHS Trust, Birmingham, UK

Benjamin Burrows Family Practice Western College, Bristol, UK

Bristol, North Somerset and South Gloucester Clinical Commissioning Group, Western College, Cotham, Bristol, UK

Felicia Elena Buruiana Pan Birmingham Gynaecological Cancer Centre, Birmingham, UK

Matthew Evans Black Country Pathology Services, Wolverhampton, UK

Editors and Contributors

Indrajit N. Fernando University Hospitals Birmingham NHS Foundation Trust, Birmingham, UK

Rakesh Garg Department of Onco-Anaesthesiology and Palliative Medicine, Dr BRAIRCH, All India Institute of Medical Sciences, New Delhi, India

Rajendra Gujar Pan Birmingham Gynaecological Cancer Centre, Birmingham, UK

Bindiya Gupta Department of Obstetrics & Gynecology, University College of Medical Sciences & Guru Teg Bahadur Hospital, Delhi, India

Howard Joy Sandwell and West Birmingham Hospitals NHS Trust, Birmingham, UK

Ashwin Kalra Wolfson Institute of Population Health, Queen Mary, University of London, London, UK

Audrey Fong Lien Kwong Pan Birmingham Gynaecological Cancer Centre, City Hospital, Birmingham, UK

Aarti Lakhiani Pan Birmingham Gynae Cancer Centre, Birmingham, UK

Elaine Leung Pan-Birmingham Gynaecological Cancer Centre, Birmingham City Hospital, Birmingham, UK

Ranjit Manchanda Wolfson Institute of Population Health, Queen Mary, University of London, London, UK

Anca Oniscu Royal Infirmary of Edinburgh, Edinburgh, UK

Jennifer Pascoe Oncology Department, Queen Elizabeth Hospital, University Hospital Birmingham NHS Foundation Trust, Birmingham, UK

Andrew Phillips Derby Gynaecological Cancer Centre, University Hospitals of Derby and Burton, Royal Derby Hospital, Derby, UK

Dan Reisel Department of Women's Cancer, Institute for Women's Health, University College London, London, UK

Shweta Sharma University College of Medical Sciences and Guru Teg Bahadur Hospital, Delhi, India

Kavita Singh Pan Birmingham Gynaecology Cancer Centre, City Hospital, Birmingham, UK

Seema Singhal Department of Obstetrics and Gynaecology, All India Institute of Medical Sciences, New Delhi, India

Monika Sobocan Wolfson Institute of Population Health, Queen Mary, University of London, London, UK

Catherine Spencer Pan Birmingham Gynaecological Cancer Centre, City Hospital, Birmingham, UK

Sudha Sundar Pan Birmingham Gynaecological Cancer Centre, City Hospital, Birmingham, UK

University Hospitals Birmingham NHS Foundation Trust, Birmingham, UK

Michael Tilby Oncology Department, Queen Elizabeth Hospital, University Hospital Birmingham NHS Foundation Trust, Birmingham, UK

Anastasios Tranoulis The Pan-Birmingham Gynaecological Cancer Centre, City Hospital, Birmingham, UK

Josefa Vella Birmingham Women's and Children's NHS Trust, Birmingham, UK

Nawaz Walji Arden Cancer Centre, University Hospitals Coventry and Warwickshire NHS Trust, Coventry, UK

Anthony Williams Birmingham Women's and Children's NHS Foundation Trust, Birmingham, UK

Sarah Williams Oncology Department, Queen Elizabeth Hospital, University Hospital Birmingham NHS Foundation Trust, Birmingham, UK

Approach to a Case of Gynae Oncology

Bindiya Gupta and Kavita Singh

1.1 Introduction

The overall burden of cancer incidence and mortality is on a rise worldwide. According to GLOBOCAN 2020, worldwide, an estimated 19.3 million new cancer cases and almost 10.0 million cancer deaths occurred in 2020 [1]. Gynaecological cancers are amongst the top 10 cancers worldwide. Amongst all gynaecological cancers, cervical cancer is the most common with age standardized incidence rate of 13.3/100,000 and is closely followed by uterine and ovarian cancer with incidence of 8.7/100,000 and 6.6/100,000 respectively.

In order to ensure uniform cancer treatment outcomes throughout the country and take care of the rising incidence of cancer, The Calman-Hine report in 1995 provided guidance for delivery of cancer care in UK [2]. The reorganized and restructured cancer delivery structure in UK is a hub and spoke model (Fig. 1.1) as follows:

1. Primary care: main focus of care
2. Cancer units (spokes): In district general hospitals to support clinical teams with sufficient expertise and facilities to mange the commoner cancers.
3. Cancer centers (hubs): provide expertise in management of all cancers and ones referred from cancer units. These provide specialized diagnostic services and treatment including radiotherapy.

The NHS cancer plan [3] takes care of issues in cancer care like allotment of funds, recruitment of specialists, strategies for cancer prevention, setting target times for waiting for diagnosis and treatment, provision of new equipment for imaging and treatment, introduction and availability of newer cancer drugs, developing NICE guidelines, cancer research, cancer services collaborative, partnership with charities for palliative care and training in communication skills.

1.2 The Diagnostic Pathway

Once the patient visits primary care; there are certain red flag signs and symptoms (Table 1.1) which warrant an urgent referral to specialist oncology care. The national target for referral for suspected cancer, is currently 2 weeks. **The oncology practitioner**, trained in sub-specialty of oncology, is pivotal in ensuring the success of cancer care. The oncologist should be well versed in evaluating the patient coming to the facility; be it a unit or a cancer center and should make individualized or

B. Gupta
Department of Obstetrics & Gynecology, University College of Medical Sciences & Guru Teg Bahadur Hospital, Delhi, India

K. Singh (✉)
Pan Birmingham Gynaecology Cancer Centre, City Hospital, Birmingham, UK
e-mail: kavitasingh@nhs.net

© The Author(s), under exclusive license to Springer Nature Switzerland AG 2022
K. Singh, B. Gupta (eds.), *Gynecological Oncology*, https://doi.org/10.1007/978-3-030-94110-9_1

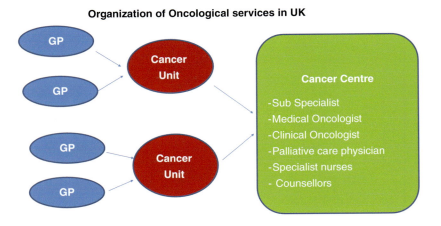

Fig. 1.1 Oncology service in UK: hub and spoke model

patient tailored treatment decisions in context of evidence based guidelines. They must understand the components of the patient visit which includes a comprehensive history and examination, advise appropriate investigations, make a tentative treatment plan and try to make the patient understand the likely course of the disease. Once the patient presents to a specialist gynae oncologist, the treatment should be started within 4 weeks.

All patients with suspected or confirmed cancers are discussed in multidisciplinary (MDT) team meetings, where gynae oncologist, clinical oncologists, pathologists, radiologists, nursing and other healthcare professionals collaboratively discuss individual patients and make recommendations for their treatment based on the available scientific evidence. MDT's help in better and quicker clinical decision-making, improved clinical outcomes, recruitment to clinical trials, and health professional satisfaction. Recommendations for treatments made in the meetings are then discussed with the patients and directly influence the decision-making process between patients and their clinician.

Besides considering traditional parameters to guide treatment like tumor characteristics, extent of spread and presence of metastasis; a holistic approach is essential. The latter includes consideration of socio economic factors, psychotherapy, social support system, positive reinforcements and predictive treatment like future implications on fertility and familial cancer risk. As soon as cancer is confirmed in a patient, specialist cancer nurses or cancer nurse specialists are assigned to the patients. These nurses help throughout the course of treatment, help the patient to understand the treatment options, provide emotional and psychological support, arrange patient care and follow up appointments in the hospital. They support the complex need of patients and also assist the specialists in decision making.

This chapter will outline the basic aspects of patient evaluation and diagnostic approach of gynaecological cancer.

1.3 History and Physical Assessment

This is the first step in evaluation of patients to reach a provisional diagnosis. The history of present illness tells about the presenting signs and symptoms; their onset, location, duration, characteristics, aggravating and relieving factors and the temporal sequence of events. In case of patients referred to specialist center, previous records of investigations and treatment should be analyzed in detail.

A full obstetric history including parity, desire for future fertility, use of contraception and history for infertility should be taken. Details about presence of chronic medical conditions like hypertension, diabetes etc., history of previous surgeries, blood transfusions etc. is also noted.

Table 1.1 Symptoms and signs of gynaecological malignancy

Cervical cancer
Abnormal vaginal bleeding: Intermenstrual, post menopausal, post coital
Vaginal discharge often malodourous, blood stained
Advanced cases: Pelvic pain, bowel and bladder pressure symptoms, passage of urine or faeces pervaginum
Examination: Presence of cervical growth, fistula in advanced cases, pyometra
Endometrial cancer[a]
Heavy menstrual bleeding, post menopausal bleeding
Advanced cases: Abdominal lump (pyometra, hematometra), ascites
Ovarian cancer
Early stage: Non specific and vague gastrointestinal, abdominal, and urinary symptoms[b]
Advanced cases: Abdominal mass, pain abdomen, ascites
Hormone producing tumours: Signs of virilization, post menopausal bleeding
Vulvar cancer
Vulva growth (warty, fleshy ulcerproliferative), bleeding, discharge, dysuria
Long standing and persistent vulval itching
Vulval skin discolouration or leucoplakia
Vaginal cancer
Vaginal discharge, often blood stained
Abnormal vaginal bleeding: Intermenstrual, post menopausal, post coital
Occasionally prior history of treatment for invasive or preinvasive disease of cervix or prior history of pelvic radiation
Fallopian tube cancer
Usually non specific and general symptoms like ovarian cancer
Triad: Pelvic mass, pelvic pain, profuse watery vaginal discharge
Systemic signs and symptoms (common to all cancers)
Weight loss, loss of appetite
Symptoms of metastatic disease: Lymphadenopathy (supraclavicular, axillary nodes, groin nodes), liver enlargement, umbilical nodule, dyspnea, bony pains, headaches, paraplegia, blindness and seizures

[a]Women are usually obese with history of metabolic syndrome in one-third cases
[b]Goff symptom index: occurrence of any of the eight symptoms including pelvic/abdominal pain, urinary urgency/frequency, increased abdominal size/bloating, and difficulty eating/feeling full more than 12 times a month for less than 1 year may be considered positive for ovarian cancer [4]

Physical assessment includes a comprehensive general physical, breast, respiratory, cardiovascular and abdominal examination. Important findings to be assessed are cachexia, presence and severity of pallor, lymphadenopathy (supraclavicular, axillary and inguinal) pedal edema, thyroid swelling, breast lump or nipple discharge, abdominal lump or organomegaly and presence of ascites.

A detailed pelvic and rectal examination helps to ascertain the nature of pelvic pathology and site of origin of the cancer of. Findings suggestive of malignancy include growth (cervical, vulval vaginal), enlarged uterus with restricted mobility, adenexal masses (unilateral or bilateral, more than 10 cm, fixed or restricted mobility), nodules in Pouch of Douglas and thickening of parametrium. Associated findings like vesicovaginal and rectovaginal fistula maybe present in advanced cervical cancer.

The common symptoms and signs of malignancy are summarized in Table 1.1.

Patient's level of functioning should also be assessed in terms of their ability to care for themselves, daily activity, and physical ability (walking, working, etc.). One of the measurements commonly used was developed by the Eastern Cooperative Oncology Group (ECOG) in 1982 and is available for public use (Table 1.2) [5].

At all times, during the patient interview, core therapeutic competencies that should be present include respect, empathy and genuineness. It establishes a bond with the patient and her relatives and gives positive reinforcement which is important for treatment success. The patient should be prepared mentally

Table 1.2 ECOG performance status

Grade	ECOG performance status
0	Fully active, able to carry on all pre-disease performance without restriction
1	Restricted in physically strenuous activity but ambulatory and able to carry out work of a light or sedentary nature, e.g., light house work, office work
2	Ambulatory and capable of all self care but unable to carry out any work activities; up and about more than 50% of waking hours
3	Capable of only limited self care; confined to bed or chair more than 50% of waking hours
4	Completely disabled; cannot carry on any self care; totally confined to bed or chair
5	Dead

from the first visit that the treatment may be multimodality and may require frequent hospital visits and follow ups.

1.4 Nutritional Assessment

Malnutrition is common in oncology patients especially elderly and in certain cancers like ovarian cancer and has a significant impact on patient's post operative recovery. Symptoms at presentation like nausea, vomiting, pain abdomen, diarrhoea should be enquired as they alter the patient food intake. Detail must be known about the women medical and surgical history, co morbidities, life style and dietary habits to assess the nutrition status. Majority of women with cancer have loss of appetite; hence detail must be obtained about daily calorie and protein intake and the deficit must be calculated. Percentage of weight loss in the last month is important and more than 5% is considered significant [6].

Body Mass Index (Weight in kg/Height in m^2) is an important tool to guide nutrition status. According to World Health Organization (WHO) criteria, the classification of undernourished, normal, overweight and obese are ≤ 18.5 kg/m^2, 18.5–24.9 kg/m^2, 25–29.9 9 kg/m^2 and ≥ 30 kg/m^2 respectively [7]. Other findings on examination that guide nutritional assessment include presence of ascites, presence of muscle wasting and cachexia, loss of subcutaneous fat and ankle or sacral edema.

Estimation of haemoglobin and serum albumin levels is an important nutritional guide. World Health Organization (WHO) has defined the normal values, mild moderate and severe anemia as ≥ 12 g/dl, 11–11.9 g/dl, 8–10.9 g/dl and ≤ 8 g/dl respectively [8]. The cut off values for serum albumin are >3.5 gm/dl, 3–3.5 g/dl, 2.1–2.9 g/dl and ≤ 2 g/dl for normal levels, mild, moderate and severe hypoalbunemia respectively [9].

Various validated screening tools like Patient Generated Global Assessment Tool (PG-SGA) [10], Malnutrition Universal Screening [11] and Mini Nutritional Assessment tools [12] and nutritional indices like serum ferritin, transferrin etc. are used in a research context.

Once a baseline nutritional assessment is done, measures like dietician referral, correction of calorie deficit, protein and iron supplementation should be undertaken to improve post operative outcomes. This is the right time to reinforce physical measures like deep breathing, stretching exercises, walking and mental relaxation techniques.

1.5 Assessment of Hereditary and Genetic Factors

All gynae oncologists should keep a low threshold of initiating a genetic assessment risk while evaluating a case of gynaecologic cancer. A detailed history should be taken regarding personal and family history (maternal or paternal lineage) which may suggest hereditary cancer. Some features in history that may suggest hereditary cancer are summarized in Table 1.3. These patients can then be referred for genetic counselling for detailed analysis, risk assessment and genetic testing.

Table 1.3 Features suggestive of hereditary cancer [13, 14]

- Early age (e.g., premenopausal breast cancer)
- Multiple primary cancers in a single individual (e.g., colorectal and endometrial cancer)
- Bilateral cancer in paired organs or multifocal disease (e.g., bilateral breast cancer or multifocal renal cancer)
- Clustering of the same type of cancer in close relatives (e.g., mother, daughter, and sisters with breast cancer)
- Cancers occurring in multiple generations of a family
- Occurrence of rare tumors (e.g. adrenocortical carcinoma, granulosa cell tumor of the ovary)
- History of epithelial ovarian, fallopian tube, or primary peritoneal cancer
- Unusual presentation of cancer (e.g. male breast cancer)
- Uncommon tumor histology (e.g. medullary thyroid carcinoma)
- Geographic or ethnic populations known to be at high risk of hereditary cancers

1.6 Psychological and Social Assessment

Diagnosis of cancer can lead to manifestation of psychological problems and exacerbation of underlying psychiatric disorder. Upto 50% of patient's experience adjustment disorders, anxiety and depression following diagnosis [15]. Psychological morbidity is associated with reduction in quality of life, impaired social relationships, increased risk of suicides, longer rehabilitation time, poor compliance and a shorter survival [16].

It is important for the treating doctor to screen for such conditions by asking specific questions affecting individual's vulnerability like enquiring about life events, chronic stress, social and family support, health attitudes, addictions etc. Language, ethnicity, race, religion should be kept in mind while addressing such issues. It is useful to counsel and ask the patients in the presence of a close relative. The treating physician should be empathetic while breaking bad news and should ensure the person is accompanied with a close relative or friend. A clear idea should be obtained about the patient and family perception of the illness, coping mechanism and psychological response to cancer diagnosis.

In cases where the person has an underlying psychiatric disorder, she should be referred for proper consultation and treatment. Assessment should be made regarding patient social support system and cases should be referred to community nursing services for continuous supportive care. In special situations help of special support services like stoma care nurses, counsellors, cancer support groups can be obtained.

1.7 Investigations

Investigations are directed towards confirmation of diagnosis, ascertaining the stage and spread of tumour, treatment planning, surveillance and detection and treatment of recurrence during follow up. Investigations include haematological tests, tumor markers, urine examination (routine, microscopy and culture), imaging and specialized diagnostic test like colposcopy, endoscopy etc.

1.7.1 Hematological Investigations

Routine preoperative investigations include a hemogram, baseline coagulation profile, blood sugar (fasting/post prandial), Liver and kidney function tests. Serum albumin is an important measure of the nutritional status of the patient.

1.7.2 Tumor Markers

Tumor markers are used for screening, diagnosis, prognosis, assessing therapeutic response, and detecting recurrence. They are also important during surveillance post treatment. Serial rise in the values after normalization may indicate recurrence, while persistence of tumor marker post treatment indicates persistence disease.

Tumor markers play an important role in ovarian cancer. CA125 is the most common used marker for ovarian epithelial cancers and plays an important role as an adjunct to imaging in diagnosis of epithelial ovarian cancers (EOC). It is a part of the Risk of Malignancy index (RMI) algorithm

Table 1.4 Risk of Malignancy index

RMI = U × M × CA-125
The **ultrasound score** is calculated by awarding 1 point for each of the following characteristics: Multilocular cyst; Evidence of solid areas; Evidence of metastases; Presence of ascites; Bilateral lesions U = 0, if none of the above listed features is found U = 1, for ultrasound score of 1 U = 3, for ultrasound score ≥ 2 **CA-125** = serum CA-125 in kU/l **Menopausal status** (M = 1 if premenopausal and M = 3 if postmenopausal)

Table 1.5 Simple IOTA rules for predicting benign or malignant ovarian tumors

Rules for predicting malignant tumor (M-rules)	Rules for predicting a benign tomor (B-rules)
M1: Irregular solid masses	B1: Unilocular cyst
M2: Presence of ascites	B2: Presence of solid portion (maximum diameter < 7 mm)
M3: Minimum four papillary structures	
M4: Irregular multiolocular solid tumors (maximum diameter ≥ 100 mm)	B3: Presence of acoustic shadows
	B4: Smooth multilocular tumor (maximum diameter < 100 mm)
M5: Abundant blood flow signals (colour score 4)	B5: Without blood flow signal (colour score 1)

(Table 1.4) which is a triage tool for evaluation of adnexal masses. Using an RMI cut-off of 200, a sensitivity of 70% and specificity of 90% can be achieved in prediction of malignancy [17].

All cases with RMI of more than 200 should be presented in multidisciplinary tumor board meeting and should be operated by a gynae oncologist. Other markers used for evaluation of EOC are Carcinoembryonic antigen (CEA) and Carbohydrate antigen 19–9 (CA19–9). An elevated CEA may indicate a gastrointestinal primary while CA19–9 is increased in primary mucinous adenocarcinoma of ovary or secondary tumours from pancreas, gastrointestinal tract and appendix. CA15–3 is elevated in primary breast cancer.

Beta-hCG, alpha-fetoprotein, lactate dehydrogenase (LDH) have proved to be useful markers for ovarian germ cell tumours. Alpha fetoprotein is elevated in endodermal sinus tumours while beta-HCG is elevated in non gestational choriocarcinoma. Beta HCG is also increased in some cases of dysgerminoma, embryonal carcinomas, polyembryomas and mixed cell tumours. LDH and placental alkaline phosphatase are elevated in dysgerminomas.

There is not much role of tumor markers in endometrial cancer, but an elevated CA125 indicates advanced disease, extrauterine spread and poor prognosis. It may be useful to monitor treatment response if it was elevated prior to treatment. Beta HCG is also elevated in gestational trophoblastic disease.

An elevated inhibin level in a postmenopausal woman is suggestive of a granulosa cell tumor. Squamous cell antigen in cancer cervix is not used routinely; its use is mainly restricted for research purposes.

1.7.3 Imaging

Imaging can identify the primary tumor, assess localized spread and distant metastasis, lymph node assessment, provide guidance for radiation ports, monitor treatment response, and post-treatment surveillance to detect recurrent disease. The main modalities of imaging are ultrasonography (gray scale and doppler), Contrast enhanced computed tomography (CECT), magnetic resonance (MR) imaging and PET–CT scan (Positron enhanced computed tomography).

Ultrasound is the first tool to evaluate adnexal masses and the International Ovarian Tumor Analysis (IOTA) have developed simple, diagnostic algorithm to characterize adnexal mass. It has defined ten simple ultrasound rules (five benign and five malignant signs) (Table 1.5) which have a sensitivity 91.66% and specificity 84.84% to characterize malignant and benign masses [18].

Transvaginal sonography is also the first tool for evaluation of postmenopausal bleeding and the endometrial thickness cut off used is 4 mm.

Local staging of uterine and cervical malignancies is primarily done with MR imaging whereas ovarian malignancies are typically staged by CT scan of chest abdomen and pelvis. Newer tools such as DWI and dynamic contrast-enhanced imaging may result in improved lesion characterization and staging but are not routinely used. The relevant radiological investigations and their indications for gynaecological cancers are summarized in Table 1.6 [19–22].

Table 1.6 Radiological investigations according to cancer site

Cervical cancer
MRI:
– **First line investigation** for staging: assess tumor size, parametrial extension (presence of intact stromal ring), suspected bladder or rectal involvement
– Fertility sparing surgery (radical trachelectomy)[a], surveillance post tracehlectomy
– Post chemoradiation to assess reponse to treatment
– Recurrent disease (pelvic recurrence: planning for pelvic exenteration, salvage surgery)
PET CT scan (preferred)/Contrast enhanced Computed Tomography Chest + abdomen + pelvis):
– Treatment planning: adjuvant radiation, stage II and above when patient is for primary chemoradiation
– Suspected distant metastasis

Endometrial cancer
MRI:
– **First line investigation** to assess site of tumor origin, size, myometrial invasion, extension to cervix and surrounding pelvic tissue
– Fertility sparing treatment (Planning and surveillance)
– Recurrent disease (pelvic recurrence)
– MRI brain: symptoms s/o brain metastasis, or lung metastasis on Chest CT
Transvaginal sonography:
Primary investigation for post menopausal bleeding, can also be used to assess tumor origin, growth size, and diagnose myometrial/cervical invasion where MRI is not available or contraindicated
CECT chest + abdomen + pelvis
– High grade endometrioid cancer, non endometrioid histology to exclude metastasis and lymph node spread
– Recurrent disease with abdominal or pulmonary symptoms
CECT chest: Suspicious findings on X ray chest
PET CT scan:
– Adjuvant radiation treatment planning
– Recurrent disease with abdominal or pulmonary symptoms

Ovarian cancer
CECT chest + abdomen + pelvis
First line investigation to evaluate extent of disease
Treatment decision: Primary debulking versus neo adjuvant chemotherapy[b]
Assessment of response to chemotherapy
Post treatment surveillance (based on clinical symptoms, examination findings, rising CA125 levels)
Recurrent ovarian cancer (disseminated versus oligo metastatic disease; planning secondary cytoreduction)
Image guided biopsy
MRI brain: If chest CT suggestive of lung metastasis
Transvaginal + transabdominal sonography
Morphological assessment of adnexal masses[c]
Ascitic tapping/image guided biopsy

Vulvar cancer
Contrast enhanced computed tomography chest + abdomen + pelvis
– Large tumours (>4 cm)
– Tumours involving vagina, urethra, anal canal
– Pelvic/abdominal/pulmonary symptoms
– Suspicious findings on X ray chest: chest CT scan

Uterine sarcoma
CECT chest + abdomen + pelvis
To assess tumor size, local and abdominal spread
Post treatment surveillance
Incidental diagnosis post TAH done for fibroid uterus especially with history of intraoperative morcellation or specimen fragmentation
PET CT scan
Suspected distant metastasis

[a] Determine tumor size, length of cervix, distance of tumor from internal os
[b] Indicators of neoadjuvant chemotherapy: Multiple liver parenchymal metastasis, disseminated high volume disease with involvement of small bowel, bulky porta hepatis disease, involvement of coeliac trunk, mesenteric infiltration or retraction, retrocrural or suprarenal RP nodes), Stage IV disease with lung, mediastinum and brain metastasis
[c] MRI may be done occasionally in indeterminate adnexal masses. PET is typically reserved for indeterminate lesions on CT/MR that would preclude primary surgery or in the recurrent setting

1.7.4 Histopathology and Cytology

Histopathological evaluation is the final confirmation of the type and grade of cancer. An endometrial and cervical punch or loop biopsy is required to confirm endometrial and cervical cancer respectively. Vulval biopsy using either a keye's punch biopsy or wedge biopsy is done to confirm vulval cancer. In case of ovarian cancer, cytological evaluation of ascitic fluid can be done. Sometimes when the results are inconclusive or in absence of ascites, an image (CT or ultrasound) guided biopsy is usually taken from the omental mass, nodal mass or peritoneal nodules. Biopsy from ovarian mass is usually avoided, especially in early stages. Occasionally, when image guided biopsy is inconclusive, a diagnostic laparoscopy may be done to confirm cancer.

A detailed histologic assessment of the surgical specimen according to standard reporting protocols is vital in all cancers, as it confirms the final stage of cancer and helps to guide adjuvant treatment.

1.7.5 Other Investigations

Upper and Lower GI endoscopy may be done in conditions where there are bilateral masses, mucinous in nature or high levels of CEA and CA19–9 in order to exclude a GI primary. Mammography may be done to exclude breast primary. In cases with positive cervical cancer screening tests, colposcopy is done to rule out microinvasive cervical cancer.

1.8 Conclusion

1.8.1 Cancer Care: The Holistic Approach!!

To conclude, treating cancers is not only diagnosing and treating a disease, but it is patient tailored application of evidence based therapeutics by an expert team of specialized professionals along with psychological and social support, ensuring both physical and mental well being of the patient. In this era of diagnostics, the art of detailed history and physical examination should not be forgotten and investigations should be chosen wisely according to the disease.

Key Points

1. In order to take care of the rising incidence of gynaecological cancer and to ensure uniformity in delivery of cancer care, the reorganized and restructured cancer delivery structure in UK is a hub and spoke model which consists of primary care, cancer units (spokes) and cancer centers (hubs).
2. In UK, the national target for referral for suspected cancer, is currently 2 weeks. Once the patient presents to a specialist gynae oncologist, the treatment should be started within 4 weeks.
3. Patient evaluation consists of a detailed history, detailed examination, nutritional assessment, genetic and hereditary factors and psychological and social assessment.
4. Investigations are directed towards confirmation of diagnosis, ascertaining the stage and spread of tumour, treatment planning, surveillance and detection and treatment of recurrence during follow up.
5. Tumour markers are used for screening, diagnosis, prognosis, assessing therapeutic response, and detecting recurrence. CA125 is the most important tumour marker in gynaecologic oncology
6. Transvaginal sonography is the first tool for evaluation of postmenopausal bleeding and adnexal masses (IOTA B and M signs). Local staging of uterine and cervical malignancies is primarily done with MR imaging whereas ovarian malignancies are typically staged by CT scan of chest abdomen and pelvis.

7. A detailed histologic assessment of the surgical specimen according to standard reporting protocols is important, as it confirms the final stage of cancer and helps to guide adjuvant treatment.
8. A holistic approach in cancer care is required to ensure both physical and mental well being of the patient. Treatment approaches should be individualised in context of latest scientific evidence.

References

1. Sung H, Ferlay J, Siegel RL, Laversanne M, Soerjomataram I, Jemal A, Bray F. Global cancer statistics 2020: GLOBOCAN estimates of incidence and mortality worldwide for 36 cancers in 185 countries. CA Cancer J Clin. 2021;71(3):209–49.
2. Munro AJ. Forum for applied cancer education and training. Eur J Cancer Care (Engl). 2001;10(3):212–20.
3. The NHS Cancer Plan. Available at: https://www.thh.nhs.uk/documents/_Departments/Cancer/NHSCancerPlan.pdf. Accessed 13 Mar 2021.
4. Goff BA, Mandel LS, Drescher CW, Urban N, Gough S, Schurman KM, et al. Development of an ovarian cancer symptom index: possibilities for earlier detection. Cancer. 2007;109:221–7.
5. Oken M, Creech R, Tormey D, et al. Toxicity and response criteria of the Eastern Cooperative Oncology Group. Am J Clin Oncol. 1982;5:649–55.
6. Beghetto MG, Luft VC, Mello ED, Polanczyk CA. Accuracy of nutritional assessment tools for predicting adverse hospital outcomes. Nutr Hosp. 2009;24:56–62.
7. Ali SM, Lindstrom M. Socioeconomic, psychosocial, behavioural, and psychological determinants of BMI among young women: differing patterns for underweight and overweight/obesity. Eur J Pub Health. 2006;16:325–31.
8. WHO, Haemoglobin concentrations for the diagnosis of anaemia and assessment of severity. 2001. [Last accessed on 2021 Feb 28]. Available from http://www.WHO/NMH/NHD/MNM/11.1
9. Lai CC, You JF, Yeh CY, Chen JS, Tang R, Wang JY, et al. Low preoperative serum albumin in colon cancer: a risk factor for poor outcome. Int J Color Dis. 2011;26:473–81.
10. Ottery FD. Definition of standardized nutritional assessment and interventional pathways in oncology. Nutrition. 1996;12:S15–9.
11. Chao PC, Chuang HJ, Tsao LY, Chen PY, Hsu CF, Lin HC, Chang CY, Lin CF. The Malnutrition Universal Screening Tool (MUST) and a nutrition education program for high risk cancer patients: strategies to improve dietary intake in cancer patients. Biomedicine (Taipei). 2015;5(3):17.
12. Vellas B, Guigoz Y, Garry PJ, Nourhashemi F, Bennahum D, Lauque S, Albarede JL. The mini nutritional assessment (MNA) and its use in grading the nutritional state of elderly patients. Nutrition. 1999;15(2):116–22.
13. Randall LM, Pothuri B, Swisher EM, et al. Multidisciplinary summit on genetics services for women with gynecologic cancers: a Society of Gynecologic Oncology White Paper. Gynecol Oncol. 2017;146(2):217–24.
14. Committee on Practice Bulletins–Gynecology, Committee on genetics, Society of Gynecologic Oncology. Practice bulletin no 182: hereditary breast and ovarian cancer syndrome. Obstet Gynecol. 2017;130(3):e110–26.
15. Grassi L, Caruso R, Sabato S, Massarenti S, Nanni MG. The UniFe psychiatry working group coauthors. psychosocial screening and assessment in oncology and palliative care settings. Front Psychol. 2015;7(5):1485.
16. Mitchell AJ, Chan M, Bhatti H, Halton M, Grassi L, Johansen C, Meader N. Prevalence of depression, anxiety, and adjustment disorder in oncological, haematological, and palliative-care settings: a meta-analysis of 94 interview-based studies. Lancet Oncol. 2011;12(2):160–74.
17. RCOG, Royal College of Obstetricians and Gynaecologists. Ovarian cysts in postmenopausal women. Guideline no. 34. 2016.
18. IOTA Simple Rules and SRrisk calculator to diagnose ovarian cancer. Available at: https://www.iotagroup.org/iota-models-software/iota-simple-rules-and-srrisk-calculator-diagnose-ovarian-cancer. Accessed 25 Mar 2021.
19. NCCN guidelines.
20. Devine C, Viswanathan C, Faria S, Marcal L, Sagebiel TL. Imaging and staging of cervical cancer. Semin Ultrasound CT MR. 2019;40(4):280–6.
21. Faria SC, Devine CE, Rao B, Sagebiel T, Bhosale P. Imaging and staging of endometrial cancer. Semin Ultrasound CT MR. 2019;40(4):287–94.
22. Orr B, Edwards RP. Diagnosis and treatment of ovarian cancer. Hematol Oncol Clin North Am. 2018;32(6):943–64.

Multidisciplinary Decision Making in Gynaeoncology: Guidance, Conduct and Legalities

Andrew Phillips and Benjamin Burrows

2.1 Introduction

Prior to the 1995 Calman-Hine report [1] the care of cancer patients in England and Wales was extremely disjointed. Individual clinicians with varying levels of expertise, experience, and caseload took patients through from diagnosis to treatment in accordance with their own beliefs and processes, often in isolation to other expert healthcare professionals. Whilst collaborative expert decision-making occurred in some cancer types, this was not typical across all cancers. Such care, in the hands of a single clinician, often lacked pathways, missed opportunities for treatment and ultimately generated poorer outcomes for patients [2]. The problem with a single clinician fully determining care was that it was at their discretion whether or not to utilize any input from an extended group of professionals (such as medical or clinical oncology) whose earlier involvement may have changed the nature of that patients pathway. The lack of involvement from others, and the missed opportunity for alternative strategies to be discussed, meant that the opinions and beliefs of that one individual remained unchecked, resulting in a lack of quality assurance. In the absence of formalized meetings with documented outcomes, there was limited ability to generate meaningful outcome data at a local or national level pertinent to cancer care. Hospitals were therefore unable to assess how disease was being managed and there was no ability to quantify the outcomes of treatment. Finally, communication to patients was at the discretion of the treating clinician, potentially resulting in less patient centered treatments for a less well informed and less empowered patient group.

The publication of the Calman-Hine report [1] set the scene for a revolution in the management of cancer patients. Central to the recommendations was the formulation of multi-disciplinary team (MDT) meetings, a regular event with a defined group of specialist members who would evaluate the evidence and recommend what they collectively believed to be the optimal management of that specific patients' cancer in that specific patients' situation. This proposed treatment remained only ever a recommendation with final management decided between the patient and the treating clinician. However, with the formulation of the MDT, decision making became more transparent, evidence-based, consistent and allowed consideration of the breadth of treatment options.

A. Phillips (✉)
Derby Gynaecological Cancer Centre,
University Hospitals of Derby and Burton,
Royal Derby Hospital, Derby, UK
e-mail: Andrew.phillips6@nhs.net

B. Burrows
Family Practice Western College, Bristol, UK

Bristol, North Somerset and South Gloucester Clinical Commissioning Group, Western College, Cotham, Bristol, UK

These MDTs rapidly became the standard of care for cancer services in England. Following the National Health Services (NHS) cancer plan in 2000 which further confirmed and refined the central role of MDTs so that "all patients have the benefit of the range of expert advice needed for high quality care" [3], the proportion of patients discussed in MDT meetings increased from less than 20% in 1994 to more than 80% in 2004 [4]. Not only were MDTs an organisational and governance success but, as expected, they objectively improved patient outcomes by reducing treatment variation and maintaining standards [5–11].

MDTs have therefore been a critical aspect of cancer care in England for the last two decades yet questions still remain regarding the future of the MDT and the value that they bring. Those not in favour might argue that as treatment variation still exists, the MDTS either lack power to maintain standards or are limited in their abilities to reduce variation. Furthermore, some have suggested that the perceived improvement in patient outcomes following the creation of MDTs is strongly confounded by the societal and therapeutic changes over the same time period [12].

Such questions remain to be answered and perhaps it would be difficult to truly unravel the benefit of such a mainstream yet expensive resource to an individuals' care. Despite the difficulties in identifying the value of the MDT in its own right, we know that MDTs change and refine decisions and assure quality of the treatment given. Indeed, the MDT is recognized as the "gold standard" with regards to cancer management [13]. The activity of this gold standard has steadily expanded with increasing patient numbers and patient complexity as well as the transition from managing initial to recurrent disease alongside performance evaluation and educational roles [4]. The MDT is therefore under increasing pressure to deliver quality decisions based upon ever greater time pressures. Despite these concerns MDTs have flourished locally and internationally [14] and expanded outside of cancer care with increasing use in chronic benign conditions (such as diabetes or ischaemic heart disease) over the last 25 years. Whilst the terminology describing such a team of specialists may vary between MDT, multi-disciplinary meetings, multi-disciplinary cancer conferences, or tumour boards, the principles of accountable, complete, expert led, evidence-based decision making remain the hallmark.

The chapter is written in accordance with national guidelines for multidisciplinary teams (MDTs) working in England. As such we discuss how the decisions arising from the MDT should be applied in view of the English legal system. Whilst the principles of MDT decision making, conduct and the legal position regarding MDT recommendations will have similar themes worldwide, international readers need to be aware that there may be variations in the specific legal requirements and the remit of the MDT depending on which country the MDT functions within.

2.2 Characteristics of a Good MDT

Whilst the concept of a collaborative team was an early objective for improving cancer care, it was only with the publication of the Characteristics of an Effective Multidisciplinary Team [2] that a statement on the qualities of participants, facilities, resources and conduct were specified. As the MDT strives to encourage high value opinions from the range of members to enable patients to be treated as individuals, certain process and behaviors need to established. Crudely these can be summarized as the information given to the MDT, the outputs generated by the MDT and the personal, behavioral and structural aspects of the MDT as a whole.

It is self-explanatory that patients need to be discussed on basis of correct information. As such, the treating clinician is best positioned to present the case to the MDT. If they are not available, an accurate record of the present situation should be submitted and increasingly MDTs are using proformas to ensure that key information datasets are presented. However, the details provided should not only be framed from a clinical perspective but also adopt a more holistic approach addressing the psychosocial issues of that patient as well considering any palliative or other supportive measures. Increasingly there have been moves to involve the patients themselves in the MDT meeting supporting the adage of "no decisions about me without me". The patients' medical records and previous MDT outcomes (if relevant) need to be available as well as both present and historical radiological images and any relevant histopathological samples. In situations where incomplete information is supplied, the discussion of that case should be postponed until further clinical information is sought, or, if an MDT recommendation is required to be made in absentia, limitations of the clinical information should be clearly documented on the MDT outcome.

The decision-making unit of the MDT should consist of an eclectic group of medical experts with knowledge of the breadth of treatment options for the specific cancer type being treated. What makes a specialist opinion varies but for the purpose of this chapter we consider it to be granted by some form of accreditation for the services supplied by that professional. As such in a Gynaecological cancer MDT, core members would include Gynaecological Oncologists, Clinical Oncologists and Medical Oncologists but other specialists may be included if their input is considered valuable such as palliative physicians or surgeons from other disciplines. Additionally, MDTs need to have the correct information presented to them and as such specialist gynaecological radiologists and pathologist are also essential. To ensure that the clinical question is correctly presented, the clinician treating the patient should ideally be in attendance as should the clinical nurse specialist who is the key worker for that patient. The final team member is the MDT coordinator who is tasked with preparing the meeting, recording discussions and releasing outputs.

Following the discussion, an MDT output should be generated prospectively in real time with the conclusions able to be checked by all team members. This is best accomplished by projection onto a screen that all can see. This forms the recommendation from the MDT. The final decision regarding treatment rests between the treating clinician and the patient but should take into consideration the MDTs recommendations. The MDT recommendation therefore needs to be fed back to all those involved in the patients care and in turn if the given management deviates significantly from it, the reasons for this should be revealed to the MDT to enable their decision-making processes to improve. Part of the outcome should record any relevant high-quality trials suitable for that patient, appropriate sources of information pertinent to their condition and any key national outcome date.

2.3 People and Processes

As the MDT can be characterized as a meeting of knowledge and opinions formed from accurate clinical details, it is important that all members have dedicated in work time to travel to and attend for any cases for which they are needed. The discourse should be respectful and productive even when the cases discussed generate strong feelings or emotions. As such, there should be mutual respect and an equal voice for all MDT members. Examples of such respectful productive behavior would be to silence mobile phones during the meeting or if a call is absolutely necessary, taking it outside of the MDT environment. More obvious failings, such as aggressive language and belittling, are clearly inappropriate and conflict should be actively resolved and debate constructive. All parties should enter into discussions in good spirits without personal agendas working to share best practice and generate effective decision making. Beyond the clinical expertise of MDT members, there are certain key positions that are required to be held to ensure a smooth running of the MDT. These roles are the Chair, the Leader and the Coordinator of the MDT. Whilst the roles of Chair and Lead may be performed by the same person, there should be a deputation system in place for situations where the Chair is unable to attend.

The Chair is responsible for the smooth running of the MDT meeting. The Chair does not need to be fixed and may change for different MDT sessions and, whilst in the authors' experience they are often a Gynaecological Oncologist, this is by no means essential and MDTs are often Chaired effectively by Clinical Nurse Specialists or other members of the MDT. The Chair sets the tempo of the MDT, discussing cases from an agenda agreed with the Coordinator. They make sure that the meeting is quorate (and taking action if it is not) and keep a register of attendance. They ensure that all cases are discussed in a focused, respectful and relevant way and that the treatment suggested is evidence-based and patient-centred. Finally, they ensure that outcomes are complete, any relevant trials have been considered, treatment recommendations are correctly documented and that all essential demographic and/or clinical data is recorded before moving on to the next patient. Certain people and personalities are more natural fits for the role of Chair but, in general, welcome attributes include being excellent at people management, a good listener and communicator with the ability to manage disruptive personalities. Additionally, the Chair should be aware of the limitations of the MDT members and be prepared to introduce any new or transient members if particular expertise is required. The Chair should be able to build a consensual clinical decision in a timely fashion and should have an approach if any conflict occurs. This later scenario is particularly damaging to MDT function and we suggest that defaulting to a vote in order to determine recommendations should be avoided in almost all situations. If a collaborative decision cannot be made, a number of options should be presented for the treating clinician to discuss with the patient.

The **Lead**, who may or may not also be the Chair, is responsible for the organisation and governance of the MDT and represents the MDT to the wider hospital organisation. They should ensure that the MDT is appropriately funded and raise concerns to the organisation of any issues that may affect the functioning of the MDT function. Additionally, they should be involved in updating the operational policy which should contain information regarding who the MDT members are, how the membership can evolve, what the standard management policies are (including how they conform to national policy and when they are due to be updated) and how information will be communicated following the MDT meeting. The operational policy along with the behaviour of the Lead should form the governance structure of the MDT.

Finally, the MDT **Coordinator** is responsible for the administrative preparation of the MDT. They should ensure that radiological, pathological and clinical resources are available, and present the final agenda for consideration to the Chair. They ensure that MDT decision-making and key demographic data are recorded and thus need to be positioned so that they can see and hear all contributions from all members during the meeting so that they can record MDT decisions in an accurate and real-time manner. They should ensure that the MDT agenda, listed in a logical order, is distributed prior to an agreed cut-off date to allow members to prepare for the meeting and to allow tracking of patients through the treatment process. Additionally, they should circulate the agreed outcomes back to the relevant clinical teams within an agreed time frame.

2.4 Environment

For a specialist team to function effectively it needs to have appropriate facilities. Whilst traditionally these consisted of a dedicated, sound-proofed room large enough for all members to be able to sit, hear and engage with the conversation, increasingly, and especially during the coronavirus pandemic, video conferencing has been utilized allowing social distancing and effective engagement. Irrespective of the medium of the meeting histopathological slides, radiological images and the prospectively recorded MDT outcome need to be projected clearly. The purpose of having the MDT outcome projected is to allow attendees to correct any inaccuracies as they are discussed. Whilst it has always been encouraged that an any technology utilized in the MDT is kept up to date to allow efficient use of clinical time and to ensure data security, the growth of video-conferencing additionally means that hospitals need to ensure that their data connection speeds and the video conferencing platforms are sufficient for the MDTs needs. Finally, a move towards greater video conferencing is yet another push towards complete electronic records to enable all members to have access to a complete clinical picture.

2.5 Governance and Responsibilities

The remit of the MDT in England has developed significantly over the last 25 years. It has grown from being an organized meeting of specialized individuals into a coordinated meeting of an extended patient pathway with a mandate to document outcomes, evaluate services and educate professional teams and patients alike. Such a wide-ranging brief may however not be appropriate for all MDTs internationally. As such, thought needs to be put into which patients should be discussed and which clinical questions are appropriate for the MDT to address. Examples of this include whether or not to discuss only newly diagnosed patients or all patients including those with recurrences? And what about private patients?

Such a wide-ranging role of the MDT makes it a vital yet expensive resource. As such, there needs to be organizational support for what has been recognized as being the gold standard [13] of cancer care. This requires investment in people, time and equipment. To quality assure the service, the outcomes of the MDT need to evaluated using both internal and external audits of outcomes and survival. The purpose of these audits is to both educate and improve the MDT functioning but also to allow good practice to be shared across a number of MDTs as an adjunct to improve cancer care for patients outside of the gynaecological MDT. Patient satisfaction surveys asking questions relevant to the MDT again allows reflective improvement of services. Increasingly the MDT are involved with identification of poor outcomes and critical events.

2.6 Legal Position of MDT Recommendations

There are many scholarly articles covering the different ethical theories behind the doctor patient relationship. Historically this relationship was often a paternalistic interaction with the learned doctor imparting their opinion on the passive patient. As healthcare has transitioned from patients to the current vogue term of clients, the perception of our interaction has also undergone a role reversal to a now more passive doctor acquiescing to the demands of a now learned patient. The GMC guidance and legal framework which instructs our interactions has however remained largely consistent throughout this long-needed move away from paternalism. Whether that interaction is between a single doctor and a patient or a group of clinicians and a patient the rules remain the same.

As there is no special regulatory or legal position attached to the MDT, the majority of our regulatory guidance can be found within the GMC's Good Medical Practice [15]. The essential message here can be distilled down to one of co-operation and respect. The clinician is now tasked with understanding the patients' narrative, what their life means to them and how their healthcare journey has been and likely will be framed by their current health needs. The clinician then has to integrate this into the MDT process, ensuring that the integrity of clinical opinion is maintained but whilst also ensuring that the option or options presented are acceptable, or at the very least debatable with the patient.

Where debate does occur, the majority are, from experience, resolvable with minor changes which are usually agreeable to both clinician and patient. Where views or positions remain entrenched it is usually worth remembering the following key elements.

It has been our experience that occasionally there is concern about the sharing of sensitive patient data between the primary clinician and the wider MDT team. Where after discussion patients can still not be assured that this is a necessary aspect of the clinical process and that only the minimum amount of essential data will it shared, it may be necessary to refer to legislation in order to proceed. The General Data Protection Regulation 2018 (GDPR) article 21 does provide patients with the right to object to the processing of their data, but this right is not an absolute one. Where the patient continues to seek clinical care despite objecting to the sharing of their health data, the NHS trust may need seek to rely on the Health and Social Care Act 2012 (HSCA). The HSCA requires public bodies to deliver safe care and suggests that the sharing of essential data is necessary for this. The HSCA should therefore provide justification for this data to be shared even in the face of an objection. A full and thorough explanation should still be provided to the patient, and the trust would be advised to seek legal advice in this unusual circumstance.

The GMC have also provided guidance on the requirement for information sharing between clinicians. If the patient does object to the sharing of any necessary information, then guidance states it is always advisable to discuss this with the patient first, to find out their concerns and where possible allay those, and once agreed share the data. If however, the patient continues to refuse to share their information, and you feel that this is an essential requirement for the provision of safe care, the GMC advises that you should explain that you cannot continue to assist the patient. We have never experienced this ourselves however and have often found where there is concern about data sharing, this is usually resolved through either dialogue or the explanation of the impact of not being able to share.

The final aspect to consider, and perhaps the one most of us are likely familiar with to some degree, is where the demands of the patient, their representative or family are either not clinically appropriate or worse may present a danger to the patient or others. The key message is that no doctor can be compelled to provide care they do not feel is in the patients interests or which they know or believe may even be harmful [16]. Where this issue arises, and we do have experience of this, the clinicians should present the appropriate treatment plan or plans to the patient for discussion. The patient's role is to then select from the presented options the plan most acceptable to them. It must be emphasised that all appropriate plans must be discussed and that the clinician can not simply provide only the plan they feel is correct [17].

Where the patient still wishes to pursue a plan not offered or recommended by the MDT then they are generally free to do so. This includes refusing all treatment, placing their faith in a higher power or seeking an alternative healthcare practitioner, we must remember that what we may see as a poor choice is usually still a valid choice [18]. The main caveats here are that this generally applies only to an adult with capacity to make such a decision, most other cases, for example children or those lacking capacity to make the relevant decision, would likely require an application to the Court of Protection for a decision. Where an advanced directive for healthcare is in place, it must be remembered that the scope for this is somewhat more restrictive and discussion of all eventualities is beyond the scope of this discussion.

2.7 Limitations of the MDT

We described the success of the MDT in terms of hospital engagement and the central role it now has in the management of cancer patients and the associated improvements in outcomes. The MDT has however become a victim of its own success. In line with the improvement in diagnostics and treatment, the MDT is increasingly having to manage more older and complex patients and more patients with recurrent disease and they do this using more individualized treatment options than ever before.

Because of this, Cancer Research UK [4] performed an analysis of 624 patient discussions in order to see if any areas of the MDT process were suboptimal. During their review, the mean duration of discussion of each patient was 3.2 min with over half of all MDT discussions being less than 2 min. Despite this, the MDT meeting could still last up to 5 h. Within those patient discussions, although between 7 and 14 members attended, the majority of verbal communication occurred between only 2 and 3 individuals with the Clinical Nurse Specialists only contributing in 75% of cases. Such a rapid turnover of cases and limited engagement is perhaps unsurprising: whilst Gynaecological Oncologists may only attend one MDT a week, the clinical and medical oncologist, radiologists and pathologists are likely to have to attend numerous different meetings which has a significant impact on their available clinical time. However, with such a rapid turnover, with limited collective engagement, there remains a risk that the quality of the MDT recommendation is subservient to the volume of the MDT workload. Cancer research UK noted that increasingly the MDTs were used to rubber stamp decisions that could be made earlier face-to-face with the patient—arranging biopsies before discussion for example. Their conclusions were that MDTs were losing the breadth of specialist consideration and debate, most likely a reflection of the work load put upon them. From this study, a number of recommendations, amongst others, were put forward [4]:

1. The use of a standardized proforma for cases submitted to the MDT to ensure that all clinical details are provided
2. A pre-MDT triage meeting for patients with full clinical information available in which a standard treatment pathway is required
3. A focused specialist group (for example only two rather that three Gynaecological Oncologists) to enable a quality assessment and key decisions to be made but simultaneously permit other clinical activity to continue

These recommendations collectively strive to return the quality to the MDT discussion. Standardized proformas enable all clinical details to be available, and, in part, reduce the ease of a reflex referral to the MDT for issues that could be managed outside of the MDT setting. A pre-MDT triage meeting (identifying patients who can be managed by protocol) should remove the patients having a brief "sign off" management of their cancer enabling more time to be available for more complex patients. Finally, by focusing the expert group, the MDT becomes a more economical resource, maintaining an expert decision without unnecessarily pulling surplus clinicians away from their other clinical duties.

The future of the MDT is likely, we suggest, to change further, with a move to a more extensive discussion about more complex patients, a greater impetus on quality outcomes and quality assurance of treatment outcomes with a protocol led, but patient-centered, standardized management plan for patients who clearly conform to a standard process.

2.8 Conclusion

We hope to have described how the concept of an MDT has developed over the last 25 years in England. Internationally, similar concepts have evolved over the same time period and the centralization of expert decision-making has now be enshrined as the gold standard of cancer management. Such expert discourse requires certain logistic and behavioral considerations, but when it can be achieved, such decision making appears to be associated with improved patient outcomes. The success of the MDT however remains one of its weaknesses with increasing pressures on the volume and complexity of patients to be discussed. It is likely therefore that the MDT will evolve over the next 10 years with more a specific focused MDT discussion on certain types of patients and a more streamlined validation, protocol led pathway for more routine cases. Whatever path the new era of MDT brings, it is certain that they will remain at the center of decision-making in Gynaecological and other cancers.

Key Points

1. Multidisciplinary team meetings have been increasingly influential in improving care of patients with cancer.
2. For meetings to have value, the constituent members of the MDT need to have expertise in their specific area and specialists representing the range of diagnostic and treatment specialties should be represented.
3. A productive MDT requires key managerial roles to be held and certain processes and behaviors be respected.
4. MDT decisions guide, but do not determine, the agreed treatment plan finalized between clinician and patient.
5. MDT's need to be able to respond to increasing complexity of both patient and treatment factors yet still deliver an expert led comprehensive treatment recommendation.

References

1. Expert Advisory Group on Cancer. A policy framework for commissioning cancer services—the Calman–Hine Report. A Report by the Expert Advisory Group on Cancer to the Chief Medical Officers of England and Wales. Department of Health. 1995.
2. National Cancer Action Team. The characteristics of an effective Multidisciplinary Team (MDT). 2010.
3. Department of Health. The NHS Cancer Plan. 2000.
4. Cancer Research UK. Meeting patients' needs: improving the effectiveness of multidisciplinary team meetings in cancer services. 2017.
5. Kesson EM, Allardice GM, George WD, et al. Effects of multidisciplinary team working on breast cancer survival: retrospective, comparative, interventional cohort study of 13 722 women. BMJ. 2012;344:e2718. https://doi.org/10.1136/bmj.e2718.
6. Morris E, Haward RA, Gilthorpe MS, et al. The impact of the Calman-Hine report on the processes and outcomes of care for Yorkshire's colorectal cancer patients. Br J Cancer. 2006;95(8):979–85. https://doi.org/10.1038/sj.bjc.6603372.
7. Birchall M, Bailey D, King P, et al. Effect of process standards on survival of patients with head and neck cancer in the south and west of England. Br J Cancer. 2004;91(8):1477–81. https://doi.org/10.1038/sj.bjc.6602118.
8. Coory M, Gkolia P, Yang IA, et al. Systematic review of multidisciplinary teams in the management of lung cancer. Lung Cancer. 2008;60(1):14–21. https://doi.org/10.1016/j.lungcan.2008.01.008.
9. Bydder S, Nowak A, Marion K, et al. The impact of case discussion at a multidisciplinary team meeting on the treatment and survival of patients with inoperable non-small cell lung cancer. Intern Med J. 2009;39(12):838–41. https://doi.org/10.1111/j.1445-5994.2009.02019.x.
10. Junor EJ, Hole DJ, Gillis CR. Management of ovarian cancer: referral to a multidisciplinary team matters. Br J Cancer. 1994;70(2):363–70. https://doi.org/10.1038/bjc.1994.307.
11. Stephens MR, Lewis WG, Brewster AE, et al. Multidisciplinary team management is associated with improved outcomes after surgery for esophageal cancer. Dis Esophagus. 2006;19(3):164–71. https://doi.org/10.1111/j.1442-2050.2006.00559.x.
12. Croke JM, El-Sayed S. Multidisciplinary management of cancer patients: chasing a shadow or real value? An overview of the literature. Curr Oncol. 2012;19(4):e232–8. https://doi.org/10.3747/co.19.944.
13. Independent Cancer Task Force. Achieving world-class cancer outcomes: a strategy for England 2015–2020 UK. 2015.
14. Saini KS, Taylor C, Ramirez AJ, et al. Role of the multidisciplinary team in breast cancer management: results from a large international survey involving 39 countries. Ann Oncol. 2012;23(4):853–9. https://doi.org/10.1093/annonc/mdr352.
15. General Medical Council. Good medical practice. 2019.
16. Re L (Medical treatment: benefit), 2005 1 FLR 491.
17. Montgomery v Lanarkshire Health Board 2015 UKSC 11.
18. Re C (Adult: Refusal of Treatment), 1994 FD.

Consent and Communication Skills in Management of Gynaeoncology

Aarti Lakhiani and Sudha Sundar

3.1 Introduction

Effective communication is key to a successful doctor–patient relationship and the delivery of safe patient care. Communication is defined as the act of imparting knowledge and encompasses the exchange of information, ideas and feelings [1]. It is a two-way, relational process that is influenced by context, culture, words, and gestures, and it is one of the most important ways that clinicians influence the quality of medical care that patients and their families receive [2]. Traditionally, this has been verbal but, increasingly, women are expecting written communication from the clinician, summarising their consultation and regarding any relevant results.

Gynaecological malignancy has an immense impact on the well-being of women. In order to help women clearly understand their disease, investigations, treatment options and prognosis, it is essential that we provide high-quality information in an appropriate manner and environment. The median survival for women with gynaecological malignancies has increased over the years and it is now not uncommon for patients to experience remission and recurrence multiple times during the course of their illness. Each recurrence can be a crisis in which the patient received bad news again and must endure the rigors of further treatment, and uncertainty about the outcome. In these instances, the application of effective communication skills in the context of a long standing relationship with the patient can reduce anxiety, facilitate patient coping and assist in providing the patient with hope [3, 4].

3.2 Flaws in Communication

Most complaints by patients about doctors' are regarding problems of communication and not clinical competency [5]. Patient surveys have consistently shown that they want better communication with their doctors [6]. Patients want more and better information about their problem and the outcome, more openness about the side effects of treatment, relief of pain and emotional distress, and advice on what they can do for themselves [7]. A study by Rodriguez et al., for example, showed significantly fewer complaints for doctors who explained things clearly, gave enough information, were perceived as caring

A. Lakhiani (✉)
Pan Birmingham Gynae Cancer Centre, Birmingham, UK
e-mail: aartilakhiani@nhs.net

S. Sundar
University Hospitals Birmingham NHS Foundation Trust, Birmingham, UK
e-mail: s.s.sundar@bham.ac.uk

© The Author(s), under exclusive license to Springer Nature Switzerland AG 2022
K. Singh, B. Gupta (eds.), *Gynecological Oncology*, https://doi.org/10.1007/978-3-030-94110-9_3

and kind, knew the medical history and spent enough time with the patient [8].

Patient dissatisfaction can also lead to low understanding and recall of information, poor compliance, lengthier recovery periods, and increased complication rates [9]. Cancer patients often have poor information recall especially during the early phase of diagnosis due to high levels of anxiety [10]. As a consequence, they can often feel they lack information, which can lead to uncertainty, anxiety and depression. A review of the literature suggests that patient-centred approaches generally are associated with greater satisfaction, compliance, feelings of being understood, and resolution of patient concerns [11].

We know, through the work published by National Voices, that patients expect 'person centred coordinated care' based on good communication and teamwork. This includes helping them to understand their care and navigate different services across health and social care boundaries. Patients expect support to help them understand their treatment options and to be involved in decisions about their care [12]. With a more integrated approach, doctors will have to start working differently. Doctors will have to increasingly take on more proactive roles to help patients understand care options and to teach them how to manage their own health.

3.3 Best Practices for Communication

The General Medical Council (GMC) emphasises that for a relationship between a doctor and patient to be effective, it should be a partnership based on openness, trust and good communication. Good communication skills in general and knowing how to impart bad news in particular are considered central to being a good doctor [13]. Equally, good interprofessional communication is essential for effective and co-ordinated care. When patients and doctors communicate well during cancer care, patients are more satisfied with their care, feel more in control and are more likely to follow through with treatment [14].

According to the GMC, effective communication involves:

- listening to patients, take account of their views, and responding honestly to their questions.
- giving patients the information, they want or need to know in a way they can understand. Arrangements should be made, wherever possible, to meet patients' language and communication needs.
- being considerate to those close to the patient and being sensitive and responsive in giving them information and support.
- being readily accessible to patients and colleagues seeking information, advice or support.

Standards have been set by the Royal College of Obstetricians and Gynaecologist (RCOG) with regard to communication both in Obstetrics and in Gynaecology [15]. These include emphasis on effective communication between team members and each discipline, as well as with women and their families and imparting training to all healthcare professionals on how to communicate in an effective and sensitive manner. Some of the other standards include:

- Offering information to each patient in a form that is accessible to them.
- Providing interpreting services to women whose first language isn't English for all appointments and avoiding reliance on family members.
- Women should receive written information regarding their clinic visit. Information should include the type of healthcare professional they will see, the expected duration of the appointment and anything they need to bring with them.

There are a number of ways of summarising and simplifying clinical consultations. The CLASS protocol identifies five essential components of the clinical consultation. They are Context (the physical context or setting), Listening skills, Acknowledgment of the patient's emotions, Strategy for clinical management, and Summary

Table 3.1 The CLASS protocol

C—**Physical context** or setting	
L—**Listening** skills	
A—**Acknowledge** emotions and explore them	
S—**Management strategy**	
S—**Summary**	

(Table 3.1) [16]. It is easy to remember and to use in clinical practice. Furthermore, it offers a relatively straightforward, technique-directed method for dealing with emotions. This is important, because one study showed that most oncologists (more than 85%) believe that dealing with emotions is the most difficult part of any clinical interview [17].

3.4 The CLASS Protocol (CLASS: A Protocol for Effective Communication)

The various components of CLASS protocol Are briefly described below.

3.4.1 C: Context (Setting)

Physical Space
- Choose an area where you can have a private conversation.
  - Your eyes should be at the same level as the patient and/or family member (sit down if you need to).
  - There should be no physical barriers between you.
  - If you are behind a desk, have the patient and/or family members sit across the corner.
  - Have a box of tissues available.

Family Members/Friends
- The patient should be seated closest to you.

Body Language
- Present a relaxed demeanour.
  - Maintain eye contact except when the patient becomes upset.

Touch
- Only touch a non-threatening area (hand or forearm).
  - Be aware of cultural issues that may not allow touching.

3.4.2 L: Listening Skills

Be an effective listener.

Open Ended Questions
- "Can you tell me more about your concerns?"
  - "How have you been feeling?"

Facilitating
- Allow the patient to speak without interrupting them.
  - Nod to let the patient know you are following them.
  - Repeat a key word from the patient's last sentence in your first sentence.

Clarifying
- "So, if I understand you correctly, you are saying…"
  - "Tell me more about that."

Time and Interruptions
- If there are time constraints, let the patient know ahead of time.
  - Try to prepare the patient if you know you will be interrupted
  - Bleeps and phone calls—don't answer, but if you must, apologise to the patient before answering.

3.4.3 A: Acknowledge Emotions

Explore, Identify, and Respond to the Emotion
- Identify the emotion.
  - Identify the cause of the emotion.
  - Respond by showing you have made the connection between the emotion and the cause.
  - "That must have felt terrible when…"

- "Most people would be upset about this."
- You don't have to have the same feelings as the patient.
- You don't have to agree with the patient's feelings.

3.4.4 S: Strategy

Propose a Management Plan that the Patient Will Understand
- Appraise in your mind or clarify with the patient their expectations of treatment and outcome.
  - Decide what the best medical plan would be for the patient.
  - Recommend a strategy on how to proceed.
  - Evaluate the patient's response.
  - Collaborate and agree on the plan.

3.4.5 S: Summary

Closing the Interview
- Summarize the discussion in a clear and concise manner.
  - Check the patient's understanding.
  - Ask if the patient has any other questions for you.
  - If you don't have time for further questions, suggest that they can be addressed at the next appointment.

3.5 Communication with Vulnerable Patients

A vulnerable adult is a patient who is or may be for any reason unable to take care of him or herself, or unable to protect him or herself against significant harm or exploitation [18]. When communicating with a patient who may be considered vulnerable, for example, an elderly patient who is visually impaired, it is important to take the time and be really clear. This will help your patient gain a better understanding and be understood. Things to consider trying in vulnerable adults are

- Allow more time for consultation.
- Sit nearby the patient and their carer
- Talk directly to the patient and make eye contact
- Involve a medical interpreter rather than a family member when there is a language barrier.
- Work out how much understanding the patient has at your first meeting.
- Talk to the patient in a manner that they can understand.
- Tell the patient and their carer what is going to happen in the consultation.
- Check frequently for understanding

Language differences alone can be a significant barrier to doctors' information sharing, contributing to suboptimal communication along with feelings of frustration for patients. Cultural differences can also make it difficult for even experienced doctors to appropriately understand and interpret the meaning behind the patient's words [19]. True cultural competence starts with cultural curiosity, which relies on asking questions, actively listening, and acknowledging when additional resources (such as interpreters) are necessary [20]. This cultural curiosity should be manifest from the onset of the doctor-patient relationship, thus serving as a foundation for all communication, not just difficult conversations.

3.6 Communication with Other Specialities

Caring for cancer patients involves working with a number of different specialists and health care professionals- oncologists, pathologists, radiologist, cancer nurse specialists etc. Due to the large number and range of specialities involved, there is a potential for poor communication and poor co-ordination of care.

Multidisciplinary teams (MDTs) meeting is key enabler in the provision of high-quality care for cancer patients. MDTs improve communication, coordination and decision making between the healthcare professionals. Patients managed by MDTs are more likely to receive appropriate staging, evidence-based management, and timely treatment [21]. Other benefits of MDTs include consistency in the standard of patient management offered, increased recruitment into clinical trials, improved job satisfaction of team members and a teaching element for junior doctors [22].

3.7 Breaking Bad News

Bad news can be defined as "any news that seriously adversely affects the patient's view of her future" [23]. The manner in which clinicians break bad news to patients affects both the way in which they adjust to the situation and their wellbeing. In gynaecologic oncology, bad news could take the form of communicating: (1) initial diagnosis; (2) disease progression; (3) disease recurrence; (4) development of new complications; and (5) change from curative to palliative care. It could also involve explaining the need for often complex therapeutic options and their debilitation side-effects and the eventual uncertainty about optimum treatments and dismal prognosis. It is necessary to have a communication model that will function in all of these circumstances.

Several task-based communication models have been developed incorporating research findings to help doctors break bad news and cope with patient grief. One such model is the Kaye's Model, which is a 10-step task centred model developed by Peter Kaye, a Consultant in Palliative Care (Table 3.2) [24].

Table 3.2 Kaye's 10-step model for breaking bad news

1. Preparation
Know all the facts before the meeting, find out who the patient wants present, and ensure privacy and chairs to sit on. Introduce yourself to the patient
2. What does the patient know?
Ask for a narrative of events by the patient e.g. "how did it all start?", use open ended questions
3. Is more information wanted?
Test the waters, but be aware that it can be very frightening to ask for more information (e.g. "would you like me to explain a bit more?")
4. Give a warning shot
E.g. "I'm afraid it looks rather serious"—then allow a pause for the patient to respond
5. Allow denial
Denial is a defence, and a way of coping. Allow the patient to control the amount of information they receive
6. Explain (if requested)
Narrow the information gap, step by step. Details may not be remembered but the way you explain will be
7. Listen to concerns
Ask: "What are your concerns at the moment?" and then allow space for expression of feelings
8. Encourage ventilation of feelings and acknowledge them
This is the KEY phase in terms of patient satisfaction with the interview, because it conveys empathy
9. Summary and plan
Summarise concerns, plan treatment, and foster hope
10. Offer further information or availability
Most patients need further explanation (the details will not have been remembered) and support (adjustment takes weeks or months) and benefit greatly from a family meeting

as the risks, benefits and alternatives to the proposed therapy, including no treatment. It should be free from coercion and the patient should have medical decision-making capacity, i.e. capacity to understand and communicate, the capacity to reason and deliberate, and the possession of a set of values and goals [25, 26].

3.8 Informed Consent

Informed consent is both an ethical and legal obligation of health professionals and originates from the patient's right to be involved in decisions about their treatment and care. In order for informed consent to be valid, a patient must receive accurate, meaningful and relevant information regarding the nature and purpose of the treatment, as well

3.8.1 Types of Consent

Implied Consent This is generally considered acceptable for minor or routine investigations or treatments if the healthcare professional is satisfied that the patient understands what one proposes to do and why. An example of this would be a patient offering her arm for venepuncture.

Express Consent This could either be oral or written. Express consent should be obtained for any procedure that carries material risk, and therefore, patient-specific agreement must be obtained before the procedure starts. Oral consent is valid, but it is usual to obtain written consent for major procedures. If it is only possible to obtain oral consent, it is good practice to make an entry in the patient's clinical notes to confirm advice was given and oral consent obtained, as well as the name and designation of any witnesses [27].

3.8.2 Model for Obtaining Consent

Consent ideally should usually be taken by the healthcare professional who recommends that the woman should undergo the intervention or by the person carrying out the procedure. However, as per GMC guidance on consent, it may also be delegated to a healthcare professional who is suitably trained and qualified, is sufficiently familiar with the procedure and possesses the appropriate communication skills. It is important that all the options available should be discussed with the women [28]. This should include doing nothing, initiating investigations, watchful waiting and providing treatment. A woman's understanding of the discussion of treatment and consent should be documented separately to the completion of the consent form, within her notes. A model for obtaining consent is shown in Fig. 3.1.

3.9 Montgomery Ruling

The 2015 Supreme Court decision on Montgomery vs. NHS Lanarkshire has significant implications for doctor–patient communications, information sharing and informed consent [29]. The implication of the Montgomery ruling is that healthcare professionals must:

(a) clearly outline the recommended management strategies and procedures to their patient, including the risks and implications of potential treatment options.
(b) discuss any alternative treatments.
(c) discuss the consequences of not performing any treatment or intervention.
(d) ensure patients have access to high-quality information to aid their decision-making.
(e) give patients adequate time to reflect before making a decision.
(f) check patients have fully understood their options and the implications.
(g) documented the above process in the patient's record

3.10 Reviewing Decisions

Before providing treatment or care, it is important to check that the patient still wants to ahead. Any new questions or concerns must be responded to especially if a significant time has passed since the initial decision was made, there has been a change in the patient's condition, any aspect of the chosen treatment or care has changed or new information has become available about the potential benefits or risks of harm of any of the options that might make the patient choose differently.

If treatment is ongoing, it is imperative to make sure there are clear arrangements in place to review decisions regularly allowing patients opportunity to ask questions and make decisions at each stage. A decision to take no action should also be reviewed regularly.

3.11 Conclusion

When patients and doctors communicate well during cancer care, patients are more satisfied with their care, feel more in control and are more likely to follow through with treatment. Patient-centred approaches are associated with greater satisfaction, compliance, feelings of being understood, and resolution of patient concerns. Patient dissatisfaction can lead to low understanding and recall of information, poor compliance, lengthier recovery periods, and increased complication rates. Ideally, consent should usually be taken by the healthcare professional who recommends that

Fig. 3.1 Model for taking consent

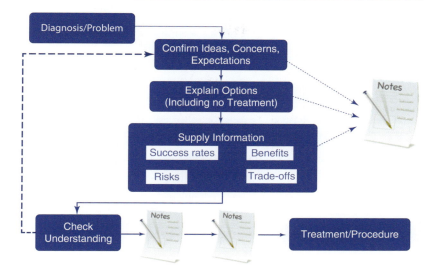

the woman should undergo the intervention or by the person carrying out the procedure. Informed consent is both an ethical and legal obligation of health professionals. It is important to ensure that patients have fully understood their options and the implications.

Key Points
1. Communication is the act of imparting knowledge and encompasses the exchange of information, ideas and feelings and is the key to delivery of safe patient care.
2. The CLASS protocol identifies five essential components of the clinical consultation i.e. Context (the physical context or setting), Listening skills, Acknowledgment of the patient's emotions, Strategy for clinical management, and Summary
3. Communication skills must take into account individual vulnerability, language and cultural barriers
4. Cancer care involves a multidisciplinary approach and Multidisciplinary teams (MDTs) meeting is key enabler in the provision of high-quality care for cancer patients.
5. Several task-based communication models have been developed incorporating research findings to help doctors break bad news and cope with patient grief like Kaye's Model
6. Consent can be implied or expressed; the latter should be obtained for any procedure that carries material risk
7. Before providing treatment or care, it is important to check that the patient still wants to ahead and the decision must be reviewed and discussed with the patient.

References

1. ACT Academy. SBAR communication tool—situation, background, assessment, recommendation. NHS Improvement.
2. Back AL. Patient-clinician communication issues in palliative care for patients with advanced cancer. J Clin Oncol. 2020;38:866–76.
3. Sardell AN, Trierweiler SJ. Disclosing the cancer diagnosis. Procedures that influence patient hopefulness. Cancer. 1993;1993(72):3355–65.
4. Zachariae R, Pedersen CG, Jensen AB, et al. Association of perceived physician communication style with patient satisfaction, distress, cancer-related self-efficacy and perceived control over the disease. Br J Cancer. 2003;88:658–65.
5. Richards T. Chasms in communication. BMJ. 1990;301(6766):1407–8. https://doi.org/10.1136/bmj.301.6766.1407.

6. Duffy FD, Gordon GH, Whelan G, et al. Assessing competence in communication and interpersonal skills: the Kalamazoo II report. Acad Med. 2004;79(6):495–507.
7. Meryn S. Improving doctor-patient communication. Not an option, but a necessity. BMJ. 1998;316(7149):1922. https://doi.org/10.1136/bmj.316.7149.1922.
8. Rodriguez H, et al. Relation of patients' experiences with individual physicians to malpractice risk. Int J Qual Health Care. 2008;20(1):5–12.
9. Zachariae R, Pedersen CG, Jensen AB, Ehrnrooth E, Rossen PB, von der Maase H. Association of perceived physician communication style with patient satisfaction, distress, cancer-related self-efficacy, and perceived control over the disease. Br J Cancer. 2003;88(5):658–65.
10. Nguyen MH, Smets EMA, Bol N, et al. Fear and forget: how anxiety impacts information recall in newly diagnosed cancer patients visiting a fast-track clinic. Acta Oncol. 2019;58(2):182–8.
11. Ong LM, de Haes JC, Hoos AM, Lammes FB. Doctor–patient communication: a review of the literature. Soc Sci Med. 1995;40:903–18.
12. National Voices. Person centred care 2020: calls and contributions from health and social care charities. September, 2014. https://www.nationalvoices.org.uk/publications/our-publications/person-centred-care-2020.
13. General Medical Council. Good medical practice. Manchester: GMC; 2013.
14. PDQ® Supportive and Palliative Care Editorial Board. PDQ Communication in Cancer Care. Bethesda, MD: National Cancer Institute. Updated 02/01/2018. Available at: https://www.cancer.gov/about-cancer/coping/adjusting-to-cancer/communication-hp-pdq.
15. Royal College of Obstetricians and Gynaecologist (RCOG). Standards for gynaecology: providing quality care for women. London: RCOG; 2016.
16. Buckman R. Communication in palliative care: a practical guide. In: Doyle D, Hanks GWC, MacDonald N, editors. Oxford textbook of palliative care. Oxford: Oxford University Press; 1998. p. 141–56.
17. Baile WB, Glober GA, Lenzi R, Beale EA, Kudelka AP. Discussing disease progression and end-of-life decisions. Oncology. 1999;13:1021–31.
18. Boland B, Burnage J, Scott A. Protecting against harm: safeguarding adults in general medicine. Clin Med (Lond). 2014;14(4):345–8. https://doi.org/10.7861/clinmedicine.14-4-345.
19. Sisk BA, Mack JW. How should we enhance the process and purpose of prognostic communication in oncology? AMA J Ethics. 2018;20(8):E757–65.
20. Kodjo C. Cultural competence in clinician communication. Pediatr Rev. 2009;30(2):57–64.
21. Scott R, Hawarden A, Russell B, Edmondson RJ. Decision-making in gynaecological oncology multidisciplinary team meetings: a cross-sectional, observational study of ovarian cancer cases. Oncol Res Treat. 2020;43(3):70–7.
22. Fleissig A, Jenkins V, Catt S, Fallowfield L. Multidisciplinary teams in cancer care: are they effective in the UK? Lancet Oncol. 2006;7(11):935–43.
23. Buckman R. Breaking bad news: why is it still so difficult? BMJ. 1984;288:1597–9.
24. Kaye P. Breaking bad news: a 10-step approach. Northampton: EPL; 1996.
25. Grisso T, Appelbaum PS. Assessing competence to consent to treatment: a guide for physicians and other health professionals. Oxford: Oxford University Press; 1998.
26. Royal College of Obstetricians and Gynaecologists. Obtaining valid consent. Clinical Governance Advice No.6. London: RCOG; 2015.
27. British Medical Association. Confidentiality and disclosure of health information tool kit. London: BMA; 2009.
28. General Medical Council (GMC). Decision making and consent. 2020.
29. Cheung E, Goodyear G, Yoong W. Medicolegal update on consent: "The Montgomery Ruling". Obstet Gynaecol. 2016;18(3):171–2.

Holistic Approach Towards Managing Patients in Case Management in Gynaeoncology

Audrey Fong Lien Kwong, Catherine Spencer, and Sudha Sundar

4.1 Introduction

Nearly 21,000 women are diagnosed with a gynaecological malignancy every year in the United Kingdom [1]. Overall cancer survival has been steadily improving over the past 20 years and is expected to continue to increase due to innovative therapies and earlier diagnosis [2]. It is important to concentrate our efforts to optimise the quality of life, improve care satisfaction, support self-management, and minimise distress from cancer survivors. A key priority for care is to identify the holistic needs of cancer survivors and facilitate access to relevant cancer rehabilitation services to promote patient independence and ease their adaptation to the considerable life changes attached to a cancer diagnosis [3]. Women with a gynaecological malignancy have unique physical and psychosexual needs including a loss of femininity and sexual function due to their disease and its treatment. Addressing these complex needs represents a challenge for healthcare professionals. In the UK, the Clinical Nurse Specialist in Gynaecological Oncology (CNS) plays a vital role and acts as a bridge between patients, their general practitioner (GP), hospitals, and the community where most of the patient's care takes place. The role of the nurse specialist includes but is not limited to addressing the information and support needs, offering emotional support, and facilitating referral to relevant specialists, support groups and local services.

4.1.1 Holistic Needs

A diagnosis of cancer will have an impact on the physical, psychological, social, economic, and spiritual wellbeing of women. The magnitude and nature of these needs not only differ from patient to patient but will also vary at different milestones along the cancer journey within the same patient. These holistic needs may be [4]:

- **Informational**—related to the need for accurate information and guide decision-making.
- **Physical**—related to patient comfort, optimal symptom management and ability to complete daily activities.
- **Psychological**—related to emotional wellbeing, preservation of self-esteem, and ability to cope with stressful situations.
- **Socioeconomic**—related to upholding relationships and addressing legal and financial difficulties.
- **Spiritual**—related to a way of life where patients reflect on their existence.

A. F. L. Kwong (✉) · C. Spencer · S. Sundar
Pan Birmingham Gynaecological Cancer Centre, City Hospital, Birmingham, UK
e-mail: audrey.kwong@nhs.net; catherinespencer1@nhs.net; sudha.sundar@nhs.net

4.1.2 Recovery Package

The UK National Cancer Survivorship Initiative (NCSI) has commissioned key initiatives, which are incorporated into a Recovery Package, to improve the outcome of patients living with and beyond cancer. The recovery package comprises of four key elements including a Holistic Needs Assessment (HNA), Treatment Summary, Cancer Care Review and Education and Support Elements [5, 6].

- **Holistic Needs Assessment (HNA)**—is a semi-structured questionnaire that is completed with the patient at the earliest contact or whenever the patient or healthcare professional deems it to be necessary. The patient is encouraged to complete a HNA questionnaire with the help of their CNS. The assessment may also require input from allied health professionals such as physiotherapists, dieticians or occupational therapists depending on the patient's needs. This is then followed by a conversation with a health professional and together a personalised care plan is agreed upon, often by facilitating access to the appropriate support services. The care plan is then copied to the GP to highlight the patient's concerns and support needs.
- **Treatment Summary**—at the completion of treatment, an outline of treatment received, its side effects, the contact details of keyworkers and signs of recurrence, should be shared with the patient and their GPs to enable a smooth transition from hospital to community-based care.
- **Cancer Care Review**—the GP should be notified of the cancer diagnosis and arrange a review within 6 weeks to initiate patient support in the community.
- **Education and Support Elements**—patients and their carers should be encouraged to attend health and wellbeing events which focus on promoting a healthy and active lifestyle and accessing the appropriate services.

4.2 Global Needs Following a Cancer Diagnosis

The needs of women with a gynaecological cancer are strongly patient and disease-dependent. We will consider how the holistic needs of cancer survivors evolve as they progress along the cancer journey.

4.2.1 The Cancer Journey

4.2.1.1 Support at Diagnosis

Most women will experience shock, confusion, and helplessness after being told that they have cancer. Whilst some women may already have many symptoms at the time of diagnosis, e.g., in advanced ovarian cancer, others may have mild or no symptoms. The healthcare professional can lessen patient anxiety by providing accurate information and involving the woman at every step in the decision-making process, while ensuring that she has the emotional resources to cope with the new diagnosis. Studies have shown that trust and close collaboration between patients and healthcare providers are associated with higher levels of patient satisfaction, better adherence to treatment, and improved quality of life [7]. Browall et al. proposed that the chief information needs of women recently diagnosed with ovarian cancer were related to the probability of cure, disease stage and what treatment options were available [8]. Concerns related to sexual attractiveness were comparatively more prevalent in younger women. They recommended that the information should therefore be tailored to the patient's age, educational level, socio-cultural background, and that women should be supported to access validated and approved information resources to fulfil their expectations and facilitate future decisions.

4.2.1.2 Support During Treatment

Some women may already have inconvenience due to their symptoms of the disease, whilst others may develop de novo ailments after initiating cancer treatment. A study by Ferrell et al.

suggested that the side-effects of multimodal treatments can potentially be more aggressive that those associated with the disease itself [9]. Postoperative pain and fatigue, or nausea and vomiting associated with adjuvant therapies are some of the most common symptoms reported by cancer patients. Treating the reversible causes of fatigue (e.g., anaemia, lack of sleep, suboptimal pain control) can lead to a significant improvement in the patient's quality of life [10]. Likewise, identifying the underlying causes of nausea and vomiting and selecting an appropriate antiemetic, on its own or in combination with alternative therapies may be helpful.

The effects of cancer treatment may persist for years after its initial diagnosis. Early recognition of the longer-term side-effects of multimodal therapies is therefore essential to articulate patient care and optimise cancer survivorship. Premenopausal women may be rendered menopausal following the removal of their ovaries or because of chemoradiotherapy. These women will experience a barrage of symptoms such as low mood, sexual dysfunction, vasomotor symptoms, accelerated loss of muscle mass, skeletal brittleness, and loss of cardiovascular protection. Although healthy lifestyle changes including weight loss, exercise, reducing alcohol consumption and smoking cessation may be beneficial, some women may still require pharmacological therapies. Whilst it is reasonable to consider hormone replacement therapy (HRT) in women with non-hormone dependent malignancies (cervical, vulval cancers), further discussion is necessary in those who have been treated for ovarian, or advanced stage endometrial cancers. Authors of a Cochrane review on the effectiveness and safety of HRT in women with an endometrial cancer concluded that while HRT does not appear to be associated with recurrence in early-stage endometrial cancer, this conclusion cannot be extrapolated for women with advanced disease. Similarly, there is a lack of high-quality evidence to support or contest the safety of HRT in women with epithelial ovarian cancer [11, 12]. This conundrum has fuelled a drive to explore alternatives to HRT. Pharmacological and non-pharmacological measures such as Cognitive Behaviour Therapy (CBT) may be helpful to address symptoms of the menopause. The *British Menopause Society (BMS)* describes a list of prescribable medications including gabapentin, pregabalin and clonidine on its website but warns that their efficacy may be offset by their side-effects [13]. An individualised plan should therefore be agreed with the woman.

The after-effects of radiation may be self-limiting or persist for years after completion of radiation therapy. Radiation inflicts ischaemic, ulcerative or inflammatory damage to soft tissues. Clinical indicators of late radiation cystitis include urinary frequency and urgency, pain or bleeding on urination, urinary incontinence, and a propensity to fistulation. The risk of radiation cystitis depends on the radiation techniques (volume irradiated, dose and fractionation, mode of irradiation such as brachy- or external beam therapy) and patient factors (concurrent medications and comorbidities). Further research is required to demonstrate the effectiveness of non-surgical therapies in alleviating or reversing the effects of late radiation cystitis [14]. Similarly, chronic radiation-induced gastrointestinal (GI) side-effects such as loose stools, faecal urgency or incontinence, rectal bleeding can have a devastating impact on the woman's quality of life [15]. Up to 9 in 10 women will experience a permanent change in their bowel habits and 4 in 10 women describe a lasting impact on their quality of life [16]. While gastrointestinal toxicity can be minimised through precision delivery methods such as Intensity-Modulated Radiation Therapy or brachytherapy, the evidence for pharmacological interventions remains sparse. Nutritional and dietary modifications may play a role in neutralising the effects of radiation induced GI toxicity and input from a multidisciplinary team of oncologists, gastroenterologists and dieticians could be beneficial for this population.

Most women will be affected both emotionally and physically by the removal of their reproductive organs, irrespective of their age or the cancer site. The psychological ramifications following cancer treatment may be substantial and 9 in 10 women may experience some sexual dysfunction and lack of desire for intimacy at some point [17]. In practice, the sexual needs of women largely remain unattended. Fulfilment of an active sex life is not achievable for many due to organic or psychological sequelae of cancer and its treatments. Vaginal shortening and denervation following surgery e.g., radical hysterectomy or chemoradiotherapy will alter the woman's anatomy and may lead to a loss of sensation over erogenous areas such as the clitoris. Women also experience a perceived loss of desirability and subsequently may become refractory to intimacy following cosmetic changes in the manifestation of alopecia, lymphoedema, bowel and urinary incontinence, and stomas, amongst others [17].

Although some of the organic causes of sexual dysfunction can be improved with the help of HRT, dilators and lubricators, patients should be counselled that restoring sexual function to their pre-diagnosis level may never be achieved. Extensive preoperative counselling, early input from a psychologist and referral for CBT may enable a smoother adjustment to these considerable life changes. The PLISSIT model (Annon, 1974) offers an excellent structure to facilitate discussion around sensitive subjects, including sexuality, for the non-specialist. This model of intervention and interaction (Permission, Limited Information, Specific Suggestions, and Intensive Therapy) offers a concise means of discussing sexual issues and enables clinicians from all levels to elicit the patient's concerns, offer effective advice or make a specialist referral to a counsellor for more comprehensive support.

The envisaged loss of fertility with cancer treatments can potentially be more devastating than the disease itself for women of childbearing age. In fact, the desire for motherhood has been positively viewed as a motivator for improved adherence to treatment [18]. Select women who are eligible for fertility preservation should therefore be supported to make informed choices and counselled about the implications of cancer treatment, the risks of fertility preserving therapies, their chances of achieving a successful pregnancy and the subsequent obstetric risks. Recognised methods of mitigating the impact of gonadal toxicity include ovarian transposition prior to radiotherapy, or fertility-sparing surgeries such as trachelectomies with conservation of the ovaries. Women who will be receiving gonadotoxic chemotherapy should be supported to discuss their fertility preservation choices (e.g., egg retrieval, in-vitro fertilisation, embryo storage and future reimplantation) in advance with a fertility specialist. Options such as surrogacy and adoption should also be considered.

Doctors often focus their efforts on alleviating the physical burden of cancer at the detriment of the psychological or spiritual aspects of the disease. A lack of expertise in the recognition of the psychosocial needs of cancer survivors and a fear of upsetting patients may discourage doctors from addressing the psychosocial burden of disease and its treatment [19]. Common psychological themes to consider in women with a gynaecological cancer include morbid anxiety and depression, sexual inferiority complex and worries surrounding genetic testing. Whilst most women will turn to their friends, family, and partners for support, some of them will warrant professional input from a counsellor, psychologist or from the mental health team. A comprehensive risk assessment is therefore essential to identify those women at higher risk of psychological morbidity e.g., women with a history of mental ill-health.

Most women who are offered genetic testing following a new cancer diagnosis will encounter a precarious scenario since the outcome of the test is likely to have significant prognostic (e.g., eligibility for chemotherapeutic agents such as PARP-inhibitors) and psychological implications for the woman herself, but also for her family. A positive result uncovers the brutal reality of living with a cumulative risk of other types of cancers. Women with BRCA mutations or Lynch syndrome subsequently face the dilemma of having to choose between risk-reducing surgery and lifelong surveillance. Studies have also shown that patients may experience guilt and regret at the prospect of conveying a faulty genetic legacy to their children, especially to their daughters [20]. The importance of careful pre-test counselling cannot be overemphasised.

A cancer diagnosis will have a considerable impact on the patient's socio-economic circumstances. Many women who have been recently diagnosed with cancer may need to be off-work for extended periods to attend their appointments and recuperate. Although patients with cancer are protected by law and should be supported to remain in work (Equality Act 2010), this is not always achievable. For many however, return to work is an important step toward rebuilding their lives. The inability to do so will further impact upon the patient's physical, emotional, and social wellbeing. Timely assistance in accessing local services such as benefits, social care, or employment advice should therefore be optimised to minimise disruptions to the patient's quality of life.

4.2.1.3 Remission

On completion of their treatment, many women tend to live well and celebrate their victory over cancer. Being in remission provides them with the time and opportunity to process their cancer experience, to consider the changes that cancer has brought, to contemplate what life will be like going forward by aiming to live well after cancer. Once active treatment has ceased, these women gradually adapt to life changes resulting from their diagnosis and adjust to a new normal life. On the other hand, less optimistic women may feel isolated and report fear and anxiety related to uncertainty now that they are no longer under regular surveillance [21]. Hodgkinson et al. found that 1 in 5 women with a gynaecological cancer will experience post-traumatic stress disorder which is manifested as intrusive thoughts, hyper-arousal, and avoidance behaviours [22]. Between 15 and 25% of women will report depressive symptoms such as a loss of interest in hobbies, a lack of energy and a lasting feeling of hopelessness. Fear of cancer recurrence is a common concern expressed among cancer survivors [23]. It is particularly prevalent among patients with ovarian cancer and contributes to significant psychological distress. The provision of ongoing psychosocial assessment by a multidisciplinary team and prompt access to the appropriate services including reintegration into the cancer pathway should therefore be accommodated to support women during the survivorship phase.

4.2.1.4 Recurrence

When women are diagnosed with a recurrence, they will either be offered surgery, chemoradiotherapy, participation in trials, or best supportive care. In some women, being told that their disease has come back may not be unexpected, especially if they have been suffering with evocative symptoms such as pain, bleeding, weight loss, ascites, or the appearance of a new lesion. For many with more subtle symptoms and who had slowly started to move on with their lives, being told the cancer has come back can bring back a flood of emotions such as anger, self-doubt, hopelessness, and devastation. This sudden change in disease status is accompanied by anxiety over what lies ahead for them and for their families, especially for those who had undergone multimodal therapies for cancer in the past: the gruelling treatments and their side-effects, the long road to recovery, significant disruptions to their life trajectory, and more importantly, a rekindled sense of death awareness. Feelings of inner turmoil may oscillate between a sense of demoralisation, grief, and spiritual distress where women question their faith and the reason for their existence [24]. Healthcare professionals should therefore remember that women who have relapsed may experience even greater psychological distress than at first diagnosis as their initial optimism for a chance of cure becomes even more remote.

4.2.1.5 Palliation and End of Life

When cancer becomes incurable, women will experience grief and may struggle to come to terms with their mortality as they realise that they will eventually succumb to their disease. It is impossible for a single individual to address the physical, emotional, and spiritual needs of the patient and her family in these situations. Palliative care is intensely reliant on efficient teamwork among doctors, nurse specialists, and social workers. Women become more and more afflicted by a range of physical ailments as their disease progresses [25]. Pain is one of the dominant issues reported by all patients with advanced cancer. Understanding the type of pain and its effect on the patient's quality of life will allow the clinician to select the most appropriate painkiller regime. Steroids are occasionally prescribed as an appetite stimulant if this will improve the patient's quality of life. Special care should be paid to patient hygiene, especially if they suffer with urinary and bowel incontinence to protect their self-esteem and reduce the risk of further complications such as fistulae and wound infections. As the disease progresses, oedema in the form of lymphoedema or ascites becomes more apparent. Supportive therapies such as compression stockings or an ascitic drain may be considered for some patients after discussion with the woman and her family. The complications of advanced disease such as bowel obstruction in ovarian cancer or vaginal bleeding in advanced cervical cancer become increasingly difficult to manage. Multidisciplinary team input is essential to balance the risk of further surgery and its complications against rapid symptomatic improvement, especially when pharmacological alternatives are limited. Women at the end-of-life may experience and exhibit distressing symptoms such as agitation, shortness of breath, delirium and noisy breathing due to secretions. Anticipatory medicines such as cyclizine, morphine, midazolam, levomepromazine and hyoscine hydrobromide, should be prescribed with the help of the Palliative Care team in response to the woman's needs [26].

Being diagnosed with incurable cancer is an emotionally challenging time for women and some of them may find it useful to confide in someone outside of their family e.g., their GP, keyworker, counsellor, or chaplain. Women should be made aware that their judgement and ability to think clearly will become compromised as their disease progresses and should therefore be offered help to plan and take important decisions in advance. Some examples of the available support include assistance in communicating their wishes about when and how they would like to be cared for at the end of their lives, as well as legal and financial advice such as entrusting legal power of attorney to someone else to take important decision about their health and wealth.

Women and their families should also be encouraged to discuss and plan the funeral service in advance, so that their final wishes can be taken into consideration and the necessary arrangements made to help cover the cost of this service. Emotional support is crucial for the family during these times as they witness the gradual decline in mental and physical capacities of their loved ones.

4.2.2 Coping Mechanisms

Many cancer patients are tempted to give up as they constantly have to overcome physical, social, and emotional obstacles while being confronted to a future marred by uncertainties. Hope for these patients rests in the philosophy that a positive outcome lies ahead. For this reason, agreeing what constitutes a positive outcome is key. Clinicians can support this process through communication and understanding of who the woman is and understanding what her aspirations and goals are. For example, women who have been newly diagnosed must have hope that they can be cured. For those who cannot be cured, there is hope that their symptoms will be controlled, and the cancer's progression contained. Women who have reached the end of their cancer journey can remain hopeful that they will pass on in dignity and without pain.

Many women embrace spirituality as a coping mechanism and engage in prayers, meditation, or joining religious group to expand their support network. There is widespread recognition that the spiritual needs of patients are often sub-optimally addressed by healthcare professionals who feel uneasy about broaching this subject [3]. These women should be referred to a support group with the appropriate expertise. Similarly, cancer patients often become frustrated with the numerous side effects of conventional therapies and the perceived futility at finding a cure and may decide to explore complementary therapies such as reflexology, acupuncture, or aromatherapy due to their lower toxicity profile [9]. Although there is currently a lack of evidence to support the role of complementary medicine in improving patient symptoms, clinicians should acknowledge that women have a right to fair information and be supported to access these services if they wish to do so [3]. One notable example is cannabidiol (CBD) oil. CBD oil can be purchased legally as a food supplement in the UK. Its potential as an anti-cancer drug and in the relief of cancer symptoms has generated widespread interest. Clinical trials in these field are still ongoing, and patients should be offered the opportunity to join a suitable clinical trial where they will have access to CBD oil in a monitored setting [27].

4.2.3 Support for Families and Carers

'Family survivorship' is an integral aspect of cancer care. Caring for a relative with a new cancer diagnosis is a stressful life event, especially for family members who suddenly find themselves propelled into this new role. Conflict may arise due to the reorganisation of the family structure, emotional pressures, and the need to prioritise resources [28]. Regular contact between the keyworkers, the cancer patient and those looking after her is necessary to enable the ongoing assessment of their holistic needs. Providing daily care for a relative living with cancer may not only be labour-intensive but also stressful for carers, who may eventually find themselves at the cusp of physical and emotional breakdown. Respite care offers carers the opportunity to take a temporary break to look after their own health and wellbeing. Different options may be available depending on the desired level of help (e.g., overnight care for terminally ill patients) or the duration of the intended break (e.g., sitting services, day centres, hospice, or home) [29].

4.3 Conclusions

A multidisciplinary approach to address the felt-needs rather than expert-defined needs of women with a gynaecological cancer will result in the best outcomes. This can only be achieved if healthcare professionals, patients and their carers come together and work in partnership. Greater education for healthcare professionals to identify and treat the non-physical needs of women living with cancer is essential to support them to live as well as possible.

Key Points

1. Women living with and beyond cancer have unmet physical, emotional, social and psychosexual needs.
2. Support from a multidisciplinary team is essential to optimise patient independence and adaptation to life-changes after a cancer diagnosis.
3. A holistic needs assessment is an essential tool to promote a shift from expert-defined to patient-centred care.
4. Further training is needed to equip clinicians with the expertise to address the non-physical needs of cancer survivors.
5. Effective communication among healthcare professionals, GPs, and social services is a key feature of an integrative care pathway aiming to improve the quality of life of cancer survivors.
6. Gynaecological cancer survivors are particularly vulnerable to the impact of a cancer diagnosis on their sexuality and desire for motherhood.
7. The needs of carers and family members should always be considered alongside those of the cancer patient.

References

1. Cancer Research UK. Clinical research on gynaecological cancer [online]. Available from https://crukcambridgecentre.org.uk/patient-care/clinical-research/gynaecological#:~:text=These%20five%20cancers%20are%20womb,%2C%20cervical%2C%20vaginal%20and%20vulval.&text=Womb%20cancer%20is%20sometimes%20called,cell%20the%20cancer%20started%20in
2. Cancer Research UK. Cancer survival statistics for all cancers combined [online]. Available from https://www.cancerresearchuk.org/health-professional/cancer-statistics/survival/all-cancers-combined#heading-One
3. NICE. Improving supportive and palliative care for adults with cancer. Cancer service guideline [online]. 2004. Available from https://www.nice.org.uk/guidance/csg4

4. Fitch MI. Supportive care framework. Can Oncol Nurs J. 2008;18(1):6–24.
5. National Cancer Survivorship Initiative. Living with and beyond cancer: taking actions to improve outcomes [online]. 2013. Available from https://assets.publishing.service.gov.uk/government/uploads/system/uploads/attachment_data/file/181054/9333-TSO-2900664-NCSI_Report_FINAL.pdf
6. Macmillan Cancer Support. The recovery package [online]. 2015. Available from https://www.macmillan.org.uk/_images/recovery-package-sharing-good-practice_tcm9-299778.pdf.
7. Snowden A, Young J, White C, Murray E, Richard C, Lussier MT, MacArthur E, Storey D, Schipani S, Wheatley D, McMahon J, Ross E. Evaluating holistic needs assessment in outpatient cancer care—a randomised controlled trial: the study protocol. BMJ Open. 2015;5(5):e006840.
8. Browall M, Carlsson M, Horvath GG. Information needs of women with recently diagnosed ovarian cancer—a longitudinal study. Eur J Oncol Nurs. 2004;8(3):200–7. discussion 208-10
9. Ferrell B, Smith S, Cullinane C, Melancon C. Symptom concerns of women with ovarian cancer. J Pain Symptom Manag. 2003;25(6):528–38.
10. Tabano M, Condosta D, Coons M. Symptoms affecting quality of life in women with gynecologic cancer. Semin Oncol Nurs. 2002;18:223–30.
11. Saeaib N, Peeyananjarassri K, Liabsuetrakul T, Buhachat R, Myriokefalitaki E. Hormone replacement therapy after surgery for epithelial ovarian cancer. Cochrane Database Syst Rev. 2020;1(1):CD012559.
12. Edey KA, Rundle S, Hickey M. Hormone replacement therapy for women previously treated for endometrial cancer. Cochrane Database Syst Rev. 2018;5(5):CD008830.
13. British Menopause Society. Tools for clinicians. Prescribable alternatives to HRT [online]. Available from https://thebms.org.uk/wp-content/uploads/2020/07/02-BMS-TfC-Prescribable-alternatives-to-HRT-July2020-01B.pdf
14. Denton AS, Clarke N, Maher J. Non-surgical interventions for late radiation cystitis in patients who have received radical radiotherapy to the pelvis. Cochrane Database Syst Rev. 2002;2002(3):CD001773.
15. Lawrie TA, Green JT, Beresford M, Wedlake L, Burden S, Davidson SE, Lal S, Henson CC, Andreyev HJN. Interventions to reduce acute and late adverse gastrointestinal effects of pelvic radiotherapy for primary pelvic cancers. Cochrane Database Syst Rev. 2018;1(1):CD012529.
16. Andreyev HJ, Davidson SE, Gillespie C, Allum WH, Swarbrick E. Practice guidance on the management of acute and chronic gastrointestinal problems arising as a result of treatment for cancer. Gut. 2012;61(2):179–92.
17. Stabile C, Gunn A, Sonoda Y, Carter J. Emotional and sexual concerns in women undergoing pelvic surgery and associated treatment for gynecologic cancer. Transl Androl Urol. 2015;4(2):169–85.
18. La Rosa VL, Garzon S, Gullo G, et al. Fertility preservation in women affected by gynaecological cancer: the importance of an integrated gynaecological and psychological approach. Ecancermedicalscience. 2020;14:1035.
19. Fagerlind H, Kettis Å, Glimelius B, Ring L. Barriers against psychosocial communication: oncologists' perceptions. J Clin Oncol. 2013;31(30):3815–22.
20. Kenen R, Arden-Jones R, Eeles R. Living with chronic risk: healthy women with a family history of breast/ovarian cancer. Health Risk Soc. 2004;5:315–31.
21. Foster C, Fenlon D. Recovery and self-management support following primary cancer treatment. Br J Cancer. 2011;105(Suppl 1):S21–8.
22. Hodgkinson K, Butow P, Fuchs A, Hunt GE, Stenlake A, Hobbs KM, Brand A, Wain G. Long-term survival from gynecologic cancer: psychosocial outcomes, supportive care needs and positive outcomes. Gynecol Oncol. 2007;104(2):381–9.
23. Ozga M, Aghajanian C, Myers-Virtue S, et al. A systematic review of ovarian cancer and fear of recurrence. Palliat Support Care. 2015;13(6):1771–80.
24. Vehling S, Kissane DW. Existential distress in cancer: alleviating suffering from fundamental loss and change. Psychooncology. 2018;27(11):2525–30.
25. Cancer Research UK. Care planning. Advanced care planning [online]. Available from https://www.cancerresearchuk.org/about-cancer/coping/dying-with-cancer/making-plans/care-planning
26. Marie Curie. Care and Support through terminal illness. Anticipatory medicines [online]. Available from https://www.mariecurie.org.uk/professionals/palliative-care-knowledge-zone/symptom-control/anticipatory-medicines
27. Cancer Research UK. Cannabis, CBD oil and cancer [online]. Available from https://www.cancerresearchuk.org/about-cancer/cancer-in-general/treatment/complementary-alternative-therapies/individual-therapies/cannabis
28. Koldjeski D, Kirkpatrick MK, Everett L, Brown S, Swanson M. The ovarian cancer journey of families the first postdiagnostic year. Cancer Nurs. 2007;30(3):232–42.
29. Marie Curie. Care and Support through terminal illness. Respite and taking a break [online]. Available from https://www.mariecurie.org.uk/help/support/being-there/support-carers/respite-care

Clinical Evidence in Gynaeoncology: Sources and Application

Elaine Leung and Sudha Sundar

5.1 Introduction

Clinical practice is evolving fast with the technological advances, improved understanding of cancer biology and clinical complexity with an aging population. Each clinician ought to use the current best evidence to inform care decisions- the basis of evidence-based medicine (EBM). EBM promotes practices that confers clinical benefits and abandonment of practices that confer no clinical benefits, which ultimately improves quality of care and its cost-effectiveness. For example, the Lymphadenectomy in Ovarian Neoplasms (LION) trial [1] assessed the benefits of systematic pelvic and paraaortic lymphadenectomy in patients with newly diagnosed advanced ovarian cancer with clinically normal lymph nodes and demonstrated that lymphadenectomy was associated with higher morbidities and no significant difference in overall and progression-free survival.

Institutions also have a duty to mandate evaluation of surgical innovation and improve the conduct of research. For example, the Idea, Development, Exploration, Assessment, Long-term follow-up (IDEAL) network has proposed a framework for the evaluation of surgical intervention at each stage of its development [2], which should be considered when a new surgical technique or device is developed.

Acknowledging the skills required to practice EBM is crucial. EBM is meant to tailor the best-available evidence to the needs and preferences of an individual patient. Evidence-based practice requires clinical judgement and the understanding of the existing evidence and the quality and comprehensiveness of this evidence to the specific clinical scenario to avoid a one-size-fits-all approach to clinical management.

In this chapter, we explore the components of evidence-based practice based on the Sicily statement in 1990s on evidence-based practice [3], with selected studies and examples relevant to gynaeoncologists. The statement proposed a five-step model of EBM (often referred as "the 5As" of EBM): Ask, Acquire, Appraise, Apply and Audit. We have also suggested relevant resources to help embed EBM into everyday practice to complement the concurrent development of clinical and technical skills.

5.2 Structured Questions (Ask)

Asking a well-structured question is key to the practice of EBM. Different tools exist to help develop structured questions to enable effective literature search [4]. The five-component approach by identifying the relevant population, intervention, comparison, outcome and design

E. Leung (✉) · S. Sundar
Pan-Birmingham Gynaecological Cancer Centre,
Birmingham City Hospital, Birmingham, UK
e-mail: E.Leung@bham.ac.uk; S.S.Sundar@bham.ac.uk

(PICOD) is commonly used for asking clinical questions. An example based on the aforementioned Laparoscopic Approach to Cervical Cancer (LACC) Trial [5] is summarised in Table 5.1. Although this approach may seem contrived at first, its routine use will provide a methodological approach to ask searchable questions related to individual clinical scenarios.

5.3 Searching for Evidence (Acquire)

5.3.1 Hierarchy of Evidence

Evidence is not equal. The early adopters of EBM suggested a hierarchy of evidence exists and was previously portrayed as a pyramid with study designs that have high risk of bias (internal validity) and low applicability (external validity) at the bottom (Fig. 5.1) [6]. However, the design of a study is not the only factor that determines the reliability of the estimated effects [7]. This will be further discussed in the next section on critical appraisal.

Table 5.1 The PICOD summary based on the LACC trial [1]

Participants/Population	Women with early-stage cervical cancer
Intervention	Minimally invasive surgery (laparoscopic or robot-assisted)
Comparator	Open surgery
Outcomes	Primary: Disease-free survival Secondary: Recurrence rate, overall survival
Design	Randomised control trial

More recently, the injudicious placement of all systematic reviews and meta-analyses at the top of the pyramid has been challenged [6]. Substantial effort has been made since the early history of EBM to improve the methodology and reporting of systematic reviews and meta-analyses (SR/MA) [8]. Some advocated the removal of SR/MA from the pyramid and treat these as tools to support the use of evidence by stakeholders [6]. The sources of evidence has also been described as a hierarchical pyramid (Fig. 5.2) [9], with more clinically usable sources at the top (e.g. computerized decision support systems incorporating guideline recommendations).

5.3.2 Examples of Primary Research Studies

All types of primary research studies have practice-changing potential. In this chapter, we use different examples to challenge the common perception that certain types of research are more important than others, before we further explore the best way to appraise each study.

5.3.2.1 Randomised Control Trials (RCT)

Evidence-based practice matters. RCTs are often regarded as the gold-standard for evaluating the effectiveness of an intervention. In an RCT, a number of similar people are randomly assigned to two or more groups to test a intervention, with at least one experimental group in which participants are given the intervention being tested.

Design	General description
SR/MA	Summarises previous studies and statistically combined the results
RCT	Randomly selects participants to receive an intervention versus a comparator
Cohort	Follows a group to track risk factors and outcomes over time
Case-control	Compares histories of participants with and without an exposure or a condition
Cross-sectional	Assesses the prevalence of an outcome in a broad population at a specific time point

Fig. 5.1 The EBM pyramid, adapted from Murad and co-workers [6], and general description of each study design. *SR/MA* systematic reviews and meta-analyses

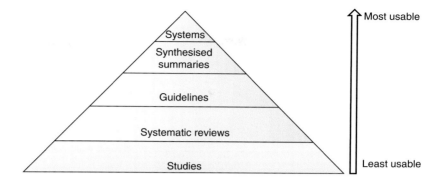

Fig. 5.2 The pyramid of sources of evidence, adapted from Alper and co-workers [9]

Participants of all groups are followed up in the same manner to compare the benefits and harm observed in each group.

Before the availability of high-quality evidence, minimally invasive surgery was widely adopted as an alternative to open surgery for radical hysterectomy in patients with early-stage cervical cancer. Two reports in 2018 [5, 10], a RCT and a large population-based dataset, provided initial high-quality evidence demonstrating minimally invasive in this group was associated with poorer recurrence rate and overall survival than open surgery, sent shock waves within the community of gynaeoncologists, and open surgery was re-established as the norm for early stage cervical cancer. Whilst the debate surrounding the best surgical approach in this context continues [11], this recent example emphasises the potential harm when clinical practice moves forward without evaluation and the need arises for systematic evaluation of existing clinical practice to support best care.

RCT is the best method for treatment evaluation. In 1990, the Advanced Ovarian Cancer Trialists Group (AOCTG) held a consensus meeting to discuss the results of their review on chemotherapy in advanced ovarian cancer [12] and the Ovarian Cancer Meta-Analysis Project [13]. The AOCTG recommended two specific questions related to adjuvant chemotherapy in patients with ovarian cancer to be addressed by large RCTs, which initiated a series of International Collaborative Ovarian Neoplasm (ICON) RCTs (Table 5.2) [23]. The early landmark trials have transformed practice and formed the basis of platinum-based chemotherapy for epithelial ovarian cancers (EOC).

5.3.2.2 Observational Studies

Observational studies identify associations between causes and effects; they dominate the literature. They investigate and record exposures (e.g. interventions or risk factors) and observe outcomes (e.g. cancer recurrence or death) as they occur. The different types of observational studies are summarised in Table 5.3. Observational studies are often used to evaluate a hypothesis when the knowledge is poor, and to formulate and test hypotheses in preparation of future trials.

They are illustrated by the evaluations of the role of secondary cytoreductive surgery (CRS) in ovarian cancer. In 1998, the Second International Ovarian Cancer Consensus Conference collated expert opinions and suggested potential criteria for selecting suitable patients for secondary CRS [24]. The panel also recognised the lack of evidence supporting surgical decision making in this context, and suggested an initial exploratory observational study to address this evidence gap. This formed the basis of the Arbeitsgemeinschaft Gynaekologische Onkologie Ovarian Committee Descriptive Evaluation of preoperative Selection KriTeria for OPerability in recurrent OVARian cancer (AGO DESKTOP OVAR) trials (Table 5.4).

The first DESKTOP study retrospectively determined factors associated with complete resection, now known as the AGO score, which included three factors- complete resection at initial surgery, Eastern Cooperative Oncology Group performance status (ECOG PS) of zero and ≤500 ml of ascites at recurrence [25]. Concurrently, the Memorial Sloan-Kettering Cancer Center also published its selection criteria

Table 5.2 A summary of ICON trials with the timing of key publications

	Year	Participants (n)	Comparison(s)	Overall survival
ICON1 [14]	2003	Early EOC; adjuvant chemotherapy (n = 447)	Adjuvant P versus observation	HR 0.66, 95%CI: 0.45–0.97, p = 0.03
ICON2 [15]	1998	First line chemotherapy (n = 1526)	Carboplatin versus CAP	HR 1.00, 95%CI: 0.86–1.16, p = 0.98
ICON3 [16]	2002	First line chemotherapy (n = 2074)	CP versus carboplatin/CAP	HR 0.98, 95%CI: 0.87–1.10, p = 0.74
ICON4/AGO-OVAR-2.2 [17]	2003	Platinum-sensitive relapsed (n = 802)	P versus P + paclitaxel	HR 0.82, 95%CI: 0.69–0.97, p = 0.02
GOG0182-ICON5 [18]	2009	Advanced EOC; first line chemotherapy (n = 4312)	Five arms comparing CP versus CP + a third cytotoxic agent	No difference between arms
ICON6 [19]	2016	Platinum-sensitive relapsed EOC (n = 486)	P versus P + concurrent or maintenance cediranib (3-arm)	HR 0.85, 95%CI: 0.66–1.10, p = 0.21
ICON7 [20]	2011	All EOC; first line chemotherapy (n = 1528)	CP versus CP + bevacizumab	HR 0.85, 95%CI: 0.69–1.04, p = 0.11
ICON8 [21]	2019	All EOC; first line chemotherapy (n = 1566)	Three-arm comparisons of CP dosing regimes	No difference between arms
ICON9 [22]	2020	First platinum-sensitive relapsed EOC (n = 618)[a]	Maintenance olaparib alone versus olaparib + cediranib	Ongoing

P platinum-based chemotherapy, *CAP* cyclophosphamide, doxorubicin, and cisplatin, *CP* Carboplatin and paclitaxel, *HR* hazard ratio, *95%CI* 95% confidence interval
[a]Projected number of participants

Table 5.3 Common types of observational studies in clinical research

	Description	Strengths	Weaknesses
Case-control study	Two groups identified by case status (e.g diseased or not) and compare factors with potential influence of outcomes	Inexpensive Individualised data Asssess multiple confounders and exposures Useful for rare disease	Cannot assess incidence, prevalence or temporality Assess a defined outcome Selection bias Recall bias
Cohort study	A group of patients are monitored over a period of time	Individualised data Can demonstrate temporality Asssess multiple onfounders, exposures and outcomes	Relatively expensive Time consuming Loss to follow-up Impractical for rare diseases
Cross-sectional study	Data collection from a population or a representative subset at a specific time point	Inexpensive Individualised data Asssess multiple confounders and outcomes	Cannot demonstrate temporality Can be impractical for rare diseases
Longitudinal study	Repeat observations of the same variables over a period of time	Participant variables do not affect data Ability to measure the pattern of change	Relatively expensive Time consuming Loss to follow-up Logistical challenges of long follow-up

for secondary CRS in patients with recurrent EOC [31]. It concluded that low volume disease (≤0.5 cm), longer disease-free interval (particularly in those who had a progression-free interval of >30 months) and fewer recurrence sites (e.g. single site recurrence) should be used as selection criteria for offering secondary CRS.

The second DESKTOP study prospectively validated the predictive significance of the AGO score after secondary CRS [26], which confirmed the AGO score predict improved surgical outcome in recurrent ovarian cancer. The Shanghai Gynaecologic Oncology Group developed its own 6-variable risk model (iMODEL; a score of 0–11.9) based on their retrospective data. The variables included in iMODEL are cancer stage, residual disease after primary surgery, progression-free interval, CA-125 levels, ECOG PS and ascites at recurrence [27]. The AGO score and iMODEL have been used to select suitable patients for the DESKTOP III [29] and SOC-1 [30] RCTs, respectively. In contrast to the earlier GOG-0213 RCT, in which any patients with investigator-determined resectable recurrent platinum-sensitive EOC were randomised to receive secondary CRS with adjuvant chemotherapy versus chemotherapy alone [28], DESKTOP III and SOC-1 suggested that secondary CRS with chemotherapy only improved survival in selected patients with platinum-sensitive recurrent EOC, compared to chemotherapy alone (Table 5.4). Together, these examples highlight the important role observational studies played to generate practice-transforming evidence.

5.3.2.3 Translational Research

Translational research aims to speed up the bidirectional move between bench discoveries and bedside observations, with explicit human health and economic benefits in mind. The definitions of translational research has evolved overtime and often described as phasic definitions. A recent systematic review by Fort and co-workers [32] has described translational research in five phases (T0–T4). From basic research to early testing in humans (T1) to the establishment of effectiveness in humans and clinical guidelines (T2), with implementation and dissemination research (T3), additional focus on outcomes and effectiveness in populations (T4) and research (e.g. multi-omic data) that could be linked back to further basic research. Clinical trials are an integral part of

Table 5.4 A summary of AGO DESKTOP OVAR and related trials with the timing of key publications

	Year	Participants (n)	Comparison(s)	Outcomes	Design
DESKTOP OVAR [25]	2006	Relapsed platinum-sensitive EOC who underwent secondary CRS (n = 267)	Not applicable	Complete resection associated with longer survival (HR 3.71, 95%CI: 2.27–6.05, p < 0.0001); AGO-score positive associated with improved R0 rate	Retrospective cohort study
AGO-DESKTOP II [26]	2011	Relapsed platinum-sensitive EOC managed based on the AGO score (n = 516)	Not applicable	261 (51%) were AGO-score positive; 129 of 261 (49%) them were operated on. R0 rate = 76%	Prospective cohort study
Tian and co-workers [27]	2012	Relapsed platinum-sensitive EOC who underwent secondary CRS (n = 1075)	Not applicable	Development of a 6-variable risk model (iMODEL; a score of 0 to 11.9). R0 rate = 53% versus 20% in low-risk and high-risk women, respectively (p < 0.0001)	Retrospective cohort study
GOG-0213 [28]	2019	Relapsed platinum-sensitive EOC who underwent secondary CRS (n = 267)	Secondary CRS + P versus P alone; no selection model used	Median survival: 50.6 versus 64.7 months. OS HR 1.29, 95%CI: 0.97 to 1.72, p = 0.08. R0 rate = 67%	RCT
DESKTOP III [29]	2021	First platinum-sensitive relapsed EOC (n = 407)	Secondary CRS + P versus P alone Selected by AGO-score	Median survival: 53.7 versus 46.2 months. OS HR 0.65, 95%CI: 0.52 to 0.81, p < 0.001. R0 rate = 74%	RCT
SOC-1 [30]	2021	First platinum-sensitive relapsed EOC (n = 357)	Secondary CRS + P versus P alone; Selected by iMODEL cut-off and PET-CT	PFS HR 0.58, 95%CI 0.45–0.74, p < 0.0001 (OS pending). R0 rate = 77%	RCT

OS overall survival, *PFS* progression-free survival, *P* platinum-based chemotherapy, *R0* Complete Gross Resection translational research (T1 and T2), with phase 1 clinical trials for assessing the safety and dosage of new interventions, phase 2 clinical trials to assess their effectiveness and phase 3 clinical trials (e.g. RCTs) to confirm their effectiveness, monitor side effects and compare the new interventions with existing standard of care treatments. Here, we use the discovery of human papillomavirus (HPV) and poly ADP ribose polymerase (PARP) inhibitor as early and recent examples of translational research.

Professor zur Hausen first published the identification of HPV DNA in cervical cancer and genital wart biopsies in 1974 [33]. His early work recognised that genital HPVs are distinct from those in non-genital warts, and later isolated the high-risk HPV subtypes (HPV-16 and HPV-18) in the cervix [34]. His group then illustrated that HPV DNA was integrated into the host genome in cervical cancer cell lines and that the viral E6 and E7 oncogenes are preferentially retained and expressed in cervical cancers [35]. This seminal work demonstrating HPV as a cause of cervical cancer has formed the basis of primary HPV screening and the development of HPV vaccines, and led to his award of the Nobel Prize in Physiology or Medicine in 2008.

Translational research has catalysed the use of new knowledge on cancer biology to discover new cancer treatments. One of the recent successes is the development of PARP inhibitors, which is now in routine clinical use and being further evaluated in large RCTs, such as ICON9 [22] (see Table 5.2). Two preclinical studies [36, 37] published in 2005 by different research teams independently concluded that *BRCA*-deficient cells were selectively sensitive to PARP inhibition (Table 5.5). In collaboration with pharmaceutical companies and academic clinicians, these research teams evaluated two drugs (olaparib and rucaparib) in clinical trials. The landmark first-in-class phase I trial demonstrated that olaparib was safe and had anti-tumoural potential [38]. Later, dosage and efficacy of PARP inhibitors in ovarian cancer were demonstrated by a number of phase II and III studies, leading to their approval for routine clinical settings (Table 5.5). Ongoing clinical trials now aim to better define the role of PARP inhibitors in the standard of care for ovarian and other cancers, particularly in those without evidence of homologous recombination repair defects.

Together, these examples demonstrate the essential roles of carefully designed pre-clinical translational studies in transforming gynaecological cancer care.

5.3.2.4 Diagnostic Test Accuracy (DTA) Studies

DTA studies are essential for assessing the ability of a test to identify a condition correctly. Studies to evaluate diagnostic test accuracy require different designs compared to those for treatment evaluation. There are two main types of DTA studies (1) those that allow direct comparisons of index, comparator and reference standard tests performed independently in the same group of participants (Table 5.6); (2) RCTs in which participants are randomised to the index and comparator tests and all received the reference standard test.

For example, in the context of primary HPV testing in the United Kingdom, Cuzick and co-workers first conducted two cross-sectional studies on HPV testing [49, 50] of ~5000 women attending for routine smears. All women were assessed by HPV testing (index test) and cervical cytology (comparator test). If indicated, they were also assessed by colposcopically-directed biopsy (reference standard) to detect high-grade cervical intraepithelial neoplasms (CIN; target condition). The sensitivity, specificity, positive and negative predictive values of HPV testing, compared to cervical cytology, were presented (Table 5.6). Based on the results of these two cross-sectional studies, a multicentre screening RCT of 11,085 women aged 30–60 years was performed (the HART study) [51]. In the HART study, women with either borderline cytology or negative cytology with high-risk HPV were randomised to immediate colposcopy or repeat HPV testing, cytology, and colposcopy at 12 months. The study suggested that HPV testing was more sensitive than cervical cytology (97.1% versus 76.6%, $p = 0.002$) but less specific (93.3 vs. 95.8%, $p < 0.0001$) for detecting histologically-

Table 5.5 A summary of selected key studies in the development of PARP inhibitors

	Year	Participants (n)	Comparison(s)	Outcomes	Design
Farmer 2005 [37]	2005	Wild type versus BRCA-deficient cell lines	KU0058684 and KU0058948 versus mock	BRCA-deficiency sensitizes cells PARP inhibition; development of olaparib	Pre-clinical
Byrant 2005 [36]	2005	Mouse V-C8 xenografts	NU1025 and AG14361 versus mock	Three of five mice responded (1 complete remission); development of rucaparib	Pre-clinical
Fong 2009 [38]	2009	First-in-human clinical trial (n = 60)	Single agent olaparib (no comparator)	Few adverse effects; anti-tumour activity in cancer associated with BRCA1 or BRCA2 mutation	Phase I clinical trial
Study 19 (NCT00753545) [39]	2012	Platinum-sensitive relapsed EOC (n = 265)	Maintenance olaparib versus placebo	PFS HR 0.35, 95%CI 0.25–0.49, p < 0.001; OS HR 0.73, 95%CI 0.55–0.96, p = 0.025); median OS was 29.8 versus 27.8 months	Phase II clinical trial
Study 42 (NCT01078662) [40]	2015	Germline BRCA1/BRCA2 mutations EOC after ≥3 lines of prior therapies (n = 193)	Single agent olaparib (no comparator)	ORR was 34% (46/137, 95%CI 26–42) and median DoR was 7.9 (95%CI 5.6–9.6) months	Phase II clinical trial
Study 10 (NCT01482715) [41]	2017	First-in-human clinical trial (n = 82)	Single agent rucaparib (no comparator)	Few adverse effects; anti-tumour activity in cancer associated with BRCA1 or BRCA2 mutation	Phase I/II clinical trial
ARIEL2 [42]	2017	Platinum-sensitive relapsed EOC after ≥1 line of prior therapy (n = 206)	Single agent rucaparib based on HRD status versus LOH low subgroup	PFS- BRCA mutant: HR 0.7, 95%CI 0.16–0.44, p < 0.0001; LOH high: HR 0.62, 95%CI 0.42–0.90, p = 0.01	Phase II clinical trial
ARIEL3 [43]	2017	Platinum-sensitive relapsed EOC after ≥2 line of prior therapy (n = 567)	Single agent rucaparib versus placebo based on HRD status	PFS- BRCA mutant: HR 0.23, 95%CI 0.16–0.34, p < 0.0001; LOH high: HR 0.32, 95%CI 0.24–0.42, p < 0.0001; intention-to-treat: HR 0.36, 95%CI 0.30–0.45, p < 0.0001	Phase III RCT
SOLO-2 [44, 45]	2017	Platinum-sensitive EOC with germline BRCA1 and/or BRCA2 mutations after ≥2 lines of prior therapy (n = 295)	Maintenance olaparib versus placebo	Overall PFS HR 0.30, 95%CI 0.22–0.41, p < 0.0001; OS HR 0.74, 95%CI 0.54–1.00, p = 0.054); median OS was 51.7 versus 38.8 months	Phase III RCT
SOLO-1 [46]	2018	New platinum-sensitive EOC with germline BRCA1 and/or BRCA2 mutations (n = 391)	Maintenance olaparib versus placebo	Overall PFS HR 0.30, 95%CI 0.23–0.41, p < 0.001	Phase III RCT
PAOLA-1 [47]	2019	New platinum-sensitive EOC (n = 806)	Olaparib + bevacizumab versus Placebo + bevacizumab	Overall PFS HR 0.59, 95%CI 0.49–0.72, p < 0.001	Phase III RCT
PRIMA [48]	2019	New platinum-sensitive EOC (n = 733)	Niraparib versus placebo	Overall PFS HR 0.62, 95%CI 0.50–0.76, p < 0.001	Phase III RCT

PFS progression free survival, *ORR* overall response rate, *DoR* Duration of Response, *HRD* homologous recombination deficiency, *LOH* Loss of heterozygosity

5 Clinical Evidence in Gynaeoncology: Sources and Application

Table 5.6 Key terms used in diagnostic test accuracy studies

	Description
Index test	A diagnostic test that is being evaluated against a reference standard test in a study of test accuracy
Reference standard	The best available test or procedure used to classify patients as having The target condition or not
Comparator test	A diagnostic test that is being evaluated against the index test, which may be the reference standard or another diagnostic test that is being assessed for accuracy
Sensitivity	Measures of how often a test (e.g. HPV testing) correctly generates a positive result for participants who have the target condition, e.g. CIN
Specificity	Measures a test's ability to correctly generate a *negative* result for people who don't have the target condition
Positive predictive value	The probability that participants with a positive screening test have the disease
Negative predictive value	The probability that participants with a negative screening test don't have the disease

proven high-grade CIN, and repeat surveillance at 12 months was as effective as immediate colposcopy for detecting high-grade CIN. Moreover, none of the women who had negative HPV test results at baseline or at 12 months repeat surveillance had high-grade CIN. The HART and other related studies [52, 53] later led to the recommendation of high-risk HPV testing, instead of cervical cytology, as the primary method for cervical cancer screening throughout the United Kingdom in 2020.

5.3.3 Examples of Other Resources to Acquire Evidence

5.3.3.1 Systematic Reviews, Scoping Reviews and Meta-Analysis

Acquiring all primary studies for each structured question to inform clinical practice is unsustainable- finding clinically usable resources effectively is crucial (Fig. 5.2). Systematic and, more recently, scoping reviews have gained popularity amongst both researchers and clinicians [54]. A systematic review uses replicable methods with the aim to minimise bias and provide reliable findings for decision making related to a specific structured question [55]. A systematic review may be performed with or without a meta-analysis, which uses statistical methods to combine and summarise numerical data from multiple separate studies collated in a systematic review. In contrast, a scoping review aims to provide an indication of the volume and focus of available literature on a specific topic. Scoping reviews are useful to determine the type of existing evidence, the way research has been conducted and the specific outstanding questions that could be addressed by more specific systematic reviews or future clinical trials [56]. Munn and co-workers [54] has provided helpful comparisons between systematic and scoping reviews (Table 5.7).

Established guidance exists to support the conduct of both types of reviews. The EQUATOR (Enhancing the QUAlity and Transparency Of health Research) Network is an international initiative aims to improve the reliability of research by improving the reporting of published reports (https://www.equator-network.org/). The network has published reporting guidelines for all main study types, including systematic and scoping reviews. The Preferred Reporting Items for Systematic Reviews and Meta-Analyses (PRISMA) guidelines suggested a minimum set of items for reporting in different types of systematic reviews and meta-analyses (http://www.prisma-statement.org/). Recently, a 20-item PRISMA extension has been published specifically for scoping review (PRISMA-ScR) [57].

To learn more about conducting systematic reviews, the Cochrane Handbook for Systematic Reviews of Interventions (http://www.cochrane-handbook.org) is an essential text. Existing systematic review protocols could be found at PROSPERO (https://www.crd.york.ac.uk/prospero/), an international database of prospectively registered systematic reviews. Conducting systematic reviews require teamwork (i.e. it cannot be done by a lone researcher), skills and a structured approach. While the time required and expertise involved should not be underestimated, there are networks of support for those who are keen to embark on the journeys of conducting their first systematic reviews.

Table 5.7 Characteristics of systematic and scoping reviews, modified from Munn and co-workers [54]

	Systematic reviews	Scoping reviews
Indications	• Uncover international evidence • Compare current practice • Identify new practices • Identify and inform areas for future research • Identify and investigate conflicting results • Produce statements to guide decision-making	• Identify the types of available evidence • Clarify key concepts/definitions in the literature • Examine how research is conducted • Identify key characteristics or factors related to a concept • Precursor of systematic reviews • Identify and analyse knowledge gaps
A priori review protocol	Yes	Yes/no
Prospective registration	Yes	Yes/no
Transparent search strategy	Yes	Yes
Standardized data extraction form	Yes	Yes
Risk of bias assessment	Yes	Yes/no
Synthesis of findings from individual studies	Yes	No

5.3.3.2 Guidelines/Synthesised Summaries

Guidelines and synthesised summaries are often the first port of call sought by clinicians when making care decisions for individual patients.

The development of evidence-based guideline involves systematic reviews that are interpreted to provide systematically derived recommendations on practice in a specific context. For example, national professional bodies and learned societies (e.g. National Institute for Health and Care Excellence and the British Gynaecological Cancer Society) regularly publish evidence-based guidelines relevant for gynaeoncologists.

Synthesised summaries are frequently updated summaries of evidence and recommendations, but existing resources for synthesised summaries (e.g. BMJ Best Practice and UpToDate) vary in responsiveness and quality.

5.4 Critical Appraisal (Appraise)

Acquired literature should be assessed on both its methodology and relevance to the considered structured clinical questions. There are useful advice and appraisal instruments (often described as toolkits or checklists) to aid critical appraisal, we have elaborated on some of the support in this session.

5.4.1 The Grading of Recommendations Assessment, Development and Evaluation (GRADE) Framework

A range of factors determines the strength of evidence (Table 5.1). The GRADE Working Group developed a 4-level framework to evaluate the quality of evidence by assessing different domains of a study (also known as certainty in evidence; Table 5.8). By assessing the GRADE domains (Table 5.9), which include the risk of bias, imprecision, inconsistency, indirectness and publication bias, the certainty in evidence could be rated up or down [7]. Evidence-based guidelines for clinical practice routinely use this framework to highlight the strength of the recommendations.

5.4.2 Resources to Support Critical Appraisal

A number of organisations have published tools to support critical appraisal (Table 5.10). A three-step approach are often described to help clinicians to decide whether the research results are applicable in a local context. Firstly, the results are evaluated for validity (i.e. whether the study measures what it purports to measure). Secondly,

5 Clinical Evidence in Gynaeoncology: Sources and Application

Table 5.8 GRADE certainty of evidence, replicated from the GRADE framework [7]

Certainty	Summary
High	True effect is similar to the estimated effect
Moderate	True effect is probably close to the estimated effect
Low	True effect might be markedly different from the estimated effect
Very low	True effect is probably markedly different from the estimated effect

Table 5.9 The GRADE Domains [7]

Assessment Domain	Description
Risk of bias	The limitations in design or conduct of a study
Imprecision	Were 95% confidence intervals examined, with reference to the effect size estimates?
Inconsistency	Did the studies yield consistent results?
Indirectness	Did the studies directly compare the interventions of interest in the population of interest? Did the studies report outcomes that are critical for decision-making?
Publication bias	Are critical studies likely to be missing from the literature?

the level of precision (e.g. the interpretation of the 95% confidence interval) and clinical importance around the results are considered. Finally, the applicability of the results to the specific questions in the intended populations (e.g. the ethnic composition of the research participants) is assessed. The use of checklists often helps to complete a comprehensive appraisal and determine the certainty of evidence, especially for novice critical appraisers.

5.5 Implementing Evidence-Based Practice in Gynaeoncology (Apply)

After mastering the skills of critical appraisal, applying the evidence in practice requires understanding of the local clinical expertise, available resources and patient's expectations. Evidence-based practice should be encouraged on both individual and institutional levels.

In addition to the generation of evidence-based guidelines, each unit can benefit from evidence-based journal clubs to discuss relevant clinical questions supported by presentation of clinical scenarios and critical appraisal toolkits. For those who do not have exposure to a local journal club, virtual journal clubs may be beneficial. For example, the International Journal of Gynaecological Cancer has a monthly Virtual Journal Club delivered via an established online teleconference platform and advertised on social media as #IJGCclub.

In this digital age, the high volume of information published challenges individual clinicians to maintain evidence-based practice; institutional support of EBM is crucial. Institutions already provide resources and organise expert panels to generate evidence-based guidance. Further could be developed to support evidence-based decision making. For example, computerised decision support systems are now incorporated in day-to-day practice (e.g. electronic prescribing systems and risk assessments for venous thromboembolism), with the potential to be explored further in gynaeoncology.

Moreover, ensuring the collection of relevant outcomes of current and ongoing studies are paramount for supporting future decision making with the results. The Core Outcome Measures in Effectiveness Trials (COMET) Initiative aims to facilitate the development and application of Core Outcome Sets (COS), which are minimum standardised sets of outcomes that should be measured and reported in all clinical trials on specific healthcare topics [58]. When available, institutions should ensure individual researchers use suitable COS when designing or reporting on healthcare studies.

Table 5.10 Selected resources to support critical appraisal and evidence-based practice

Organisation	Webpage
Critical appraisal skills	
The critical appraisal skills Programme (CASP)	https://casp-uk.net/casp-tools-checklists/
The Centre for Evidence-Based Medicine	https://www.cebm.net/
The Scottish intercollegiate guidelines network (SIGN)	https://www.sign.ac.uk/what-we-do/methodology/checklists/
Resource Page of the specialist unit for review evidence at the University of Cardiff	https://www.cardiff.ac.uk/specialist-unit-for-review-evidence/resources
Evidence-based practice- guidelines/societies	
The International Federation of Gynaecology and Obstetrics (FIGO)	https://www.figo.org/committee-gynaecologic-oncology
International gynaecologic cancer society (IGCS)	https://igcs.org/
The European Society of Gynaecological Oncology (ESGO)	https://www.esgo.org/
National Cancer Intelligence Network (NCIN)	http://www.ncin.org.uk/
The British Gynaecological cancer society (BGCS)	https://www.bgcs.org.uk/
Information on clinical trials	
Gynaecological cancer InterGroup (GCIG)	https://www.gcigtrials.org/
European Organisation for Research and Treatment of Cancer (EORTC)	https://www.eortc.org/
The gynaecologic oncology group (GOG)	https://www.gog.org/
National Cancer Research Institute (NCRI)	https://www.ncri.org.uk/

5.6 Evaluation of Clinical Performance (Audit)

Even with both individual and institutional support, adherence of EBM requires continual evaluation of clinical performance. At a local level, audits of surgical outcomes and adherence to relevant evidence-based guidelines should be an integral part of practice. More importantly, systematic effort should be made at national and international levels to evaluate clinical practice across different units. For example, the Ovarian Cancer Audit Feasibility Pilot (OCAFP) in the United Kingdom, jointly funded by a national professional society and cancer charities, has provided a template for a national clinical audit and demonstrated the challenges of benchmarking clinical performance against evidence-based practice [59].

Continual evaluations and adherence to evidence-based practice are not without challenges. The applicability of existing evidence is particularly difficult when the research is not directly aligned with the clinical scenarios, for example in rarer tumours, non-Caucasian ethnicities and low-and-middle-income countries. Finally, our improved understanding of the molecular basis of cancers (Table 5.4) has started to challenge our current cancer management approach based on broad histopathology subtypes. These challenges and our desire to improve clinical care should serve as incentives to put systems in place for evaluating clinical performance as an integral part of our practice.

5.7 Summary

The future of EBM will integrate clinical evidence from a range of sources. Not only from large RCTs with clearly defined interventions and outcomes, but also high-quality annotated datasets with biological samples. Gynaecological oncology has benefitted greatly from EBM, and there are ample resources to help us achieve evidence-based practice on an individual and organizational levels. We believe the combination of evidence-based practice and excellence in clinical and surgical skills tailored to the patient is crucial for achieving the best possible care. We hope this chapter has inspired and encouraged you to start or continue the practice of EBM for our patients.

Key Points

- The "5As" of evidence-based medicine (EBM): Ask, Acquire, Appraise, Apply and Audit.
- The five-component approach by identifying the relevant population, intervention, comparison, outcomes and design (PICOD) is commonly used to formulate structured questions.
- It is important to recognise the strengths and weaknesses of each study design (hierarchy of evidence) and the usability of different sources of evidence when acquiring evidence.
- Critical appraisal of the literature could be supported by established toolkits and checklists, such as the Critical Appraisal Skills Programme (CASP) checklists.
- Applying the evidence in practice requires understanding of the local clinical expertise, available resources and patient's expectations, with reference to regular evaluations of clinical performance (audits).
- In the near future, EBM will be judiciously combined with understanding of tumour biology to develop individualized evidence-based approaches to cancer care.

References

1. Harter P, Sehouli J, Lorusso D, Reuss A, Vergote I, Marth C, et al. A randomized trial of lymphadenectomy in patients with advanced ovarian neoplasms. N Engl J Med. 2019;380(9):822–32.
2. McCulloch P, Altman DG, Campbell WB, Flum DR, Glasziou P, Marshall JC, et al. No surgical innovation without evaluation: the IDEAL recommendations. Lancet. 2009;374(9695):1105–12.
3. Dawes M, Summerskill W, Glasziou P, Cartabellotta A, Martin J, Hopayian K, et al. Sicily statement on evidence-based practice. BMC Med Educ. 2005;5(1):1.
4. Methley AM, Campbell S, Chew-Graham C, McNally R, Cheraghi-Sohi S. PICO, PICOS and SPIDER: a comparison study of specificity and sensitivity in three search tools for qualitative systematic reviews. BMC Health Serv Res. 2014;14(1):579.
5. Ramirez PT, Frumovitz M, Pareja R, Lopez A, Vieira M, Ribeiro R, et al. Minimally invasive versus abdominal radical hysterectomy for cervical cancer. N Engl J Med. 2018;379(20):1895–904.
6. Murad MH, Asi N, Alsawas M, Alahdab F. New evidence pyramid. Evid Based Med. 2016;21(4):125.
7. Alonso-Coello P, Schünemann HJ, Moberg J, Brignardello-Petersen R, Akl EA, Davoli M, et al. GRADE evidence to decision (EtD) frameworks: a systematic and transparent approach to making well informed healthcare choices. 1: introduction. BMJ. 2016;353:i2016.
8. Page MJ, McKenzie JE, Bossuyt PM, Boutron I, Hoffmann TC, Mulrow CD, et al. The PRISMA 2020 statement: an updated guideline for reporting systematic reviews. BMJ. 2021;372:n71.
9. Alper BS, Haynes RB. EBHC pyramid 5.0 for accessing preappraised evidence and guidance. Evid Based Med. 2016;21(4):123.
10. Melamed A, Margul DJ, Chen L, Keating NL, del Carmen MG, Yang J, et al. Survival after minimally invasive radical hysterectomy for early-stage cervical cancer. N Engl J Med. 2018;379(20):1905–14.
11. Hillemanns P, Hertel H, Klapdor R. Radical hysterectomy for early cervical cancer: what shall we do after the LACC trial? Arch Gynecol Obstet. 2020;302(2):289–92.
12. AOCT Group. Chemotherapy in advanced ovarian cancer: an overview of randomised clinical trials. Advanced Ovarian Cancer Trialists Group. BMJ. 1991;303(6807):884–93.
13. TOCM-A Project. Cyclophosphamide plus cisplatin versus cyclophosphamide, doxorubicin, and cisplatin chemotherapy of ovarian carcinoma: a meta-analysis. The ovarian cancer meta-analysis project. J Clin Oncol. 1991;9(9):1668–74.
14. International Collaborative Ovarian Neoplasm Collaborators. International collaborative ovarian neoplasm trial 1: a randomized trial of adjuvant chemotherapy in women with early-stage ovarian cancer. J Natl Cancer Inst. 2003;95(2):125–32.
15. ICON Group. ICON2: randomised trial of single-agent carboplatin against three-drug combination of CAP (cyclophosphamide, doxorubicin, and cisplatin) in women with ovarian cancer. Lancet. 1998;352(9140):1571–6.
16. ICON Group. Paclitaxel plus carboplatin versus standard chemotherapy with either single-agent carboplatin or cyclophosphamide, doxorubicin, and cisplatin in women with ovarian cancer: the ICON3 randomised trial. Lancet. 2002;360(9332):505–15.
17. Parmar MK, Ledermann JA, Colombo N, du Bois A, Delaloye JF, Kristensen GB, et al. Paclitaxel plus platinum-based chemotherapy versus conventional platinum-based chemotherapy in women with relapsed ovarian cancer: the ICON4/AGO-OVAR-2.2 trial. Lancet. 2003;361(9375):2099–106.
18. Bookman MA, Brady MF, McGuire WP, Harper PG, Alberts DS, Friedlander M, et al. Evaluation of new platinum-based treatment regimens in advanced-stage

ovarian cancer: a phase III trial of the gynecologic cancer InterGroup. J Clin Oncol. 2009;27(9):1419–25.
19. Ledermann JA, Embleton AC, Raja F, Perren TJ, Jayson GC, Rustin GJS, et al. Cediranib in patients with relapsed platinum-sensitive ovarian cancer (ICON6): a randomised, double-blind, placebo-controlled phase 3 trial. Lancet. 2016;387(10023):1066–74.
20. Perren TJ, Swart AM, Pfisterer J, Ledermann JA, Pujade-Lauraine E, Kristensen G, et al. A phase 3 trial of bevacizumab in ovarian cancer. N Engl J Med. 2011;365(26):2484–96.
21. Clamp AR, James EC, McNeish IA, Dean A, Kim J-W, O'Donnell DM, et al. Weekly dose-dense chemotherapy in first-line epithelial ovarian, fallopian tube, or primary peritoneal carcinoma treatment (ICON8): primary progression free survival analysis results from a GCIG phase 3 randomised controlled trial. Lancet. 2019;394(10214):2084–95.
22. Elyashiv O, Ledermann J, Parmar G, Farrelly L, Counsell N, Feeney A, et al. ICON 9—an international phase III randomized study to evaluate the efficacy of maintenance therapy with olaparib and cediranib or olaparib alone in patients with relapsed platinum-sensitive ovarian cancer following a response to platinum-based chemotherapy. Int J Gynecol Cancer. 2021;31(1):134.
23. Ghersi D, Parmar MKB, Stewart LA, Marsoni S, Williams CJ. Early ovarian cancer and the Icon trials. Eur J Cancer. 1992;28(6):1297.
24. Berek JS, Bertelsen K, du Bois A, Brady MF, Carmichael J, Eisenhauer EA, et al. Advanced epithelial ovarian cancer: 1998 consensus statements. Ann Oncol. 1999;10:S87–92.
25. Harter P, Bois A, Hahmann M, Hasenburg A, Burges A, Loibl S, et al. Surgery in recurrent ovarian cancer: the Arbeitsgemeinschaft Gynaekologische Onkologie (AGO) DESKTOP OVAR Trial. Ann Surg Oncol. 2006;13(12):1702–10.
26. Harter P, Sehouli J, Reuss A, Hasenburg A, Scambia G, Cibula D, et al. Prospective validation study of a predictive score for Operability of recurrent ovarian cancer: the multicenter Intergroup study DESKTOP II. A project of the AGO Kommission OVAR, AGO study group, NOGGO, AGO-Austria, and MITO. Int J Gynecol Cancer. 2011;21(2):289–95. https://doi.org/10.1097/IGC.0b013e31820aaafd.
27. Tian WJ, Chi DS, Sehouli J, Tropé CG, Jiang R, Ayhan A, et al. A risk model for secondary Cytoreductive surgery in recurrent ovarian cancer: an evidence-based proposal for patient selection. Ann Surg Oncol. 2012;19(2):597–604.
28. Coleman RL, Spirtos NM, Enserro D, Herzog TJ, Sabbatini P, Armstrong DK, et al. Secondary surgical Cytoreduction for recurrent ovarian cancer. N Engl J Med. 2019;381(20):1929–39.
29. Du Bois A, Sehouli J, Vergote I, Ferron G, Reuss A, Meier W, et al. Randomized phase III study to evaluate the impact of secondary cytoreductive surgery in recurrent ovarian cancer: final analysis of AGO DESKTOP III/ENGOT-ov20. J Clin Oncol. 2020;38(15_suppl):6000.
30. Shi T, Zhu J, Feng Y, Tu D, Zhang Y, Zhang P, et al. Secondary cytoreduction followed by chemotherapy versus chemotherapy alone in platinum-sensitive relapsed ovarian cancer (SOC-1): a multicentre, open-label, randomised, phase 3 trial. Lancet Oncol. 2021;22(4):439–49.
31. Chi DS, McCaughty K, Diaz JP, Huh J, Schwabenbauer S, Hummer AJ, et al. Guidelines and selection criteria for secondary cytoreductive surgery in patients with recurrent, platinum-sensitive epithelial ovarian carcinoma. Cancer. 2006;106(9):1933–9.
32. Fort DG, Herr TM, Shaw PL, Gutzman KE, Starren JB. Mapping the evolving definitions of translational research. J Clin Transl Sci. 2017;1(1):60–6.
33. Hausen HZ, Meinhof W, Scheiber W, Bornkamm GW. Attempts to detect virus-specific DNA in human tumors. I. Nucleic acid hybridizations with complementary RNA of human wart virus. Int J Cancer. 1974;13(5):650–6.
34. Boshart M, Gissmann L, Ikenberg H, Kleinheinz A, Scheurlen W, zur Hausen H. A new type of papillomavirus DNA, its presence in genital cancer biopsies and in cell lines derived from cervical cancer. EMBO J. 1984;3(5):1151–7.
35. Schwarz E, Freese UK, Gissmann L, Mayer W, Roggenbuck B, Stremlau A, et al. Structure and transcription of human papillomavirus sequences in cervical carcinoma cells. Nature. 1985;314(6006):111–4.
36. Bryant HE, Schultz N, Thomas HD, Parker KM, Flower D, Lopez E, et al. Specific killing of BRCA2-deficient tumours with inhibitors of poly(ADP-ribose) polymerase. Nature. 2005;434(7035):913–7.
37. Farmer H, McCabe N, Lord CJ, Tutt ANJ, Johnson DA, Richardson TB, et al. Targeting the DNA repair defect in BRCA mutant cells as a therapeutic strategy. Nature. 2005;434(7035):917–21.
38. Fong PC, Boss DS, Yap TA, Tutt A, Wu P, Mergui-Roelvink M, et al. Inhibition of poly(ADP-ribose) polymerase in tumors from BRCA mutation carriers. N Engl J Med. 2009;361(2):123–34.
39. Ledermann JA, Harter P, Gourley C, Friedlander M, Vergote I, Rustin G, et al. Overall survival in patients with platinum-sensitive recurrent serous ovarian cancer receiving olaparib maintenance monotherapy: an updated analysis from a randomised, placebo-controlled, double-blind, phase 2 trial. Lancet Oncol. 2016;17(11):1579–89.
40. Domchek SM, Aghajanian C, Shapira-Frommer R, Schmutzler RK, Audeh MW, Friedlander M, et al. Efficacy and safety of olaparib monotherapy in germline BRCA1/2 mutation carriers with advanced ovarian cancer and three or more lines of prior therapy. Gynecol Oncol. 2016;140(2):199–203.
41. Kristeleit R, Shapiro GI, Burris HA, Oza AM, LoRusso P, Patel MR, et al. A phase I–II study of the oral PARP inhibitor rucaparib in patients with germline BRCA1/2-mutated ovarian carcinoma or other solid tumors. Clin Cancer Res. 2017;23(15):4095.
42. Swisher EM, Lin KK, Oza AM, Scott CL, Giordano H, Sun J, et al. Rucaparib in relapsed, platinum-

sensitive high-grade ovarian carcinoma (ARIEL2 part 1): an international, multicentre, open-label, phase 2 trial. Lancet Oncol. 2017;18(1):75–87.

43. Coleman RL, Oza AM, Lorusso D, Aghajanian C, Oaknin A, Dean A, et al. Rucaparib maintenance treatment for recurrent ovarian carcinoma after response to platinum therapy (ARIEL3): a randomised, double-blind, placebo-controlled, phase 3 trial. Lancet. 2017;390(10106):1949–61.

44. Pujade-Lauraine E, Ledermann JA, Selle F, Gebski V, Penson RT, Oza AM, et al. Olaparib tablets as maintenance therapy in patients with platinum-sensitive, relapsed ovarian cancer and a BRCA1/2 mutation (SOLO2/ENGOT-Ov21): a double-blind, randomised, placebo-controlled, phase 3 trial. Lancet Oncol. 2017;18(9):1274–84.

45. Poveda A, Floquet A, Ledermann JA, Asher R, Penson RT, Oza AM, et al. Olaparib tablets as maintenance therapy in patients with platinum-sensitive relapsed ovarian cancer and a BRCA1/2 mutation (SOLO2/ENGOT-Ov21): a final analysis of a double-blind, randomised, placebo-controlled, phase 3 trial. Lancet Oncol. 2021;22(5):620–31.

46. Moore K, Colombo N, Scambia G, Kim B-G, Oaknin A, Friedlander M, et al. Maintenance olaparib in patients with newly diagnosed advanced ovarian cancer. N Engl J Med. 2018;379(26):2495–505.

47. Ray-Coquard I, Pautier P, Pignata S, Pérol D, González-Martín A, Berger R, et al. Olaparib plus bevacizumab as first-line maintenance in ovarian cancer. N Engl J Med. 2019;381(25):2416–28.

48. González-Martín A, Pothuri B, Vergote I, DePont CR, Graybill W, Mirza MR, et al. Niraparib in patients with newly diagnosed advanced ovarian cancer. N Engl J Med. 2019;381(25):2391–402.

49. Cuzick J, Szarewski A, Terry G, Ho L, Hanby A, Maddox P, et al. Human papillomavirus testing in primary cervical screening. Lancet. 1995;345(8964):1533–6.

50. Cuzick J, Beverley E, Ho L, Terry G, Sapper H, Mielzynska I, et al. HPV testing in primary screening of older women. Br J Cancer. 1999;81(3):554–8.

51. Cuzick J, Szarewski A, Cubie H, Hulman G, Kitchener H, Luesley D, et al. Management of women who test positive for high-risk types of human papillomavirus: the HART study. Lancet. 2003;362(9399):1871–6.

52. Koliopoulos G, Nyaga VN, Santesso N, Bryant A, Martin-Hirsch PPL, Mustafa RA, et al. Cytology versus HPV testing for cervical cancer screening in the general population. Cochrane Database Syst Rev. 2017;8(8):CD008587.

53. Committee UNS. Consultation on modifying the NHS Cervical Screening Programmes in the four UK nations The United Kingdom: UK National Screening Committee; 2019 [cited 2021 4 April]. Available from: https://legacyscreening.phe.org.uk/cervicalcancer.

54. Munn Z, Peters MDJ, Stern C, Tufanaru C, McArthur A, Aromataris E. Systematic review or scoping review? Guidance for authors when choosing between a systematic or scoping review approach. BMC Med Res Methodol. 2018;18(1):143.

55. Higgins JPT, Thomas J, Chandler J, Cumpston M, Li T, Page MJ, Welch VA (editors). Cochrane handbook for systematic reviews of interventions version 6.2 (updated February 2021). The Cochrane Collaboration 2021.

56. Arksey H, O'Malley L. Scoping studies: towards a methodological framework. Int J Soc Res Methodol. 2005;8(1):19–32.

57. Tricco AC, Lillie E, Zarin W, O'Brien KK, Colquhoun H, Levac D, et al. PRISMA extension for scoping reviews (PRISMA-ScR): checklist and explanation. Ann Intern Med. 2018;169(7):467–73.

58. Clarke M. Standardising outcomes for clinical trials and systematic reviews. Trials. 2007;8(1):39.

59. National Cancer Registration and Analysis Service (NCRAS). Gynaecological Cancer Hub. The United Kingdom. 2020 [Last access: 14 April 2021]. Available from: http://www.ncin.org.uk/cancer_type_and_topic_specific_work/cancer_type_specific_work/gynaecological_cancer/gynaecological_cancer_hub/

Surgical Principles and Practices in Gynaecological Oncology: Achieving the Best Outcome

Janos Balega and Desmond Barton

6.1 Introduction

Humanity has been trying to remove cancers from different parts of the human body for as long as written documents are available. Surgery has evolved throughout centuries with large scale wars in Europe in particular giving surgeons and anaesthetists the opportunities and impetus to develop new techniques, and accordingly, expertise in cancer surgery also grew, particularly from the nineteenth century onward. The last 70 years have seen an exponential growth in medical technology; cancer surgery has been supported by the development of antibiotics, modern anaesthesia, imaging technologies, modern haemostatic instruments and materials, and advanced theatre technology. Surgery had been for long the only or main anticancer treatment modality for solid malignancies but with the introduction of radiotherapy and particularly systemic chemotherapy, the role of cancer surgery has evolved. Anticancer treatment has become a sophisticated discipline built on a multidisciplinary team approach.

Despite the recent advances in non-surgical anticancer treatment, surgical resection has remained the most important treatment modality in the management of the majority of solid cancers. And whilst chemo- and radiotherapy have both been greatly standardised and protocol driven, surgery has remained highly dependent on human factors. Clinical trials have been conducted in cancer treatments, especially in the fields of medical oncology and to a lesser extent in clinical oncology. Despite the key role of surgery in the treatment of cancer, clinical trials in surgery have been notable by their absence and, as such, evidence-based surgical practice has been weak.

Cancer surgery is often hampered by a chain of unexpected events, and it is, therefore, imperative to prepare both the patient and the surgical team, and to optimise the institutional circumstances well before the operation. Ideally, the right operation should be offered to the right patient by the right surgeon in the right hospital, at the right time. The same, of course, can be reiterated in other disciplines treating cancer.

Cancer treatment should not be more harmful than the cancer itself, and careful preoperative patient selection and optimisation, maximum surgical and anaesthetic effort and diligent postoperative care should always be exercised.

J. Balega (✉)
Pan-Birmingham Gynaecological Cancer Centre,
City Hospital, Birmingham, UK
e-mail: janos.balega@nhs.net

D. Barton
The Royal Marsden Hospital, London, UK
e-mail: dbarton@sgul.ac.uk

6.2 Before Operation

6.2.1 Multidisciplinary Approach

Cancer surgery is a complex process involving the preoperative period, the operation itself, and the postoperative phase. It requires surgeons to prepare their patients physically, mentally and emotionally for the operation, collaborating with multiple stakeholders in healthcare during this process. Modern cancer care is built on multidisciplinary approach: surgeons work closely with pathologists and radiologists to establish diagnosis and plan surgery; with oncologists to finalise the management plan; and they optimise patients for surgery with the expertise of the anaesthetist in particular (including intensive care), nurse specialist, nutritionalist, clinical psychologist, cardiologist, haematologist, and geriatrician, as required. Surgeons, therefore, must be proficient in different fields of medicine and must possess good understanding of pathophysiology for all patients—from the young to the elderly, from the fit to the debilitated, from those with cachexia to those with morbid obesity, to name but a few. Each patient's therapeutic planning should be done individually, tailored to the biology of the cancer, the fitness of the patient and the capabilities of the surgical team.

6.2.2 Patient Selection

One of the most difficult decisions for the surgeon to make is to decide if the patient is suitable, that is, fit for the operation. Despite the availability of numerous scoring systems to assess potential mortality and morbidity associated with surgery, it remains a challenging task to decide whether to offer an operation or not. The 'art' of patient selection greatly depends on the patient's age, clinical condition, physical reserve capacity, but is also subject to the surgeon's skill and experience level as well as the infrastructural support of the hospital. Whilst helpful and often essential, opinions from anaesthetists and geriatricians, for example, may not always take the burden of decision-making off the shoulders of the surgeon, although they can substantially share this responsibility. Second-opinion from a fellow surgical oncologist within the team or outside is not an admission of inadequate clinical acumen, but a useful tool to make the right decision for the patient.

In the decision making what must be included is thorough knowledge of prior treatments, and in particular, any previous surgery. The detailed surgery notes should be obtained rather than accepting a brief summary of what was performed mentioned in a referral letter. Case selection also involves the decision "not to operate". No amount surgery will make amends for the error in judgement to operate. Often in ovarian cancer surgery for primary and recurrent disease the decision to operate or not to operate is clear-cut; perhaps as often the decision is not that straightforward. This is where there should be recourse to the opinion of other surgeons (outside the team) and a formal second opinion. Ideally the additional opinion should be sought from an experienced surgical team.

6.2.3 Consenting

During the decision-making phase, the aim of surgery must be discussed with the patient and relatives: the goals of surgery must be clearly reasoned by the surgical team and communicated to the patient—curative, palliative, staging, or prophylactic. It is very difficult to categorise ovarian cancer cytoreductive surgery, as most patients will experience relapse of their cancer, despite 'successful' surgery and chemotherapy. The term *life-prolonging surgery*, therefore, could be used for this group of patients.

The consenting process must include the explanation of all management options including the standard treatment and its alternatives, with the associated risks and potential complications. The explanation of no treatment option is a mandatory medical and medico-legal part of the consenting process. It is good practice to use pictorial or video guidance during the discussion with the patient and patients should be provided with written information leaflets and a detailed clinic letter to enable them to have a full understanding of the procedure. The consenting should not take place on the day of the operation: the patient and her family/friends must be given adequate time to reflect on the discussions and recommendations and to ask questions. This period of reflection should ideally be in a stress-free environment—that is, not in hospital with medical staff in the vicinity.

6.2.4 Prehabilitation

There is some evidence that physical and emotional preoperative optimisation of the patient improves surgical outcomes. As part of the enhanced recovery programme, preoperative carbohydrate drinks are part of standard practice. Aiming to achieve positive nitrogen balance and an anabolic metabolic state is of particular importance in operating on patients with disseminated cancer, cachexia, sarcopenia, hypoalbuminemia [1]. Involving a nutritionalist and physiotherapist in the management of such patients could potentially increase the proportion of patients suitable for major cancer surgery and will likely improve surgical and oncological outcomes. Preoperative psychological prehabilitation seems to have a positive impact on postoperative quality of life and other patient reported measures [2, 3]. However, in ovarian cancer patients the prehabilitation period may be short. In patients scheduled for neo-adjuvant chemotherapy, prehabilitation starts then and not when the patient is referred for surgery after a few cycles of chemotherapy. One can also regard neoadjuvant chemotherapy as a prehabilitation method for debulking surgery.

6.3 In Theatre

An operating theatre is a highly complex environment with multiple levels of human-to-human and technology-to-human interactions. Whilst some of these interactions are beyond the control of the theatre team, the surgical, anaesthetic and nursing teams must aspire to have direct or indirect control over the theatre environment to maximise the safety and efficiency of the surgical procedure.

Preparation of the theatre list is a task not to be given to the most junior and inexperienced member of the team. The lead surgeon, often will have had discussions with the anaesthetic team and theatre coordinator, will plan the cases on the list, with the procedures listed, the order agreed and a reasonable expectation that the list will finish on time. At the start of the operating list, it is very distracting to learn that the list order is incorrect, or the procedures listed are inaccurate. Nevertheless, the whole team must be adept at dealing with the unexpected changes in the order of the list (for example, sudden cancellation or addition, or the patient fails to attend).

6.3.1 Teamwork

The theatre team is built up by three professional groups who should function as a cohesive unit: surgical team, anaesthetist team and nursing team. Ideally, these groups should form a permanent formation as evidence shows that disruption of teamwork by random allocation of staff adversely impacts the theatre dynamics [4]. Permanently working together as a team improves efficiency and safety in theatre and may also build team morale by establishing a mutually respectful professional relationship. Increasingly, in long and complex procedures, as is often encountered in cytoreductive surgery, more than one senior surgeon should be involved in the peri-operative care of the patient: intra-operatively this is exemplified by the "buddy-operating" team.

Preoperative team brief (WHO surgical safety checklist) provides the opportunity to all team members to understand the operating list, the order of the list, the operations, and the equipment requirements. The brief clearly allocates tasks, improves ownership of the operation, and therefore improves safety [5].

Consideration must be given to the members of the surgical team who will be present during the operation—their experience, knowledge of the case and the procedures, what their role will be and what supervised procedures they will undertake. This is a challenge when there are new and/or inexperienced team members. On occasions the lead surgeon may be faced with operating with an inexperienced team or with one less assistant than ideal—the buddy operating setup minimises the impact of such pressures on the operating team. Ideally discussion about the theatre list and "who does what, when" should take place the day before surgery or during team briefing. A key role of the lead surgeon is to instruct the junior staff about the importance of knowing in detail the patients about to be operated on, what procedures are to be performed and what is expected of each team member. Equally important is the team debriefing after the operation, especially for learning and reflection on the whole operating list.

6.3.2 Theatre Environment

Operating theatres have traditionally been quiet places to facilitate concentration and patient-related conversations. Auditory and mental distractions can lead to disruption of the flow of the operation and may yield in higher intraoperative complication rates and will reduce efficiency. Such distractions have more significant impact on less experienced surgeons. Maximising focus on the operation, therefore, requires minimising all distractions. It is important that the lead surgeon should have maximum focus on the operation as the mental readiness has been proved to be a key indicator of a successful operation [6, 7]. The most common sources of theatre distractions are related to unnecessary movements in theatre; auditory disturbances such as case-irrelevant conversations, mobile phone usage, equipment murmur; and equipment failures [8].

6.3.3 Noise Level

As modern technology has conquered the operating theatre, so has increased the background noise during surgical procedures. Patient warmer, suction device, electrosurgical equipment all contribute to a relatively high baseline noise level in theatre, which can have an impact on case-relevant conversations during surgery. To achieve maximum level of safety and efficiency, team members must have clear communication intraoperatively. Excess noise level may cause distraction and increased stress levels, which have an impact on the safety, quality, and cost effectiveness of the theatre activity [9, 10]. Prolonged surgical procedures hinder optimal theatre utilisation with resulting reduced efficiency. These problems were aggravated and highlighted during the pandemic with the wearing of heavy, cumbersome masks and visors.

6.3.4 Surgeon

Whilst working in and supported by a team of different professionals, it is the lead surgeon who must make continuous decisions critical to the outcome of the operation. To be able to encounter with such stressful situations during cancer operations and to make the best decisions to achieve the optimal outcome, the surgeon must be fully prepared mentally, physically, and emotionally. However, the decisions are only effective and will only achieve their purpose if they are communicated in a clear and timely manner to other members of the operating team. The key discussions are most often with the anaesthetist.

In general, surgical oncologists must possess the following skills:

– Stress resistance, calm
– Adequate stamina
– Thorough knowledge of surgical anatomy
– Anticipation and preparedness for aberrant anatomy
– Fine dissecting skills and good spatial orientation
– Knowledge of literature
– Full understanding of all treatment modalities
– Recognition of his/her limitations
– Situational awareness—for example, taking a break during the operation, calling for help
– Flexibility and adeptness in dealing with the unexpected

Gynaecological cancer surgery, particularly ovarian cancer cytoreduction, requires deep understanding of surgical anatomy of the whole peritoneal cavity, from the pelvis, through the retroperitoneum and up to the chest. Deepening the anatomy knowledge by continuous education in surgical anatomy, especially attending cadaveric courses is an important building brick for the preparedness of a cancer surgeon to all eventualities. Fine dissection skills and careful tissue handling are key attributes of a successful surgical oncologist and will minimise blood loss and tissue trauma. This is of particular importance during long, complex surgical procedures such as cytoreductive surgery.

Prior to the operation, the surgeon must be physically and mentally prepared for performing at the highest level of skill, for teamwork concentration and intra-operative judgement. A basic level of physical fitness is essential to have the required stamina during long operations. The surgeon should have a good level of feeding and hydration prior to the procedure and it is essential to maintain these during prolonged procedures as dehydration and low blood sugar levels impede judgment and fine motor skills. A key component of teamwork is dialogue between the surgeon, scrub team and the anaesthetist. In essence, with a routine uncomplicated procedure, the dialogue should be at a minimum as the whole team is efficient and unconsciously competent. When there is a different member of the team, or there are unexpected developments during the operation then the dialogue will be directed by the lead surgeon, anaesthetist and nursing team. There must be clear directions and instructions and the senior surgeon may need to ask for everyone to be quiet, to listen and then to give instructions. The question should be asked has everyone understood the instructions and who are responsible for following through on these.

Generic working is standard in many health care systems as per limited resources. This means that the first opportunity for the operating surgeon to meet the patient is not until the day of the operation. Whilst this may be considered a necessary part of surgical practice, it is full of potential pitfalls due to lack of adequate rapport built between the patient and the operating surgeon, and due to the potential lack of communication between the clinicians. It is, therefore, essential to check the patient's full history, examination findings, scan reports, blood test results and multidisciplinary team opinions before meeting the patient right before the operation. It is essential to review the available scans prior to surgery to ensure that all factors are considered during the operation. As a general principle, scans should be no older than 6–8 weeks (and sometimes considerably less), as per potential tumour progression. The operating surgeon must explain the rationale behind performing the operation, the details, risks and potential complications of the planned procedures, as well as all treatment alternatives. This always should be the final step of the consenting process. It is the opinion of the authors that ideally, all cases to be operated on must, with very rare exceptions (for example, sudden absence of a surgical colleague; or an emergency procedure), have met the lead surgeon before the day of surgery.

6.3.5 Operation

The 'thinking surgeon' follows the principles of cancer surgery by going through the different phases of an operation: these steps are rehearsed and analysed before surgery when the case is reviewed to discuss the history, recent imaging and pathology—in essence to ensure the decision to operate is the correct one. No surgical procedure will rectify what was, in retrospect, an error of judgement to operate.

When surgery is to go ahead as planned then the key elements for most cancer operations are:

1. Exploration
2. Decision-making
3. Resection
4. Reconstruction

6.3.5.1 Exploration

Before starting the operation, adequate positioning of the patient on the operating table is essential. Most gynaecological cancer operations are performed using a Lloyd-Davies position which provides the surgeon access to the vagina and anus throughout the operation for internal examination or for colorectal anastomosis. Careful positioning of the legs in the holding boots is of paramount importance, as pressure on the peroneus nerves or the calves may result in nerve injury or compartment syndrome, both of which are detrimental to the short and long-term postoperative recovery. The lead surgeon is responsible for the optimal positioning of the patient.

One of the most important principles of cancer surgery is to provide **adequate exposure** to gain optimal access to the surgical field. In major gynaecological cancer surgery such as staging laparotomy for pelvic masses, cytoreductive surgery for advanced ovarian cancer, and surgery for recurrent gynaecological cancers, an extended midline laparotomy remains the standard way of entry. Extending the incision from the pubic bone to the xiphisternum will allow the surgeon to access all four quadrants of the peritoneal cavity during cytoreductive surgery. **Table-mounted surgical retractors** are vital in obtaining good retraction during extensive surgical resection and ease the operation by reducing physical strain on team members. **Adhesiolysis** is an important initial step during surgery to gain access and to avoid iatrogenic injuries such as tears. **Packing** of the bowel is only effectively achieved after appropriate mobilisation of the right and left hemicolon and the small bowel from the resection field and is important not only to gain access but also to protect bowels from drying and contact with surgical instruments. With appropriate mobilisation, minimal traction is required to keep the small and large bowel from the operating field. Packing the spleen by placing wet packs between the spleen and the diaphragm will descend the spleen and will help to avoid capsular tear during omental surgery. During exploration the surgeon visualises and palpates the operative field and beyond and often performs adhesiolysis and opens up surgical planes. This part of cancer surgery is the information gathering phase that will enable the surgeon to make the right decisions about the operation.

6.3.5.2 Decision-Making

The aim of cancer surgery is almost always complete resection of the disease:

- Cervical cancer—clear microscopic margins
- Adnexal mass—complete macroscopic removal with no spillage
- Advanced ovarian cancer—complete macroscopic clearance
- Vulval cancer—clear microscopic margins
- Unifocal recurrences—clear microscopic margins
- Uterine cancer—no perforation

During the decision-making phase, the surgeon must decide if the preoperative objectives can be achieved, and should answer the following questions:

- Can the cancer be removed completely with negative macroscopic margins or with macroscopic clearance?
- How many procedures are required to achieve the goals of operation?
- Is the patient fit to undergo the required procedures?

It is often the more difficult decision to make when *not* to operate or to stop operating. A useful tool aiding decision-making is an ***intra-operative second opinion***: a second, experienced gynaecological oncologist scrubs in and assesses the tumour burden and provides help to make the optimal decision. This is one of the key benefits of buddy-operating. However, buddy operating also has the potential to lead to errors in intra-operative decision making; for example, to continue to operate when the evidence suggests otherwise. This scenario may be likely to arise when the two surgeons are very different in terms of experience and seniority. When clinical practice is regularly reviewed—such as in morbidity and mortality meetings, such scenarios should be discussed.

6.3.5.3 Resection and Reconstruction

As a general principle, resectability is disease and surgeon dependent. A cancer centre must assure that adequate level of surgical expertise is always present in theatre or if this is not possible, referral to more experienced centres should be considered. This, however, does not often happen—other centres are busy, one team may not want to admit their limitations, and there can be delays in reviewing the case.

During resection the following principles must be followed to achieve optimal outcomes:

- *Careful handling* of tissues and organs is important during surgery particularly in prolonged procedures. Avoiding bruises, haematomas, surface damage, or even more serious damage (like splenic injury during omentectomy) improves tissue healing and reduces complications such as ileus or infective complications. Careful handling of the cancer is also important to avoid spillage, particularly during staging laparotomies for adnexal masses when rupturing a cyst will have a potentially detrimental impact on oncological outcomes.
- Applying *traction-countertraction* is vital during dissection of surgical planes and reduces the risk of inadvertent injuries to underlying structures.
- *Fine dissection* will reduce blood loss and the chance of injury to underlying structures.
- *Meticulous haemostasis*. Excessive blood loss is best to be avoided by fine dissection, careful tissue handling and continuous haemostasis. Reducing blood loss will improve visibility, especially in laparoscopy, will reduce the risk of anaemia and the need for blood transfusion and will help reducing postoperative infective complications.
- *Modern energy devices*. Monopolar and bipolar diathermy, ultrasonic and other types of devices are safe and efficient in dissecting tissue planes and controlling vessels. These energy devices have become indispensable and invaluable parts of modern oncological surgery. Important to mention, that appropriate and careful use of these instruments is paramount as such hot instruments can cause significant collateral damage.
- *Plan B*. An important principle in surgical oncology is to always have a 'plan B' prior to starting the resection, should there be any significant complication developing. Buddy operating, i.e., the availability of support during surgery by an experienced colleague is safe and useful practice and reduces stress level, share the burden of decision-making, and it can also improve efficiency of the theatre.

The unexpected and serious. It is not uncommon such a situation arises during cytoreductive surgery for ovarian cancer or during complex pelvic resections. Prompt recognition, accurate communication to team members and timely interaction to limit the potential adverse consequences are essential. Staying calm is a key response of the lead surgeon and anaesthetist.

6.4 The Postoperative Period

The lead surgeon should ideally lead a debrief session after each operation, which is part of the reflective practice and serves educational purposes for the team members. This is an excellent opportunity for the trainees to maximise their learning opportunity associated with the operation.

In general, the postoperative management of gynaecological cancer patients should follow the enhanced surgical recovery principles [11]. For uncomplicated cases, once daily ward round by senior clinician is necessary but in case of complications, the lead consultant must review the patient as frequently as required. Proactive management of complications, particularly bowel anastomotic leakages and infective complications is essential to avoid more serious, even fatal outcome. Again, multidisciplinary approach with requesting second opinion if necessary is a basic principle of postoperative management.

The perioperative complications should be registered in a departmental database and should be presented in the regular morbidity and mortality meetings with case discussions of severe or rare complications.

6.5 Conclusion

To conclude surgical outcomes not only are dependent on the surgical team but depend on a multitude of preoperative, intraoperative and postoperative factors and infact starts from the very first meeting with the patient. It is very important for a surgeon to reflect on their practice, audit his or her own results, practice evidence based medicine and keep updating their skills to ensure good patient outcomes.

> **Key Points**
> 1. Cancer surgery is often hampered by a chain of unexpected events and it is, therefore, imperative to prepare both the patient and the surgical team, and optimise the institutional circumstances well before the operation.
> 2. Preoperative measures include the right patient selection, MDT decision to support surgical treatment, decide regarding route of surgery and extent of radicality, detailed consenting and patient counselling and prehabilitation.
> 3. Various scores like Alleti score, Fagotti scoring system, AGO scoring etc. assist in taking important preoperative decisions on patient selection.
> 4. In theatre, there should be conducive operating conditions, good coordination between the surgical team, anaesthetist and theatre staff.
> 5. The essential skills of a good surgical oncologist include adequate stamina, thorough knowledge of surgical anatomy, anticipation and preparedness for aberrant anatomy, fine dissecting skills and good spatial orientation, knowledge of recent literature and situational awareness.
> 6. When surgery is to go ahead as planned then the key elements for most cancer operations are Exploration, Decision-making to ensure complete clearance, Resection and Reconstruction.
> 7. Some important principles of surgery are careful dissection and handling of tumor, adequate exposure, protecting vital structures using sloops and meticulous hemostasis.
> 8. Buddy operating, i.e., the availability of support during surgery by an experienced colleague is safe and useful practice and reduces stress level, share the burden of decision-making, and it can also improve efficiency of the theatre.
> 9. Post operative care is very important and includes the principles of enhanced recovery and need a holistic care to hasten the patient's recovery for timely adjuvant treatment.

References

1. Daley J, Khuri SF, Henderson W, et al. Risk adjustment of the postoperative morbidity rate for the comparative assessment of the quality of surgical care: results of the National Veterans Affairs Surgical Risk Study. J Am Coll Surg. 1997;185:328–40.
2. Schneider S, Armbrust R, Spies C, et al. Prehabilitation programs and ERAS protocols in gynecological oncology: a comprehensive review. Arch Gynecol Obstet. 2020;301(2):315–26.
3. Tsimopoulou I, Pasquali S, Howard R, et al. Psychological prehabilitation before cancer surgery: a systematic review. Ann Surg Oncol. 2015;22(13):4117–23.
4. Carthey J, de Level MR, Wright DJ, et al. Behavioural markers of surgical excellence. Safety Sci. 2003;41(5):409–25.
5. Sotto KT, Burian BK, Brindle ME. Impact of the WHO surgical safety checklist rela-

tive to its design and intended use: a systematic review and meta-meta-analysis. J Am Coll Surg. 2021;S1072-7515(21):02141–4.
6. McDonald J, Orlick T, Letts M. Mental readiness in surgeons and its links to performance excellence in surgery. J Pediat Orthop. 1995;15:691–7.
7. Suh IH, Chien JH, Mukherjee M, et al. The negative effect of distraction on performance of robot-assisted surgical skills in medical students and residents. Int J Med Robot. 2010;6:377–81.
8. Wheelock A, Suliman A, Wharton R, et al. The impact of operating room distractions on stress, workload, and teamwork. Ann Surg. 2015;261(6):1079–84.
9. Mentis HM, Chellali A, Manser K, et al. A systematic review of the effect of distraction on surgeon performance: directions for operating room policy and Surgical training. Surg Endosc. 2016;30(5):1713–24.
10. Mcleod R, Myint-Wilks L, Davies SE, Elhassan HA. The impact of noise in the operating theatre: a review of the evidence. Ann R Coll Surg Engl. 2021;103:83–7.
11. Nelson G, Bakkum-Gamez J, Kalogera E, et al. Guidelines for perioperative care in gynecologic/oncology: Enhanced Recovery After Surgery (ERAS) Society recommendations-2019 update. Int J Gynecol Cancer. 2019;29(4):651–68.

Techniques of Enhanced Recovery in Post Operative Care

Shweta Sharma and Bindiya Gupta

7.1 Introduction

Surgery disrupts the physiologic homeostasis and induces a general stress response, altering hormonal, metabolic, immunologic, and neurologic functions. Therefore, patients undergoing major surgery are predisposed to a 20–40% decrease in functional capacity as a response to surgical stress, which can delay post-operative recovery. The recovery is further delayed in presence of perioperative complications.

For years, conventional perioperative approach like preoperative calorie restriction, use of bowel preparation, liberal administration of intravenous fluids and opioids, prolonged immobilization, and use of drains and catheters have been used in all field of surgery including gynaecologic oncology. This resulted in alteration of the normal physiological mechanisms, bowel dilatation and occasionally electrolyte imbalance.

The concept of "enhanced recovery" was introduced by Kehlet in 1990s as a comprehensive, multimodal approach to minimize the effects of surgical trauma by maintaining normal physiology perioperatively and encouraging early mobilization postoperatively [1]. Enhanced Recovery After Surgery (ERAS) is improvement in peri and post operative care by inclusion of certain clinical practices and exclusion of certain traditional practices to facilitate earlier and holistic recovery of patient after a major surgical event. It has been developed for various surgical specialties for clinical and cost benefits to health care system without increase in the complications or readmission rate. It has preoperative, intraoperative and postoperative components. This chapter will describe various components of the ERAS programme and evidence in support of its usefulness in surgical practice.

7.2 Components of ERAS Programme

7.2.1 Cancer Prehabilitation

Preparation of ERAS starts with preoperative rehabilitation or prehabilitation in order to improve or optimize baseline fitness. It has been defined as *"a process on the continuum of care that occurs between time of cancer diagnosis and the beginning of acute treatment, includes physical and psychological assessments that establish a baseline functional level, identifies impairments, and provides targeted interventions that improve a patient's health to reduce the incidence and the severity of current and future impairments"* [2].

The patient and her relative or care taker meet the team of surgeon, anesthetist, physiotherapist,

---

S. Sharma
University College of Medical Sciences and Guru Teg Bahadur Hospital, Delhi, India

B. Gupta (✉)
Department of Obstetrics & Gynecology, University College of Medical Sciences & Guru Teg Bahadur Hospital, Delhi, India

© The Author(s), under exclusive license to Springer Nature Switzerland AG 2022
K. Singh, B. Gupta (eds.), *Gynecological Oncology*, https://doi.org/10.1007/978-3-030-94110-9_7

psychologist, dietician, and nurse preoperatively and have at least three evaluation visits: at the time of diagnosis (baseline assessment), a week before surgery (preoperative), and 8 weeks after surgery (especially if they require adjuvant treatment). In patients planned for interval debulking surgery in ovarian cancer, prehabilitation is done during the time they receive neoadjuvant chemotherapy, which usually lasts for 2 months.

Baseline assessment aims to perform risk stratification by identifying the preoperative performance status which includes assessment of nutritional, physical and psychological factors. Patients can be asked to maintain a diary and document the daily activities, diet and exercise schedule [3]. Based on the result of this screening, either a home based or a supervised program is advised and it is preferable to provide an information booklet containing all instructions.

The components of rehabilitation include medical optimization, physical intervention, nutritional counselling, and psychological support. The program should be individualized according to the patient's functional status, comorbidities, and cancer type.

7.2.1.1 Medical Optimization

It targets to identify and manage preexisting comorbidities. Preoperative screening for anemia should be done and if hemoglobin level is less than 11 g/dl, oral or intravenous iron therapy needs to be given. Evaluation for chronic conditions like hypertension, chronic obstructive pulmonary disease, chronic heart disease, and diabetes is done and if diagnosed the patients should be referred to a general or specialist physician. Smoking and alcohol consumption should be stopped at least 4 weeks prior to surgery. Hospital pulmonology program which consists of behavioral support and nicotine replacement therapy can be helpful for the smokers.

Since most of the gynaecologic oncology patients are elderly, a geriatric screening scale for frailty, the G-8 scale can be used for those older than 70 years [4]. It is a screening tool that contains eight questions i.e. decrease in food intake, weight loss over last 3 months, mobility, neuropsychological problems, body mass index, intake of more than three prescription drugs per day, comparative health status and age. If the G-8 score is less than or equal to 14, then second opinion should be taken from a geriatrician.

7.2.1.2 Physical Intervention

Physical interventions include aerobic and resistance exercises and inspiratory muscle training to improve physical function and cardiorespiratory status. Physical exercises may include walking, cycling, weight training, push ups, yoga, etc. depending on patient's fitness levels, morbidity status and performance score. These exercises should preferably be under the supervision of a physiotherapist.

All patients must be advised inspiratory muscle training; 10 min sessions at least three times in a day. The patients may be asked to do deep breathing exercises, diaphragmatic breathing or use an incentive spirometer.

7.2.1.3 Nutritional Intervention

Assessment of nutritional status includes measurement of parameters like body mass index, laboratory parameters including serum albumin and hemoglobin. All efforts should be made to maintain serum albumin levels above 4 g/dl, especially in patients with ascites, post neoadjuvant chemotherapy and ovarian cancer scheduled for major debulking surgery.

The recommended dietary intake of protein is around 1.2–1.6 g/kg/day to mitigate age-related muscle depletion and for optimal muscle health in elderly [5]. Patients can be given a list of home made recipes for protein rich food, protein supplements like shakes and protein powders.

Iron supplementation and iron rich diet should be given if hemoglobin levels are below 10 g/dl.

7.2.1.4 Psychological and Social Intervention

It is one of the most important components for a holistic healing. After the diagnosis of cancer, all patients usually have a mental setback. This intervention involves extensive counselling and aims to alleviate stress, support behaviour change, and encourage overall well being. The patient also needs to be counseled and convinced about the need of her active participation in certain components of ERAS program like early ambulation, early resumption of oral intake, pulmonary physiotherapy and should be told the discharge criteria before hand. This sets her expectations, identify barriers to discharge and helps in early achievement of postoperative milestones and improved outcomes [6].

Other interventions like daily home based relaxation techniques, music therapy and meditation can be advised. Patients can contact support groups and hospitals can organize group activities so that they can perform physical activities and relaxation sessions together. In cases of patients with known psychiatric problems, they should be referred to a psychologist for personalized expert psychotherapy. The social environment plays an important role for the care and effective implementation of ERAS program. In the baseline evaluation, the social environment is assessed and if required, a social assistant should be provided.

7.2.2 Preoperative Bowel Preparation

Oral antibiotics are given 1 day prior to surgery for bowel preparation. Oral antibiotic preparation best tolerated are 1 g oral neomycin +1 g erythromycin or combination of 1 gm erythromycin and 400 mg metronidazole in evening and night before surgery [7]. In cases where colon resection is planned, bowel preparation is according to the surgeon's discretion and a mild laxative may be administered the night before surgery if the patient has constipation.

Mechanical bowel preparation like enema or laxatives which were used conventionally, are not recommended as per the ERAS protocol as preoperative dehydration and electrolyte disturbances can impair post-operative recovery. Evidence has shown that its use is not associated with decrease in overall mortality, surgical site infections rate, anastomotic leak rate, or reoperation compared with no mechanical bowel preparation [8, 9].

7.2.3 Maintenance of Peri-operative Normoglycemia

The traditional prolonged fasting of more than 12 h causes depletion of glycogen stores which leads to insulin resistance and hyperglycemia. Decreasing the preoperative fasting time and administration of an oral carbohydrate drink 2 h prior to surgery helps attenuate this catabolic response and insulin resistance and thus helps in faster healing [10].

Patients should be encouraged to eat a light meal that is non fatty, nonfried low residue preferably up until 6 h before surgery. Clear fluids can be given upto 2 h before initiation of anesthesia for surgery. A clear complex carbohydrate drink of 50 g should be given 2–3 h before surgery. If there is history of diabetes, gastro esophageal reflux disease, or morbid obesity in the patient, there should be at least 8 h of fasting and the carbohydrate drink should be omitted.

Perioperative glucose levels should be maintained below 200 mg/dl (<11 mmol/l) in diabetic as well as non-diabetic patients and monitored at 4 hourly intervals. This can be achieved by using glucose insulin drip on the morning of surgery in diabetics and/or by adding insulin infusion whenever required.

7.2.4 Venous Thromboembolism Prophylaxis

There is a high risk of venous thromboembolism (VTE) in gynaecologic oncology patients with the rate of 3–4% in cervical cancer, 4–9% in endometrial cancer, and 17–38% in ovarian cancer [11–13]. Apart from malignancy, other factors like high BMI, pelvic surgery, extra pelvic disease, pre-operative corticosteroids, receipt of neoadjuvant chemotherapy, immobility and a hypercoagulable state further increase the risk of VTE [14]. The risk of venous thromboembolism can be quantified by using Caprini [15] score which consists of 20 variables to calcultate a venous thromboembolism risk and the thromboprophylaxis is recommended based upon this score.

All patients should receive dual VTE prophylaxis (mechanical and chemoprophylaxis) for 28 days. Mechanical prophylaxis can be given with the use of pneumatic compression pumps, elastic compression stockings and graduated compression stockings. Chemoprophylaxis is done by administration of low molecular weight heparin (LMWH), like dalteparin 5000 IUsc daily, enoxaparin 40 mg sc daily, tinzaparin 3500 IUsc daily [16]. It is started preoperatively preferably 12 h before surgery and resumed 12 h after surgery after ensuring surgical hemostasis. The timing of VTE chemoprophylaxis also determines the placement and removal of epidural catheter. The scheduled dose of heparin should be delayed for 2 h after the epidural catheter removal. The catheter is removed 10–12 h after the last dose of LMWH.

7.2.5 Surgical Site Infection Reduction Bundles

Surgical site infections are defined as infections of the surgical incision or organ space that develop within 30 days of surgery. Surgical site infection reduction bundle comprises of antimicrobial prophylaxis, skin preparation, avoiding hypothermia, avoiding surgical drains, and maintaining perioperative normoglycemia.

7.2.5.1 Antimicrobial Prophylaxis

First generation cephalosporin (preferably cefazolin 1 g intravenous) should be given within 1 h before the surgical incision [17]. Increased dose should be given to obese patients. Additional doses should be given after 1.5–4 h in case of prolonged surgery (>3 h) or blood loss of more than 1500 ml. Addition of anaerobic coverage is recommended if bowel is entered during pelvic surgery. Antibiotic prophylaxis can extend to 24–48 h in the perioperative period.

7.2.5.2 Skin Preparation

In order to reduce the amount of bacterial flora on the skin prior to the surgical incision, patients should shower with a chlorhexidine based soap night before and on the morning of surgery. Part preparation is to be done by hair clipping. All patients should undergo a chlorhexidine-alcohol based skin preparation in the operating room before the surgery [18].

7.2.5.3 Normothermia

Maintenance of normothermia is crucial, as hypothermia (<36 °C) during surgery leads to a higher rate of wound infections, increase in cardiac morbidity, increased rate of coagulopathy and bleeding. Warming with warm air blankets 2 h prior and after surgery can increase the core body temperature. Interventions like fluid warming before infusion, use of forced-air infusion blankets, heating mattress pads, and circulating garment systems are effective to prevent hypothermia during surgery [19].

7.2.5.4 Drains and Catheters

Use of peritoneal drains, subcutaneous drains and nasogastric tubes should be minimized in abdominal surgeries as introduction of any foreign body can increase the chances of bacterial infection. Urinary catheters should also be removed as soon as possible, usually within 24 h of surgery or as soon as mobilization is established.

7.2.6 Minimizing Surgical Insult

A key component of enhanced recovery is the focus minimally invasive surgery. Role of minimally invasive surgery (MIS) has been established in surgery for endometrial cancer and is associated with improved patient outcomes. In the Gynaecologic Oncology Study LAP2, it was concluded that laparoscopic surgical staging of uterine cancer is more feasible and safe in terms of short term outcomes and results in fewer complications and hospital stay when compared with lapratomy [20].

However, due to recent controversy regarding the role of MIS in cancer cervix consequent to the LACC trial [21], which showed reduced survival in the MIS arm compared to open surgery; MIS is not recommended for cancer cervix. In these cases, in order to expedite recovery transverse incision like Maylard's may be used for better and faster postoperative recovery. In ovarian cancer, a midline laparotomy is still the preferred mode of surgery.

7.2.7 Standard Anaesthetic Protocol

Anaesthesia for gynaecological cancer surgery requires appropriate monitoring, adequate fluid replacement and liberal use of regional blocks for perioperative pain relief. Arterial line monitoring of blood pressure can be done and trans-oesophageal dopplers can be placed to ensure adequate fluid replacement during surgery. Regular blood gases monitoring, vasopressors for blood pressure maintenance where required, and central venous access is used for major gynaecological oncology surgery [22–24]. In the ERAS management group, the anaesthesia conduct is similar to conventional techniques except for a few modifications like (a) The intraoperative analgesia is maintained using Fentanyl 1 mcg/Kg IV injected just prior to induction, followed by dexmedetomidine 0.6 mcg/kg IV infusion and continued at 0.4 mcg/kg/hr intraoperatively. (b) For postoperative analgesia, epidural injection of bupivacaine is used to maintain VAS pain score <4. Rescue analgesia is done by using paracetamol 1 gram IV infusion. (c) Epidural catheterisation is tailored according to patient requirement and is used more frequently in ERAS protocol. (d) For postoperative nausea and vomiting prophylaxis, in addition to ondansetron 4 mg IV, dexamethasone 4 mg IV is also injected prior to reversal. (e) Intraoperative fluid management is aimed to not use liberal administration of fluids and limit the volume to minimum required (1–3 ml/Kg/hr) while ensuring patient safety.

7.2.8 Perioperative Fluid Management

The main aim is to maintain perioperative euvolemia or a zero-sum fluid balance. *Zero-sum fluid balance* means that the weight of the patient before entering the surgery should be equal to that after exiting the surgery.

This is achieved by preferring colloid administration over crystalloids. If necessary, infusion of balanced crystalloids like ringer lactate should be preferred instead to normal saline due to its lower sodium content therefore avoiding electrolyte disturbances.

The other key components of zero sum fluid balance are use of vasopressors instead of crystalloids for the treatment of hypotension in a euvolemic patient and goal-directed fluid therapy. *Goal-directed fluid therapy* is a technique to manage hemodynamics with the use of fluids and inotropes to improve tissue perfusion and oxygenation and requires minimally invasive hemodynamic monitoring [25].

Post operatively, a restrictive fluid policy is employed and enteral feeding should be started early and intravenous fluids be removed as soon as oral intake is started or post-operative day one at the latest.

For post-operative nausea and vomiting prophylaxis, in addition to ondansetron 4 mg IV, dexamethasone 4 mg IV should be injected prior to reversal of anesthesia.

7.2.9 Pain Management

Adequate pain control helps in early postoperative recovery. Opioid sparing multimodal post-operative analgesia like non-steroidal anti-inflammatory drugs, acetaminophen and gabapentin are advocated for enhanced recovery. Opioids are avoided as they cause nausea, sedation, and fatigue along with increased risk of addiction. Analgesics with different mechanisms have a synergistic effect. Oral analgesics should be started as soon as possible. However, rescue analgesia would need intravenous drugs like 1 g paracetamol infusion.

In addition, incisional infiltration of either bupivacaine or ropivacaine, thoracic epidural analgesia and transversus abdominal plane blocks are other measures that can be done for adequate pain control [26]. The local anesthetic solutions that can be used for postoperative pain control include bupivacaine (maximum dose ~150 mg, varies based on body weight), ropivacaine (maxi-

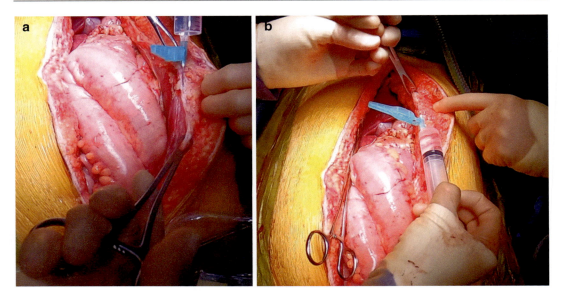

Fig. 7.1 (**a**, **b**) Rectus sheath infiltration of local anaesthetic solution

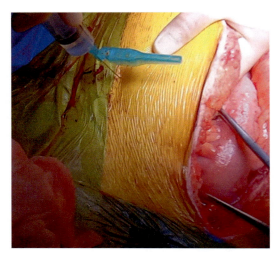

Fig. 7.2 Transversus abdominis plane (TAP) block performed by injecting local anaesthetic between internal oblique and transverse abdominis muscles, just deep to the fascial plane through which sensory nerves pass

mum dose ~300 mg, varies based on body weight), and liposomal bupivacaine (maximum dose 266 mg) [26]. When using a local anaesthetic infiltration, it is important to ensure that all the layers of the surgical incision are infiltrated under direct visualization on a controlled manner. It is best to infiltrate using a 22 gauge, 1.5 inch needle which is inserted approximately 0.5–1 cm into the tissue plane (e.g.: peritoneal, rectus sheath, musculofascial, or subdermal planes) and the local anaesthetic solution is injected while slowly withdrawing the needle to reduce the risk of intravascular injection (Fig. 7.1) [26]. Alternatively, bilateral Transversus abdominis plane (TAP) blocks can be performed by injecting local anesthetic between internal oblique and transverse abdominis muscles for midline incisions with or without ultrasound guidance and is associated with decreased pain and less opioid requirement (Fig. 7.2) [27].

7.2.10 Perioperative Nutrition

It is recommended to start a regular diet as soon as possible after the surgery preferably within 24 h.

The dietary chart should be individualized according to the patient status by the dietician. A high protein and calorie diet is preferred with up to 2 g/kg/day proteins and 25–30 kcal/kg/day [28]. In addition, nutritional supplementation like polyunsaturated fatty acids, arginine, glutamine and antioxidants can be given for improved healing.

7.2.11 Prevention of Post-operative Ileus

For prevention of post-operative ileus and to ensure early bowel return, on post-operative day one, patients can be given choices like black coffee and chewing gum. Other components of ERAS program like maintenance of euvolemia, opioid sparing multimodal analgesia, early feeding, early ambulation also prevent post-operative ileus.

Alvimopan is a FDA approved drug which is an oral selective opioid receptor antagonist that acts on the gastrointestinal tract and therefore prevents post-operative ileus. Its use is reserved for patients undergoing planned bowel resection and the first dose is given preoperatively [29].

7.2.12 Early Ambulation

It is a hallmark component of the ERAS programs. Early mobilization decreases pulmonary atelectasis, insulin resistance, prevents loss of muscle mass and helps in early return of bowel function. It is recommended that patients get out of bed and mobilize as much as possible at least for 2 h on the day of surgery and for 6 h per day until discharge.

7.2.13 Discharge

Readiness of the patient is and presence of a caretaker is mandatory for discharge. Patients can be discharged when they are ambulatory, stable vitals, able to tolerate solid food without nausea and vomiting, non-distended abdomen, passage of either flatus or stool and have adequate pain control. The patient and caretaker should be explained well about postoperative care including diet and to report to the hospital immediately in case of fever, complaints or any other complication. Emergency numbers should be provided before discharge. They can be called for suture removal in the second or third week.

The various components of ERAS are summarized in Table 7.1.

Table 7.1 Components of enhanced recovery program

Preoperative phase
Prehabilitation: Preoperative risk stratification, risk modification, and medical optimization have to be performed
Preoperative counseling of patients and care-givers
Preopeartive nutrition: Drink clear fluids until 2 h prior to and carbohydrate loading using 50 gm carbohydrate loaded drink 2 h prior to surgery provided there are no contraindications
Bowel preparation: Use antibiotics like erythromycin, metronidazole, mild laxatives. Avoid routine mechanical bowel preparation

Intraoperative phase
Goal directed fluid therapy
Multimodal opioid-sparing regimens/loco-regional analgesic techniques
Incorporating best practices of anesthetic care and techniques
Infusion of local anesthetic in the subcutaneous wound or rectus sheath prior to closure
Use of thromboprophylaxis (mechanical and chemoprophylaxis)
Use of prophylactic antibiotics
Avoidance of routine use of drains and catheters

Postoperative phase
Early feeding, early discontinuation of intravenous fluid regimes
Early mobilization
Early removal of urinary catheter and drains (if any)
Pain control with non opioid analgesia regimens
Clear postoperative discharge instructions and emergency contacts

Table 7.2 Literature review of enhanced recovery program in gynaecological oncology

Study	Design	Outcomes analyzed	Results	Remarks
Bernard L 2021 [30]	Prospective study ERAS (n = 187) versus pre ERAS implementation (n = 441)	Patient demographics, surgical variables, post operative outcomes	Mean LOS significantly shortened after ERAS from 4.7 (SD 3.8) days to 3.8 (SD = 3.2) days p = 0.0001	Overall complication rate decreased from 24.3 to 16% (p = 0.02) Significant decrease in rates of post operative infections, cardiovascular complications no increase in readmission rates
Sanchez-Iglesias JL et al. 2020 [31]	Prospective interventional RCT PROFAST ERAS (n = 50); CM (n = 49) for cytoreductive surgery in advanced ovarian cancer	Primary outcome: reduction in LOS Secondary outcome complications, readmissions rate, mortality	Results (ERAS vs. CM) Decreased median LOS (7 vs. 9 days; p = 0.0099) Decreased rate of readmission (6% versus 20%; p = 0.0334)	No difference with respect to complications, re operation rates and mortality
Gentry ZL 2020 [32]	Case control study ERAS (n = 179); controls (n = 197) for laparotomy	Primary outcome: direct and indirect costs, reduction in LOS	Overall contribution per margin encounter decreased in the ERAS group (dollar 11,619 vs. dollar 8528; p = 0.01)	LOS significantly lower in ERAS group (4.1 vs. 2.9 days; p = 0.04)
Harrison RF 2020 [33]	Retrospective cohort study ERAS (n = 213) versus conventional group (n = 58)	Difference in hospital charges	Median hospital charge significantly reduced by 15.6% in ERAS	Significantly lower charges for laboratory service, pharmacy service, room and board and material goods
Wijk L et al. 2019 [34]	Enhanced recovery after surgery audit N = 2101 patients following ERAS protocol	Length of hospital stay and complications	Every unit increase in ERAS guideline score significantly reduced LOS by 8–12% and reduced the odds of total complications by 12%	
Iniesta MD 2019 [35]	Prospective study ERAS (n = 584)	Relation between level of compliance and post operative outcomes	More than 80% compliance had significantly less complications, shorter LOS	Overall compliance 72.3% Readmission rates and re-operation dates not impacted
Agarwal R et al. 2019 [36]	Prospective interventional study ERAS (n = 45); CM (n = 45) for laparotomy in advanced ovarian cancer	Primary outcome: reduction in LOS Secondary outcome complications, readmissions rate	Decreased median LOS (6 vs. 4 days; p < 0.001) Significant reduction in moderate or severe complications (0 vs.17.8%; p = 0.003)	No difference in readmission rates

Table 7.2 (continued)

Study	Design	Outcomes analyzed	Results	Remarks
Boitano TKL et al. 2018 [37]	Retrospective study ERAS (n = 179); Controls (n = 197) in laparotomy	Primary outcome: rate of post operative ileus Secondary outcome: LOS, readmissions rate	ERAS vs. controls: Ileus rate significantly lower (2.8 vs. 15.7%; $p < 0.001$); Reduced NG tube placement (2.2% versus 7.1%)	Epidural use significantly increased ileus risk, severe morbidity LOS significantly decreased in ERAS group
Bisch SP et al 2018 [38]	Prospective study Post ERAS (n = 367); pre ERAS implementation (n = 152) in laparotomy and debulking surgery	Clinical outcomes and compliance	Decreased median LOS (4 vs. 3 days; $p = 0.001$); adjusted LOS decrease of 31.4% Significant reduction in complications from 53.3 to 36.2% post ERAS ($p = 0.0003$)	Net cost savings per patient was 956 dollars No difference in readmission rates or mortality
Berstrom JE 2018 [39]	Retrospective ERAS (n = 158) versus historical patient cohort (n = 158)	Demographics, surgical variables, post operative outcomes compared with historical patient cohort	ERAS patients required less narcotics 70.7 vs. 127.4; $p = 0.007$ and PCA use (32 vs. 50.6%, $p = 0.002$).	Significantly less pain on post op day 3 in ERAS No difference in LOS (5 days), complication rates or 30 days readmission rates
Dickson EL et al 2017 [40]	RCT ERAS (n = 51); CM (n = 52) for laparotomy in gynaecologic cancer	Primary outcome: reduction in LOS Secondary outcomes: total daily narcotic usage, time to post operative milestones complications	No difference in LOS (median = 3 days; $p = 0.36$)	No statistical significant difference in secondary outcomes
Myriokefalitaki E et al. 2016 [41]	Non randomized trial ERAS (n = 99); historic controls with traditional approach (n = 99) for all major Gynaec-oncology operations	Patient characteristics and outcomes stratification was done with respect to laparoscopic and abdominal surgery	ERAS vs. controls: Decreased mean LOS (4.29 ± 2.78 days vs. 7.23 ± 5.68 days; $p < 0.001$) Decreased rate of readmission (6 vs. 20%; $p = 0.0334$)	No difference with respect to complications, and readmission rates Maximum benefit was seen in the abdominal surgery group

7.3 Benefits of ERAS Program: Evidence in Literature

Various studies have been done to study the impact of ERAS implementation on clinical outcomes, length of hospital stay, complication and readmission rates and financial impact. The evidence is summarized in Table 7.2. Overall implementation of the ERAS protocol leads to 30% reduction in hospital stay and 40% decrease in complications and reduces overall hospital costs without increasing re-hospitalization [42]. It is also associated with earlier start of adjuvant chemotherapy in patients

> **Key Points**
> 1. Successful implementation of an ERAS program requires coordination of a multidisciplinary team including varieties of disciplines like anaesthesiologists, surgeons, trainees, hospital administrators, dieticians, physiotherapists and nurses.
> 2. Preoperative patient counselling, and prehabilitation are important part of ERAS to assess and improve patients performance status.
> 3. Mechanical bowel preparation is no longer recommended routinely and is according to the discretion of the operating surgeon if colonic resection is planned. Oral antibiotics like neomycin, erythromycin and metronidazole are given
> 4. Prophylaxis for venous thromboembolism with low molecular weight heparin for 28 days and mechanical methods is recommended for all oncology patients.
> 5. Surgical site infection reduction bundles include antibiotics, local hygiene and no or minimal use of drains and catheters.
> 6. To ensure appropriate glycaemic control, various measures include reduced preoperative fasting, perioperative normoglycemia and early initiation of oral intake.
> 7. Other components of the programme include maintenance of euvolemia, normothermia, early postoperative ambulation, multimodal analgesia and early discharge

undergoing cytoreductive surgery for advanced ovarian cancer [43].

7.4 Conclusion

Successful implementation of an ERAS program requires coordination of a multidisciplinary team including varieties of disciplines like anesthesiologists, surgeons, trainees, hospital administrators, dieticians, physiotherapists and nurses and it is essential to assess the adherence to specific ERAS components. For proper reporting, the ERAS USA and the ERAS Society have published the Reporting on ERAS Compliance, Outcomes, and Elements Research (RECOvER) Checklist [44]. This tool consists of various items including best practices for reporting clinical pathways, compliance auditing and formatting guidelines.

References

1. Kehlet H. Multimodal approach to control postoperative pathophysiology and rehabilitation. Br J Anaesth. 1997;78:606–17.
2. Schneider S, Armbrust R, Spies C, du Bois A, Sehouli J. Prehabilitation programs and ERAS protocols in gynecological oncology: a comprehensive review. Arch Gynecol Obstet. 2020;301(2):315–26.
3. Schmidt S, Vilagut G, Garin O, et al. Reference guidelines for the 12-item short-form health survey version 2 based on the Catalan general population. Med Clin. 2012;139:613–25.
4. Baitar A, Van Fraeyenhove F, Vandebroek A, De Droogh E. Groningen frailty indicator and the G-8 questionnaire as screening tools for frailty in older patients with cancer. J Geriatr Oncol. 2013;4(1):32–8.
5. Phillips SM, Chevalier S, Leidy HJ. Protein "requirements" beyond the RDA: implications for optimizing health. Appl Physiol Nutr Metab. 2016;41(5):565–72.
6. Halaszynski TM, Juda R, Silverman DG. Optimizing postoperative outcomes with efficient preoperative assessment and management. Crit Care Med. 2004;32(4 Suppl):S76–86.
7. Kumar AS, Kelleher DC, Sigle GW. Bowel preparation before elective surgery. Clin Colon Rectal Surg. 2013;26(3):146–52.
8. Pineda CE, Shelton AA, Hernandez-Boussard T, et al. Mechanical bowel preparation in intestinal surgery: a meta-analysis and review of the literature. J Gastrointest Surg. 2008;12:2037–44.
9. Slim K, Vicaut E, Launay-Savary M-V, et al. Updated systematic review and meta-analysis of randomized clinical trials on the role of mechanical bowel preparation before colorectal surgery. Ann Surg. 2009;249:203–9.
10. Nygren J, Thorell A, Ljungqvist O. Preoperative oral carbohydrate therapy. Curr Opin Anaesthesiol. 2015;28:364–9.
11. Matsuo K, Yessaian AA, Lin YG, et al. Predictive model of venous thromboembolism in endometrial cancer. Gynecol Oncol. 2013;128:544–51.
12. Levitan N, Dowlati A, Remick SC, et al. Rates of initial and recurrent thromboembolic disease among patients with malignancy versus those without malig-

nancy. Risk analysis using Medicare claims data. Medicine. 1999;78:285–91.
13. Mokri B, Mariani A, Heit JA, et al. Incidence and predictors of venous thromboembolism after debulking surgery for epithelial ovarian cancer. Int J Gynecol Cancer. 2013;23:1684–91.
14. Lyman GH, Khorana AA, Kuderer NM, et al. Venous thromboembolism prophylaxis and treatment in patients with cancer: American Society of Clinical Oncology clinical practice guideline update. J Clin Oncol. 2013;31:2189–204.
15. Golemi I, Salazar Adum JP, Tafur A, Caprini J. Venous thromboembolism prophylaxis using the Caprini score. Dis Mon. 2019;65(8):249–98.
16. Bell BR, Bastien PE, Douketis JD, Canada T. Prevention of venous thromboembolism in the enhanced recovery after surgery (ERAS) setting: an evidence-based review. Can J Anaesth. 2015;62(2):194–202.
17. Bratzler DW, Dellinger EP, Olsen KM, et al. Clinical practice guidelines for antimicrobial prophylaxis in surgery. Surg Infect. 2013;14:73–156.
18. Johnson MP, Kim SJ, Langstraat CL, et al. Using bundled interventions to reduce surgical site infection after major gynecologic cancer surgery. Obstet Gynecol. 2016;127:1135–44.
19. Wong PF, Kumar S, Bohra A, et al. Randomized clinical trial of perioperative systemic warming in major elective abdominal surgery. Br J Surg. 2007;94:421–6.
20. Walker JL, Piedmonte MR, Spirtos NM, et al. Laparoscopy compared with laparotomy for comprehensive surgical staging of uterine cancer: gynecologic oncology group study LAP2. J Clin Oncol. 2009;27(32):5331–6.
21. Ramirez PT, Frumovitz M, Pareja R, Lopez A, Vieira M, Ribeiro R, et al. Minimally invasive versus abdominal radical hysterectomy for cervical cancer. N Engl J Med. 2018;379(20):1895–904.
22. Sneyd JR, Carr A, Byrom WD, et al. A meta-analysis of nausea and vomiting following maintenance of anaesthesia with propofol or inhalational agents. Eur J Anaesthesiol. 1998;15:433–45.
23. Blaudszun G, Lysakowski C, Elia N, et al. Effect of perioperative systemic α2 agonists on postoperative morphine consumption and pain intensity: systematic review and meta-analysis of randomized controlled trials. Anesthesiology. 2012;116:1312–22.
24. Futier E, Constantin J-M, Paugam-Burtz C, et al. A trial of intraoperative low-tidal-volume ventilation in abdominal surgery. N Engl J Med Overseas Ed. 2013;369:428–37.
25. Hamilton MA, Cecconi M, Rhodes A. A systematic review and meta-analysis on the use of preemptive hemodynamic intervention to improve postoperative outcomes in moderate and high-risk surgical patients. Anesth Analg. 2011;112(6):1392–402.
26. Joshi GP, Janis JE, Haas EM, Ramshaw BJ, Nihira MA, Dunkin BJ. Surgical site infiltration for abdominal surgery: a novel neuroanatomical-based approach. Plast Reconstr Surg Glob Open. 2016;4(12):e1181.
27. Gasanova I, Alexander J, Ogunnaike B, Hamid C, Rogers D, Minhajuddin A, Joshi GP. Transversus abdominis plane block versus surgical site infiltration for pain management after open Total abdominal hysterectomy. Anesth Analg. 2015;121(5):1383–8.
28. Wischmeyer PE, Carli F, Evans DC, et al. American society for enhanced recovery and perioperative quality initiative joint consensus statement on nutrition screening and therapy within a surgical enhanced recovery pathway. Anesth Analg. 2018;126:1883–95.
29. Bakkum-Gamez JN, Langstraat CL, Lemens MA, et al. Accelerating gastrointestinal recovery in women undergoing ovarian cancer debulking: a randomized, double-blind, placebo-controlled trial. Gynecol Oncol. 2016;141:16.
30. Bernard L, McGinnis JM, Su J, Alyafi M, Palmer D, Potts L, et al. Thirty-day outcomes after gynecologic oncology surgery: a single-center experience of enhanced recovery after surgery pathways. Acta Obstet Gynecol Scand. 2021;100(2):353–61.
31. Sánchez-Iglesias JL, Carbonell-Socias M, Pérez-Benavente MA, Monreal Clua S, Manrique-Muñoz S, et al. PROFAST: a randomised trial implementing enhanced recovery after surgery for highcomplexity advanced ovarian cancer surgery. Eur J Cancer. 2020;136:149–58.
32. Gentry ZL, Boitano TKL, Smith HJ, Eads DK, Russell JF, Straughn JM Jr. The financial impact of an enhanced recovery after surgery (ERAS) protocol in an academic gynecologic oncology practice. Gynecol Oncol. 2020;156(2):284–7.
33. Harrison RF, Li Y, Guzman A, Pitcher B, Rodriguez-Restrepo A, Cain KE, et al. Impact of implementation of an enhanced recovery program in gynecologic surgery on healthcare costs. Am J Obstet Gynecol. 2020;222(1):66.e1–9.
34. Wijk L, Udumyan R, Pache B, Altman AD, Williams LL, Elias KM, et al. International validation of enhanced recovery after surgery society guidelines on enhanced recovery for gynecologic surgery. Am J Obstet Gynecol. 2019;221(3):237.e1–237.e11.
35. Iniesta MD, Lasala J, Mena G, Rodriguez-Restrepo A, Salvo G, Pitcher B, et al. Impact of compliance with an enhanced recovery after surgery pathway on patient outcomes in open gynecologic surgery. Int J Gynecol Cancer. 2019;29(9):1417–24.
36. Agarwal R, Rajanbabu A, Nitu PV 5th, Goel G, Madhusudanan L, Unnikrishnan UG. A prospective study evaluating the impact of implementing the ERAS protocol on patients undergoing surgery for advanced ovarian cancer. Int J Gynecol Cancer. 2019;29(3):605–12.
37. Boitano TKL, Smith HJ, Rushton T, Johnston MC, Lawson P, Leath CA 3rd, et al. Impact of enhanced recovery after surgery (ERAS) protocol on gastrointestinal function in gynecologic oncology patients undergoing laparotomy. Gynecol Oncol. 2018;151(2):282–6.
38. Bisch SP, Wells T, Gramlich L, Faris P, Wang X, Tran DT, et al. Enhanced Recovery After Surgery (ERAS) in gynecologic oncology: system-wide implementation and audit leads to improved

value and patient outcomes. Gynecol Oncol. 2018;151(1):117–23.
39. Bergstrom JE, Scott ME, Alimi Y, Yen TT, Hobson D, Machado KK, et al. Narcotics reduction, quality and safety in gynecologic oncology surgery in the first year of enhanced recovery after surgery protocol implementation. Gynecol Oncol. 2018;149(3):554–9.
40. Dickson EL, Stockwell E, Geller MA, Vogel RI, Mullany SA, Ghebre R, et al. Enhanced recovery program and length of stay after laparotomy on a gynecologic oncology service: a randomized controlled trial. Obstet Gynecol. 2017;129(2):355–62.
41. Myriokefalitaki E, Smith M, Ahmed AS. Implementation of enhanced recovery after surgery (ERAS) in gynaecological oncology. Arch Gynecol Obstet. 2016;294(1):137–43.
42. Bajsová S, Klát J. ERAS protocol in gynecologic oncology. Ceska Gynekol. 2019;84(5):376–85. Summer
43. Tankou JI, Foley O, Falzone M, Kalyanaraman R, Elias KM. Enhanced recovery after surgery protocols improve time to return to intended oncology treatment following interval cytoreductive surgery for advanced gynecologic cancers. Int J Gynecol Cancer. 2021;31(8):1145–53.
44. Elias KM, Stone AB, McGinigle K, et al. The reporting on ERAS compliance, outcomes, and elements research (RECOvER) checklist: a joint statement by the ERAS® and ERAS® USA societies. World J Surg. 2019;43:1–8.

Surgical Complications in Gynaecological Oncology

Kavita Singh and Bindiya Gupta

8.1 Introduction

A surgical complication is defined as 'an undesirable and unintended result of an operation affecting the patient that occurs as a direct result of the operation' [1].

Accurate recording of complications is important to guide clinical practice, patient counselling, future planning, resource allocation and compare inter-institutional performance. Complications also act as surrogate marker of surgical quality and is related to performance or conduct of a surgical procedure and may be preventable. 'To err is human' and is acceptable but not to learn or rectify one's mistakes is not acceptable in surgical practice [2]. This chapter will be focussing on why, how and when complications occur and our approach to their management and lastly a reflection on how to prevent or reduce the incidence of complications.

K. Singh (✉)
Pan Birmingham Gynaecology Cancer Centre,
City Hospital, Birmingham, UK
e-mail: kavitasingh@nhs.net

B. Gupta
Department of Obstetrics & Gynecology, University College of Medical Sciences & Guru Teg Bahadur Hospital, Delhi, India

8.2 Professional Duty of Candour [3]

This has been highlighted in Good Medical Practice Code by General Medical Council (GMC) where every healthcare professional should be open and honest in communicating to the patient or where appropriate to patient's family, carer/advocate about any complication which has happened, explain its management and discuss long term impact, if any, in a non-partial/honest way. Its is the duty of the health professional to participate and cooperate with their colleagues/organisation to take part in any investigation or review of adverse incidents/complications.

8.3 Complications Versus Adverse Effect/Sequelae of Surgery

Conditions, which are inherent to the procedure and are expected to occur (such as pain or scar formation) should be discriminated from complications and be termed 'sequelae'.

Adverse effect of surgery is an expected event during performance of surgery and depends upon extensiveness, duration and complexity of surgery. For example, upto 1 litre of blood loss is acceptable after a major cytoreductive surgical procedure for ovarian cancer but is not acceptable for laparoscopic bilateral salpingoopherectomy.

Surgical complication should also be distinguished from adverse impact of surgery. For example, inadvertent injury to ovarian vessels during surgery resulting in removal of ovaries is a complication whereas removal of ovaries to treat an invasive cancer in a young patient is an expected adverse effect. Formation of stoma after extensive cytoreductive surgery or colostomy formed to remove a pelvic mass adherent to bowel in an elderly with diverticular disease is an expected surgical outcome but a stoma formation secondary to rectal injury in pelvic surgery is a complication. Vascular injury has to be distinguished from tears in the adventitial vessels in a vessel wall during lymphadenectomy.

8.4 Factors Affecting Complications Rates

Surgical complications are inherent in gynaecological oncology surgery because of the extensiveness of surgical procedure, alteration in anatomy by the presence of large tumours and also patient related factors. Complexity of gynaecological surgery has been scored by Aletti (2007) and surgeries were classified into low complexity group (score <3), intermediate complexity group (score 4–7) and high complexity group (score >8) [4]. Intraoperative complications increased with the surgical complexity score; 2.9% for a surgical score <3 and 20% for a score of >8.

Factors influencing complication rates are summarised in Table 8.1.

Grading of surgical complications is crucial and so is their careful recording. The Clavien-Dindo classification has been universally accepted and remains the most common method for grading surgical secondary events (SSEs), Table 8.2 [6, 7].

The Memorial Sloan Kettering Cancer Surgical Secondary Events (SSE) Database modified the Clavien-Dindo classification by

Table 8.1 Factors influencing complications rates [5]

- Patient factors like age, obesity, ASA grade (1–4) previous abdominal surgery, medical co-morbidities like diabetes, VTE, cardiac disease, hypoalbuminemia, hypomagnesemia
- Disease factors
- Previous chemotherapy/radiation
- Clinical experience/expertise/skills
- Resources—Equipment/theatre time/supporting team
- Surgical approach—Laparoscopy/laparotomy/robotic
- Surgical complexity
- Blood loss
- Duration of surgery

Table 8.2 Clavien-Dindo classification of surgical secondary events

Grade	Definition
Grade I	Any deviation from the normal post-operative course not requiring surgical, endoscopic or radiological intervention. This includes the need for certain drugs (e.g. antiemetics, antipyretics, analgesics, diuretics and electrolytes), treatment with physiotherapy and wound infections that are opened at the bedside
Grade II	Complications requiring drug treatments other than those allowed for grade I complications; this includes blood transfusion and total parenteral nutrition (TPN)
Grade III	Complications requiring surgical, endoscopic or radiological intervention Grade IIIa—intervention not under general anaesthetic Grade IIIb—intervention under general anaesthetic
Grade IV	Life-threatening complications; this includes CNS complications (e.g. brain haemorrhage, ischaemic stroke, subarachnoid haemorrhage) which require intensive care, but excludes transient ischaemic attacks (TIAs) Grade IVa—single-organ dysfunction (including dialysis) Grade IVb—multi-organ dysfunction
Grade V	Death of the patient

If a patient continues to suffer from a complication at the time of discharge, the suffix "d" (for disability) is added to the respective grade of complication

defining complications by physiologic system and refined their categories to oncologic-specific procedures while retaining the five tiered grades [8] (Table 8.3).

Table 8.3 Memorial Sloan Kettering Cancer Surgical Secondary Events database classifications

Grade	Surgical secondary event requiring or resulting in
Grade 1	Bedside care or oral medications
Grade 2	Intervenous medications, transfusion
Grade 3	Radiologic, endoscopic, or operative intervention required
Grade 4	Chronic disability or organ resection
Grade 5	Death
Body systems	
Cardiovascular system	Infection
Endocrine system	Metabolic
Gastrointestinal system	Musculoskeletal system
General	Nervous system
Genitourinary system	Pain
Head and neck	Pulmonary system
Hematologic or vascular system	Wound or skin

The SSE database classifies all deviations from the expected post-operative course with a modification of the Clavien-Dindo classification

8.5 Surgical Complications in Gynae-Oncology

Complications can occur intra-operatively or postoperatively. Postoperative complications are classified into immediate (within 24 h of surgery), early (occurring within 7 days of surgery, late complications (1–6 weeks postoperatively) and delayed complications which occur after 6 weeks postoperatively like lymphedema manifesting few weeks to few months postoperatively.

Intra-operative complications include haemorrhage, injury to urinary tract (bladder, ureter), spleen, gall bladder, liver lacerations, nerve injury (obturator, femoral nerve), diaphragmatic injury and anaesthetic complications relating to cardiac and respiratory compromise or anaphylactic reaction.

Table 8.4 Terminology for incidence of surgical complications

Very common	≥1/10
Common (frequent)	≥1/100 and <1/10
Uncommon (infrequent)	≥1/1000 and <1/100
Rare	≥ 1/10,000 and <1/1000
Very rare	<1/10,000

UKGOSOC, a large prospective cohort multicentric study on data collected from 10 cancer centres in UK between 2010 and 2012 and outcome of 2948 surgical procedures was recorded [9]. Overall incidence of intraoperative complications was 4.9% (143 out of 2948); haemorrhage (28.7%) was commonest followed by bladder injury (15.4%) and small bowel injury (15.4%). Intraoperative complications were highest following ovarian cancer surgery, especially those involving bowel or upper abdomen. Surgery for cervical cancer had the second highest intraoperative complication, more in laparoscopic approach. Uterine cancer surgery had low intraoperative complication rate of 3.4% which was similar between laparoscopic and open approach. Inclusion of lymphadenectomy for endometrial cancer increased the complication rate by 1.8% and 7.3% in open and laparoscopic surgery respectively.

Iyer et al. reported a 25.9% postoperative complication rate, of which wound infection was the commonest. Vulval surgery had the highest postoperative complication rate with wound breakdown rate of 32.9% and lymphocyst/lymphedema of 35.7% following inguinofemoral lymphadenectomy [5]. Cervical cancer surgery also had high postop complication rate with no difference in open and laparoscopic approach. Ovarian cancer surgery had significantly lower complication rate 26.6% when compared to vulval and cervical cancer surgery.

Incidence of surgical complications/secondary surgical events can be expressed as very common to very rare and common descriptive terminology used to describe frequency of these events is shown in Table 8.4.

8.6 Intraoperative Complications

8.6.1 Haemorrhage

This is one of the commonest complication in gynaeoncological surgery because of the extensiveness of surgery required and hemodynamic alterations caused by malignancy. The risk of haemorrhage is increased in patients on preoperative therapeutic anticoagulation, post chemotherapy cytoreductive surgery and after major multi quadrant cytoreductive surgery.

Haemorrhage can be classified as:

- *Primary:* occurs during surgery and is related to direct surgical cause e.g. direct surgical trauma to a vascular organ like liver, spleen or vessels like aorta, pelvic vessels.
- *Reactionary:* occurs postoperatively within first 24 h and is usually caused by a rise in blood pressure at the end of the operation, which causes sealed vessels that had previously not been bleeding to start to do so.
- Secondary: normally manifests after few days/weeks and is due to infection which causes erosion of a sealed vessel.

8.6.1.1 Management of Vascular Injuries

Vascular injuries can be arterial or venous. **Arterial injuries** can be caused by blunt trauma during traction and overstretching, direct penetrating wounds or transection. Arterial laceration usually results in more serious bleeding, as retraction of the cutting edge and contraction of the intact vessel wall will further open the wound. A false aneurysm can sometimes develop at the site of the weakened arterial wall. Too much traction occasionally may result in intramural haemorrhage and thrombus formation causing luminal occlusion with subsequent distal ischaemia. Careful traction of the iliac vessels during lymphadenectomy can avoid such an injury.

Venous injuries are more common as veins are thinner and more fragile, owing to the lack of a robust muscularis layer, and their course is more variable forming plexuses and aberrant branches. Common sites of vascular injury occur at the bifurcation of the common iliac vein, as there is always a node at the bifurcation which needs to be mobilised and both external and internal iliac vein are prone to injury due to uncontrolled traction. External iliac venous injury repair is not a challenge but internal iliac venous injury can be challenging as it's a narrower vessel and oriented posteriorly.

Second common site of venous injury is in distal external iliac vein where there can be direct communication with the obturator vein (corona mortis or circle of death) which is seen in a quarter of patients and can result in profuse haemorrhage because difficulty in surgical access if patients are obese or the pelvis is deep and the vessels retract.

Presacral haemorrhage or bleeding can be encountered in cases requiring modified posterior exenteration with rectosigmoid resection. One has to avoid the presacral vascular plexus and remain in the transmesometrial resection plane. Presacral haemorrhage is difficult to control because of retraction of vessels in the sacral foramina.

In the distal inferior vena cava, 2 cm from the common iliac junction, the precaval lymph node is attached to the inferior vena cava by a short and fragile vein: the Fellow's vein. Careless lifting of the lymph nodes may cause tearing in this vein, with significant bleeding.

During mobilisation of the liver, careful attention needs to be paid to the hepatic veins draining into the inferior vena cava. Laceration of these veins has potential risk of causing fatal haemorrhage. Before mobilisation of the liver it may sometimes be useful to sloop the inferior vena cava or even the portal vein with a rubber vascular strings to enable the surgeon to stop the hepatic blood flow.

The **management** of haemorrhage depends on the cause and its severity. It includes fluid and blood product resuscitation, reversal of anticoagulant effect and surgical intervention.

Haemorrhage is quite often controlled with pressure as there is usually contraction of the vessel wall and thrombus formation. In smaller wounds, haematoma formation can provide some tamponade. Massive, uncontrolled intraoperative haemorrhage from presacral or pararectal venous bleeding can also be controlled with packing of the pelvis and leaving the abdomen open (laparostomy). The packs are removed 48 h later and the abdomen is closed.

If bleeding is profuse then hemostatic agents as shown in Table 8.5 can be used. Injectable cyclokapron (tranexamic acid) may be used per-operatively.

For controlling severe pelvic haemorrhage with no identifiable bleeder, ligation of internal iliac vessel is recommended which should be performed distal to the origin of the gluteal branches, as bilateral proximal ligation of this vessel can result in gluteal claudication, owing to the reduced blood supply to the gluteal muscles. Ligation of the inferior mesenteric artery can result in ischaemic changes in the rectosigmoid colon though marginal vessels do maintain the vascularity of the rectosigmoid but in a small percentage the marginal vessels may be absent with a potential risk of bowel ischaemia if IMA has been injured or transected during para-aortic lymphadenectomy.

The type and extent of the lesion will determine the reconstructive technique. Punctures or small lacerations can be repaired using lateral suture of interrupted 5-0 or 6-0 polypropylene suture (or 4-0 for the aorta). For Fellow's vein, 4-0 or 5-0 polypropylene figure-of-eight stitch is required to control the bleeding following manual compression. Lacerations comprising more than 30% of the vascular circumference should not be closed this way to avoid stenosis of the vessel lumen: a widening patch can be used instead. Arterial transection can be repaired with a direct end-to-end anastomosis of the divided ends or an anastomosis using a graft placement where help from vascular surgeon maybe needed. Adequate access for repair should be dissected around the vessel, following control of the proximal and distal ends of the injured vessel by vascular clamps. The distal arterial system should be irrigated with heparin to remove the distal thrombus and to prevent further thrombosis.

8.6.1.2 Management of Reactionary and Secondary Haemorrhage

Reactionary haemorrhages are not common and management depends upon the severity. If the patient becomes hemodynamically unstable, re-exploration is required. Sometimes help can be obtained from interventional radiologist for embolization if isolated discrete bleeder is identifiable on angiogram, especially if a patient is too high risk to return to theatre because of their associated medical comorbidities.

Secondary haemorrhage requires management with antibiotics. Collection at the vault if excessive, can be drained by creating an opening at the vaginal vault by excising the vault suture.

Management of haemorrhage is always greatly supported by anaesthetist in maintaining hemodynamic stability and resuscitating with blood transfusion.

8.6.2 Thrombosis and Embolism

Venous thromboembolism can be an incidental finding or symptomatic cases present as tachycardia, tachypnoea, hypoxemia, or manifestation of thrombosis with tender and swollen lower limb. CT pulmonary angiogram is performed for confirmation in cases with equivocal findings on CT chest to confirm pulmonary embolism.

Once thrombosis or embolism is suspected immediate anticoagulation is started with LMWH (low molecular weight Heparin) 1 mg/kg body weight as a single dose or in two divided doses. Support with oxygen and supportive measures like leg elevation, avoiding dehydration, analgesics are undertaken. Thrombolytic therapies are rarely required except in cases of massive embolism resulting in cardiac strain and severe hypoxemia.

Table 8.5 Hemostatic agents used for control of intraoperative haemorrhage

Product	Constituent	Mechanism of action	Salient features
A. Absorbable hemostat			**Assist in the control of capillary, venous, and small arterial haemorrhage**
(i) Surgicel original		Oxidised regenerated cellulose. Formation of a gelatinous mass upon saturation with blood, which leads to formation of a stable clot	Efficacy with bactericidal properties on even surfaces
(ii) Surgicel fibrillar		Oxidised regenerated cellulose. Pressure and matrix for clot formation	Easily separated layers are customizable allowing for precise placement in cavities
(iii) Surgicel SNoW		SNoW: structured non woven material. Oxidised regenerated cellulose provides a physical barrier to block blood flow and provides a large surface area for rapid fibrin clot formation	Conforms & adherence to tissue better in irregular surfaces

(iv) Surgicel Nu Knit		Oxidised regenerated cellulose for physical compression and rapid fibrin clot formation	High tensile strength and thickness allows it to hold suture
(v) Surgicel powder		Provides surface for platelet adhesion & aggregation, allowing endogenous clotting factors to initiate clot formation	Powder form and can be used to fill cavities—Presacral bleed
(vi) Spongoston		Absorbable gelatine sponge, swells to promote mechanical compression. Platelets trapped within the pores forms a fibrin clot	It can be used dry or can be made wet before application
B. Biological agents			
(i) Surgiflo (Ethicon)		Gelatin (porcine) with thrombin	Pressure as gelatin swells +promoter of coagulation	Preparation time of 1–2 min
(ii) Floseal (Baxter)		Gelatin (bovine) with thrombin	Pressure as gelatin swells +promoter of coagulation	Preparation time of 1–2 min
C. Biological agents through a matrix			
Tachosil	Fibrinogen and thrombin on one side of the collagen patch	Promote haemostasis by triggering the last stage of the coagulation cascade to create a fibrin clot	Sealant haemostatic over hepatic, splenic, pancreatic surface & aortic surfaces after lymphadenectomy as can seal lymphatic vessels

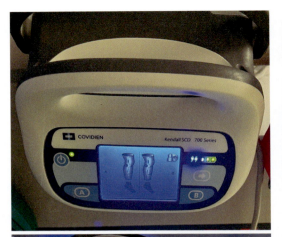

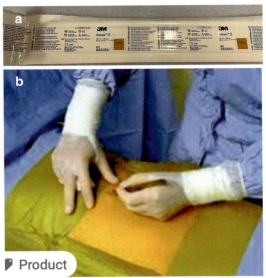

Fig. 8.2 (**a**, **b**) IO-ban adhesive surgical drape

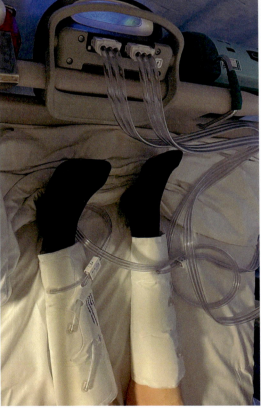

Fig. 8.1 Flowtrons boots to prevent thrombo-embolism

General measures to prevent thromboembolism includes TED (thrombo-embolic deterrent) graduated stockings, Flowtrons boots (Fig. 8.1) and prophylactic anticoagulation.

In patients on therapeutic anticoagulation due to DVT/PE, in order to reduce surgical complications and embolism risk, elective surgery is recommended after 4–6 weeks of diagnosis. However, in certain acute cases where surgery cannot wait for 4–6 weeks then an IVC filter is recommended in cases with deep vein thrombosis to prevent occurrence of embolism.

8.6.3 Infections

The most common postoperative infections are urinary tract, respiratory and wound infections. Risk factors are obesity, diabetes, chronic obstructive pulmonary disease, malnutrition and immunocompromised state related to chemotherapy.

Antibiotic prophylaxis is administered preoperatively and dose is repeated if surgery lasts more than 4 h. If any bowel resection and anastomosis have been performed, then prophylactic doses can be extended to 24 h. Usually 1.2 gm of Augmentin (Amoxycillin + clavulanic acid is administered 0.5–1 h prior to commencement of surgery or at induction of anaesthesia. If patients maintain allergy to penicillin then alternative like Clindamycin 650 mg may be administered for surgical prophylaxis.

Measures to reduce infection risk during surgery include use of IO-ban adhesive surgical drape (Fig. 8.2) which has bactericidal film and also prevents wound contamination from skin flora. Careful hemostasis, rational use of drains to avoid fluid accumulation, adequate nutrition and hydration help in reducing incidence of wound infection. Other interventions to reduce infection include active chest physiotherapy, early mobilisation, adequate hydration and early removal of catheter and drains.

Vigilance for early signs of infection is important for early intervention. C- reactive protein (CRP) assessment from third postoperative day is useful and if progressively rising (>200) in presence of bowel surgery with anastomosis or in presence of other associated signs of infection like raised white blood cell count or pyrexia >38°C; a CT scan maybe required to exclude collection or anastomotic leakage as a cause for infection. Timely intervention in such situations avoids unfavourable long term outcomes.

If wound shows signs of erythema then underlying sepsis, seroma or hematoma should be suspected and drainage is encouraged by removal of overlying staples. Vacuum dressing may be considered in wound sepsis in conjunction with tissue viability team.

8.6.4 Lymphatic Complication

Lymphadenectomy is an integral surgical procedure performed for vulval, endometrial, cervical and selected cases of ovarian cancers. Pelvic, para-aortic/paracaval and inguinal lymphadenectomy may result in local lymph collection as lymphocyst or retrograde accumulation as lymphedema. Lymphedema and lymphocyst formation is likely to be more in extensive lymphadenectomy, and use of double treatment modality (like surgery and adjuvant radiotherapy). Risk of lymphedema/lymphocyst is reduced with use of sealant devices like ultrasonic cutting devices (Harmonic Ace,Ethicon), Ligasure as these devices cut and seal the lymph channels.

8.6.5 Visceral Injuries

8.6.5.1 Ureteric Injuries

Ureters are prone to surgical trauma during pelvic surgery as they are retroperitoneal and can be mistaken for blood vessels, get entangled in tumours or their course can be altered by large pelvic tumours. Presence of a cervical fibroid, pelvic side wall endometriosis or adhesions, malignant conditions such as cervical cancer and adnexal masses involving the side wall and unmindful handling of tissues or attempts at haemostasis make the ureters vulnerable. There are three high-risk anatomical sites in the course of the ureter where injuries usually occur:

(i) **Pelvic brim:** The ureter is in close proximity to the bifurcation of the common iliac vessels and the infundibulopelvic ligament. To avoid ureteric trauma when the gonadal vessels are ligated, the retroperitoneum should be explored and the ureter visualised and palpated prior to ligation. Lifting the ovary away from the pelvic side wall also facilitates the safe ligation of the infundibulopelvic ligament.

(ii) **Level of the ureter crossing the uterine vessels**: The ureter is easy to damage with careless clamping. The uterine artery crosses the ureter from above while a number of uterine veins pass below.

(iii) **Vesicoureteric junction**: The intravesical portion of the ureter is prone to injury during bladder mobilisation and during haemostasis following release of the ureteric tunnel during radical hysterectomy. Careful stitching or the use of bipolar diathermy during haemostasis prevents such injuries.

There are several types of ureteric injury:

(i) **Deliberate:** The ureter is intentionally transected during during anterior or total exenteration or may be resected when malignant or benign conditions (endometriosis, ovarian cancer, sarcoma) are invading the ureter.

(ii) **Accidental:** crushing trauma, needle trauma, transection, ligation, avascular necrosis.
(iii) **Delayed:** fibrosis-related stenosis, neoplasia-related stenosis.

If ureteric injury is suspected, then the whole ureter is dissected and peristalsis is noted. Indigo caramine 40 mg (5 ml) can be injected intravenously and cystoscopic visualization of this dye through the ureteric orifice excludes any direct trauma.

Crushing injury of the ureter caused by clamping (with no transection) and pressure trauma requires careful intraoperative inspection. If no signs of ischaemia are identified, retrograde stenting is advised to minimise the effects of transient ureteral wall oedema. However, if the ureter has been compressed for a prolonged period and no functional peristalsis is seen over a significant length of ureter indicative of divitalized tissue, then resection may be required of the ischaemic area with end-to-end anastomosis with ureteral stenting.

Complete transection of the ureter results in obvious urine leakage. The ureteric ends need debridement and a retrograde ureteric stent is introduced immediately. The ureter is carefully mobilised to avoid tension and an end-to-end ureteroureterostomy is performed using an oblique suture line to prevent subsequent stricture.

To avoid tension on the ureteric anastomosis, the bladder can be mobilised and sutured to the psoas muscle (vesicopsoas hitch). If the residual ureter is not sufficient for primary anastomosis, the tubularised bladder wall can replace a longer segment of the ureter (Boari flap). If the ureteric injury is close to the bladder, then ureteroneocystostomy is performed.

Partial transection of the ureter may remain unrecognised during the procedure. Patients develop post operative fever, chill, pelvic tenderness or pain, abdominal distension, prolonged ileus, urine peritonitis and urine leakage from the vaginal or abdominal incision. CT urogram with intravenous contrast is helpful to demonstrate the extravasation of the contrast material and to identify the site and extent of the damage. Depending on the patient's physical status, the extent of the injury and the interval since the operation, the management of partial ureteric transection can vary from insertion of ureteric stent to re-laparotomy and surgical repair. If the patient is septic and unwell, drainage of the pelvic urinoma with percutaneous nephrostomy helps to resolve the acute clinical situation.

Ligation or acute angulation of the ureter leads to hydroureter and hydronephrosis and presents with lower back pain, tenderness and fever. In the rare case of bilateral ligature, anuria is the presenting symptom. If CT urogram with contrast confirms a complete ligation, emergency insertion of percutaneous nephrostomies is essential to avoid renal damage. Partially ligated or kinked ureter should first be stented with extreme care so as not to perforate the ureter. Subsequent surgical repair should be considered in cases of ligation. Occasionally, the injury is identified during surgery; the ligature then needs to be removed and the ureter closely observed. If no damage is identified, placement of a retrograde ureteric stent is required.

Avascular necrosis resulting in ureterovaginal fistulation is a rare complication of radical

Table 8.6 Management of urinary tract injuries

Complication	Repair	Comment
Cystotomy	Two-layer closure with absorbable suture	Stent if near ureteral orifice
Urethral injuries	Two-layered repair	Foley drainage × 10–14 days
Ureteral injury: Below pelvic brim	Ureteroneocystostomy is preferred	Avoid tension May need psoas hitch or flap Stent × 14 days
Ureteral injury: Above pelvic brim	Ureteroureterostomy, unless mobility allows ureteroneocystostomy	Avoid tension Stent × 14 days
Ureteral resection	Ureteroureterostomy if sufficient ureteral length remains transureteroureterostomy bowel interposition graft	Some tumors require large portions of ureter to be resected

hysterectomy, when the blood supply of the ureter is impaired during its release from the ureteric tunnel. Women usually present with vaginal leakage 2–3 weeks after surgery. The diagnosis of ureterovaginal fistula is confirmed by the odour of the fluid, the raised creatinine level of the discharging fluid and by demonstration on the CT urogram. In most cases, conservative management with retrograde ureteral stenting is sufficient to reduce the symptoms of leakage and enhance healing. Occasionally, surgical repair is necessary with uretero neocystostomy.

8.6.5.2 Bladder Injury

Bladder injury is a frequent complication, mostly after previous caesarean section when the bladder is morbidly adherent to the uterus. In cases of muscularis or mucomuscularis injury, the bladder wall is closed in two layers using 2-0 Vicryl® interrupted sutures or continuous sutures. Extreme care should be taken to avoid suturing close to the ureteral orifices. If in doubt, retrograde filling of the bladder using saline with methylene blue dye should be used to exclude leakage. During the early postoperative phase, overloading of the bladder should be avoided, so placement of a Foley catheter for 5–10 days is recommended.

The repair of urinary injuries is summarized in Table 8.6 [10].

8.6.5.3 Bowel Injury

Bowel injuries most commonly occur during debulking operations for advanced ovarian cancer. Needle injury to the bowel needs careful observation only in most cases with no suturing. Lacerations usually are sustained during sharp dissection of the tumour tissue off the bowel serosa, predominantly at the rectosigmoid colon or the transverse colon. En-bloc resection of the cancer with the adjacent bowel (Hudson procedure/modified posterior exenteration) and primary anastomosis should be performed to prevent bowel injury. If the bowel is lacerated and the edges are clear with no significant faecal spillage, primary closure with 3-0 polydioxalone interrupted suture is recommended.

The risk of postoperative leakage of rectosigmoid anastomoses is around 4–5%. Diabetes mellitus, hypertension, hypoalbuminaemia, smoking and previous radiotherapy are all important risk factors for leakage and defunctioning loop ileostomy may be performed to protect the anastomosis in high risk cases. Subtle symptoms such as low-grade pyrexia, abdominal tenderness with rise in white blood cell count and CRP may indicate an imminent bowel leakage. Frank leakage manifests as peritonitis with guarding, rebound and fever. When anastomotic leakage is suspected, full blood count and blood cultures should be taken and broad spectrum intravenous antibiotics commenced. Contrast CT can facilitate the diagnosis of anastomotic leakage by showing intraperitoneal collection or abscess. The cornerstone of the management is surgical exploration with consideration of revision of the anastomosis and bowel diversion (defunctioning ileostomy or colostomy) proximal to the site of leakage. Conservative management with percutaneous drainage can be considered in selected cases. Bowel lacerations that are not identified during operation have identical clinical findings and management to anastomotic leakage.

8.6.5.4 Nerve Injury

Nerve injuries are usually caused by transection or crushing impact caused by a clamp or crude handling. Transection of the genitofemoral nerve during pelvic lymphadenectomy is not uncommon, mostly seen in patients who are obese, and this does not require repair. The patchy loss of skin sensation on the anterior thigh usually recovers postoperatively. During pelvic lymphadenectomy the obturator nerve can also get damaged in the obturator fossa. In case of transection, end-to-end repair of the nerve is required. The adductor muscle function and some inner-thigh sensation may get lost but with active physiotherapy it returns in most of the cases.

The sympathetic plexus can get removed during para-aortic lymphadenectomy, causing vasodilation of the ipsilateral leg so the contralateral leg feels colder. During Wertheim's radical hysterectomy, when the hypogastric nerves are not preserved, cutting through these structures results in impaired bladder innervation and voiding difficulty. Routine use of either a Foley catheter or a suprapubic bladder catheter prevents overdistension of the bladder and ureteric reflux. This will also reduce the risk of ureteric fistulae. Nerve-sparing radical hysterectomy diminishes these complications.

8.6.6 Paralytic Ileus

Dehydration, electrolyte imbalance, prolonged surgery requiring small or large bowel dissection or resection predispose for development of paralytic ileus. Patients usually present on the second or third postoperative day with nausea, vomiting, abdominal distension and absent or sluggish bowel sounds. One should distinguish ileus from intestinal obstruction, which usually occurs later on postoperative days 5–7 and presents with similar symptoms and associated colicky abdominal pain and exaggerated bowel sounds in early stage. Plain erect abdominal X-ray shows generalised dilatation of small and large bowel loops. Management of mild paralytic ileus consists of intravenous hydration, correction of electrolyte imbalance and restricted oral intake. In severe cases presenting with profuse vomiting, nasogastric aspiration is required. Prokinetic antiemetics, such as metoclopramide, also facilitate resolution of paralytic ileus.

8.6.7 Shift in Fluid Balance

Shift in fluid balance is a unique complication of debulking surgery for advanced ovarian cancer. Constant loss of protein-rich ascitic fluid during a prolonged operation usually leads to low serum albumin, fluid shift to interstitial space resulting in intravascular dehydration, fall of blood pressure, impaired microcirculation and low urine output. Active fluid resuscitation with intensive monitoring of central venous pressure through a central line or with the recently advocated transoesophageal Doppler cardiac output surveillance is desirable for adequate recovery. There is no evidence supporting the benefit of using albumin infusion.

8.7 Late Postoperative Complications

8.7.1 Incisional Hernias

Incisional hernias are more common with vertical extended laparotomies. Predisposing factors for hernia formation are multiple previous laparotomies, increased body mass index, elderly, chronic cough, constipation, wound infection and poor nutrition, which all impair wound healing. The most common location for incisional hernias is in the periumbilical region, as this is site with the least resistance and maximum strain. Presentation is dependent upon the size, site and contents of the hernial sac. Patients may present with an asymptomatic abdominal swelling or have symptoms of abdominal pain or even signs of intestinal obstruction. Hernias become a surgical emergency if they are non-reducible, if they have alteration of colour of overlying skin or they present with features of intestinal obstruction. The management of incisional hernias depends on the severity of the symptoms and can be conservative or surgical.

8.8 Prevention of Complications

Complications can be prevented by adequate preoperative optimization of associated comorbidities by appropriate medical attention and anaesthetic review, careful and appropriate case selection for surgery from a multidisciplinary consultation, detailed clinical review of the patient to enable the right treatment for the right patient, adequate nutrition, albumin correction and availability of skilled surgical staff and team.

8.9 Conclusion

Surgical complications depend upon the type and mode of surgery required and also on patient profile with elderly and obese having a higher postoperative morbidity. A multidisciplinary approach in decision making, extreme vigilance during surgery regarding any intraoperative injury, as rectifying the injury intra-operatively

Key Points

1. Accurate recording of complications is important to guide clinical practice, patient counselling, future planning, resource allocation and compare inter-institutional performance.
2. Complications should be distinguished from adverse effects and squeal of surgery
3. Factors influencing complication rates include patient factors, disease factors, surgical approach and complexity, previous treatment, surgical expertise and available resources
4. Common complications include haemorrhage, visceral injuries, lymphatic and nerve injuries, infection, paralytic ileus and fluid imbalance
5. Vascular injuries are managed by pressure, suturing and hemostatic agents. Secondary haemorrhage usually responds to antibiotics and rarely requires drainage.
6. Preventive strategies for venous thrombosis include TED (thrombo-embolic deterrent) graduated stockings, Flowtrons boots and prophylactic anticoagulation
7. Bladder, bowel, ureteral injuries should be recognised early and require surgical repair with occasional diversion stomas
8. Common nerve injuries include injury to genitofemoral, obturator nerves and sympathetic plexus
9. A multidisciplinary approach in decision making, extreme vigilance during surgery, rectifying the injury intraoperatively, early recognition of post operative complications is of paramount importance.

has minimal postoperative complications. It is imperative to adequately and wisely allocate the right treatment for the right patient by the right team to avoid unnecessary surgical morbidity which will avoid strain on the infrastructural and healthcare resources.

References

1. Sokol DK, Wilson J. What is a surgical complication? World J Surg. 2008;32(6):942–4.
2. Institute of Medicine. To err is human: building a safer health system. Washington, DC: The National Academies Press; 1999.
3. General Medical Council. Good medical practice. 2013. https://www.gmc-uk.org/ethical-guidance/ethical-guidance-for-doctors/candour%2D%2D-openness-and-honesty-when-things-go-wrong
4. Aletti GD, Dowdy SC, Podratz KC, Cliby WA. Relationship among surgical complexity, short-term morbidity, and overall survival in primary surgery for advanced ovarian cancer. Am J Obstet Gynecol. 2007;197(6):676.e1–7.
5. Iyer R, Gentry-Maharaj A, Nordin A, Burnell M, Liston R, Manchanda R, et al. Predictors of complications in gynaecological oncological surgery: a prospective multicentre study (UKGOSOC-UK gynaecological oncology surgical outcomes and complications). Br J Cancer. 2015;112(3):475–84.
6. Clavien PA, Barkun J, de Oliveira ML, Vauthey JN, Dindo D, Schulick RD, et al. The Clavien-Dindo classification of surgical complications: five-year experience. Ann Surg. 2009;250(2):187–96.
7. Dindo D, Demartines N, Clavien PA. Classification of surgical complications: a new proposal with evaluation in a cohort of 6336 patients and results of a survey. Ann Surg. 2004;240(2):205–13.
8. Strong VE, Selby LV, Sovel M, Disa JJ, Hoskins W, Dematteo R, et al. Development and assessment of memorial sloan kettering cancer center's surgical secondary events grading system. Ann Surg Oncol. 2015;22(4):1061–7.
9. Burnell M, Iyer R, Gentry-Maharaj A, Nordin A, Liston R, Manchanda R, et al. Benchmarking of surgical complications in gynaecological oncology: prospective multicentre study. BJOG. 2016;123(13):2171–80.
10. Horvath S, George E, Herzog TJ. Unintended consequences: surgical complications in gynecologic cancer. Womens Health (Lond). 2013;9(6):595–604.

9

Minor Procedures in Gynaecological Oncology

Felicia Elena Buruiana, Rajendra Gujar, and Bindiya Gupta

9.1 Introduction

Minor surgical procedures are defined as procedures in which short surgical techniques are used in, usually under local anesthesia, require minimal equipment, are associated with minimal complications and usually done on a day care basis. These encompass a broad range of both diagnostic and therapeutic procedures. This chapter will briefly describe the various minor surgical procedures in gynaecologic oncology.

9.2 Colposcopy

Indications for colposcopy include mild dyskaryosis with positive hrHPV test, moderate or severe dyskaryosis, cytology suggestive of malignancy, glandular abnormalities, three consecutive unsatisfactory cervical cytology reports, post coital bleeding, persistent intermenstrual bleeding, suspicious cervix and repeated inflammatory cervical cytology [1].

Relevant history using a specifically designed proforma should be obtained in all women coming for colposcopy regarding menstruation, date of last menstrual period, contraception, pregnancies, smoking, previous cervical cytology, symptoms, previous treatments.

The contents of a colposcopy tray include bivalve speculum, lubricant, cotton wool balls, sponge holder forceps, cotton-tip and jumbo swabs, endocervical canal specula, biopsy forceps and pots with fixative for specimens, three small pots with saline, acetic acid (3–5%) and Lugol's iodine, haemostatic solutions (Monsel's solution) or silver nitrate sticks [1]. 3–5% acetic acid is freshly made by diluting 3 ml of glacial acetic acid in 97 ml of distilled water. Monsel's paste, a thick, sticky, fast-acting compound is made by combination of Ferric sulphate base, Ferrous sulphate powder and glycerol starch [2]. As it is a caustic product that can damage tissues if left too long, no vaginal packing should be used after application.

Sample collection bottles for liquid based or conventional smears should be available in the colposcopy clinics.

9.2.1 Procedure

The perineum and external genitalia are examined to rule out any potential abnormalities and cervix is exposed by using a speculum. If a cervical cytology sample is needed, it should be taken before acetic acid is applied. For liquid-based

F. E. Buruiana (✉) · R. Gujar
Pan Birmingham Gynaecological Cancer Centre, Birmingham, UK
e-mail: f.buruiana@nhs.net; rajendra.gujar@nhs.net

B. Gupta
Department of Obstetrics & Gynecology,
University College of Medical Sciences & Guru Teg Bahadur Hospital, Delhi, India

© The Author(s), under exclusive license to Springer Nature Switzerland AG 2022
K. Singh, B. Gupta (eds.), *Gynecological Oncology*, https://doi.org/10.1007/978-3-030-94110-9_9

cytology, the Cervex brush is rotated clockwise five times after being applied to the cervix, sampler is immersed or agitated in fixative fluid. In the case of conventional smear wooden or plastic spatula or cervical brushes are used. In both cases sampling of the endocervix is done using a cytobrush.

After application of normal saline, lesions like nabothian follicles, cervical polyps, warts, cysts and leukoplakia are identified and documented. Green filter is used to assess the vascular patterns and abnormalities. Acetic acid (3–5%) is then gently applied to the cervix with cotton balls on sponge forceps for 60 s. The transformation zone is recognised and atypical areas are noted. This is followed by application of Lugol's iodine (Schiller's test) which is optional. The test is positive when the atypical epithelium fails to take up the iodine stain as it contains a small amount or no glycogen. Normal squamous epithelium turns into mahogany brown with Lugol's iodine. Columnar epithelium fails to stain because it also contains little or no glycogen.

The findings are recorded in a standard format, according to the International Federation of Colposcopy and Cervical Pathology (IFCPC) criteria and lesion classified as minor or major (Table 9.1) [3]. A clear management plan (i.e. discharge back to GP care, further cervical smear test, follow up in colposcopy clinic, or potential

Table 9.1 International Federation of Colposcopy and Cervical Pathology (IFCPC) revised colposcopy nomenclature 2011 [3]

General assessment
Adequate or inadequate; if inadequate, for what reason (e.g. cervix obscured by inflammation, bleeding, scar)
Squamocolumnar junction visibility: completely visible, partially visible, not visible
Transformation zone types 1 (on ectocervix), type 2 (between both endo and ectocervix upper end visible), type 3 (in endocervix, upper end not visible)
Normal colposcopic findings
Original squamous epithelium: mature, atrophic
Columnar epithelium; ectopy/ectropion
Metaplastic squamous epithelium: Nabothian cysts; crypt (gland) openings
Deciduosis in pregnancy
Abnormal colposcopic findings
General principles

Table 9.1 (continued)

Location of the lesion	Inside or outside the transformation zone
	Documented by the "clock position"
Size of the lesion	Number of cervical quadrants the lesion covers
	Size of the lesion as a percentage of the cervix

Grade 1 (minor): Thin acetowhite epithelium; Irregular, geographical border; Fine mosaic; fine punctuation
Grade 2 (major): Dense acetowhite epithelium; Rapid appearance of acetowhitening; cuffed crypt openings; Coarse mosaic; coarse punctuation; Sharp border; inner border sign[a]; ridge sign[b]

Non-specific	Leukoplakia (keratosis, hyperkeratosis); erosion
	Lugol's staining (Schiller test): stained or nonstained

Suspicious for invasion
Atypical vessels
Additional signs: Fragile vessels; Irregular surface; Exophytic lesion; Necrosis; Ulceration (necrotic; Tumour or gross neoplasm
Miscellaneous findings
Congenital transformation zone; Condyloma; Polyp (ectocervical or endocervical) Inflammation; Stenosis; Congenital anomaly; Post-treatment consequence; Endometriosis

[a]Inner border sign: Low-grade and high-grade lesions may coexist, and there may be internal margins (borders) because of the abrupt change in the nature of a lesion or lesions. This is called a "lesion within a lesion" or the "inner border sign" and is a feature of high-grade neoplasia

[b]Ridge sign: If the acetowhite area is thick and elevated and is projected near the SCJ like the top of a wall or ridge, this is called the "ridge sign". The ridge sign indicates the presence of a high-grade lesion

intervention i.e. loop excision) should be documented according to the findings.

Cervical biopsy should be taken if cytology shows high-grade dyskaryosis (moderate) or worse, and/or when there is major grade or higher lesion on colposcopy [4]. Biopsy is not required in low grade cytology with negative or minor abnormalities on colposcopy and is also avoided

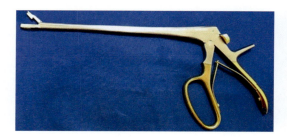

Fig. 9.1 Tischler's cervical biopsy forceps

Table 9.2 Prerequisites for ablation

- Transformation zone must be fully visible and accessible (i.e. type 1 or type 2 TZ)
- Lesion involves <75% of transformation zone (TZ)[a]
- No endocervical canal or vaginal involvement by the lesion
- No evidence of invasive cancer, no suspicion of glandular disease
- Pregnancy or less than 3 months post partum is a contraindication
- No menstrual bleeding
- No history of previous treatment
- There should be no disparity between cytology and colposcopy

[a]This prerequisite is required for cryotherapy not for thermal ablation as latter can have multiple applications to ablate the lesion

in pregnancy unless colposcopy is suggestive of invasive cancer.

Biopsy forceps (e.g. Tischler's) (Fig. 9.1) have different shapes, remove small piece of tissue of approximately 3.5 mm without distortion or crushing. Multiple biopsies from the atypical TZ give greater diagnostic accuracy compared to a single one [5]. If more than one biopsy is required, the posterior lip of the cervix should be biopsied first to avoid bleeding covering the field. In case of a frank cervical growth the biopsy should be taken from the edge of the lesion to avoid necrotic tissue. Bleeding usually stops, however if persists, silver nitrate, Monsel's solution, diathermy or vaginal packing can be used.

9.3 Ablative Techniques

Ablative methods play an important role in the treatment of cervical intraepithelial neoplasia (CIN). These are also used for *screen and treat approach* in visual inspection with acetic acid (VIA) and HPV positive cases, in low resource settings where lesion is identified and ablation is done in the same sitting, without any prior colposcopic or histopathologic confirmation [6]. If facility is available biopsy can be taken before ablating the lesion. Ablative methods include cryotherapy, thermal ablation or cold coagulation and laser ablation; out of which the first two methods are more commonly used. The depth of destruction by ablation is at least 7 mm as the deepest crypt opening is 5 mm. The major disadvantage of ablation is that the adequacy of treatment cannot be ascertained as there is no histological diagnosis of margins and depth of destruction. The essential pre-requisites to be fulfilled before ablation are summarized in Table 9.2. Follow up after ablation is done after 6–12 months.

9.3.1 Cryotherapy

It is an outpatient procedure, does not require anaesthesia and is the method of choice for low resource settings [7]. Transformation zone is ablated using Nitrous oxide (N_2O) or carbon dioxide (CO_2) at temperature of −60 °C or −80 °C.

The equipment consists of a cryoprobe of different sizes, cryo gun with trigger, compressed gas cylinder, pressure gauge, release valves and a flexible plastic tubing. At a temperature of −89 °C at the centre and −20 °C at the periphery, intracellular water undergoes crystallization along with protein coagulation causing cryonecrosis. A double freeze-thaw-freeze technique is used for 3–5–3 min respectively. Precaution should be taken not to touch the vaginal walls with the cryoprobe, and once the freeze cycle is over the probe should not be forcefully pulled from the cervix till complete thawing occurs (Fig. 9.2).

The cure rate has been reported as 92% for CIN 2 and 70–85% for CIN 3 lesions after cryotherapy [8, 9].

Side effects include profuse discharge, mild pain and rarely vasovagal symptoms.

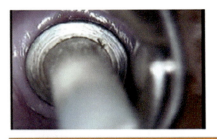

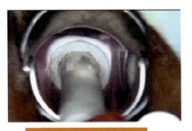

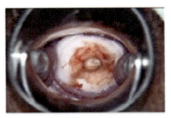

Fig. 9.2 Cryotherapy procedure

Barriers that prevent widespread implementation of this rather safe treatment are logistics of transportation of heavy tanks of gas to remote areas and sometimes these are difficult to procure [6].

9.3.2 Thermal Ablation

Thermal ablation or cold coagulation is the treatment of cervical intraepithelial neoplasia using a metallic probe heated to 100 °C. Thermal destruction of cervical tissue occurs as intracellular water reaches boiling point and the cells undergo necrosis. The instruments required are a Thermocoagulator with metallic cervical probes (Fig. 9.3), electrical connections, colposcope (when available), speculums and light source. After the patient is placed in lithotomy position, cervix is adequately exposed and delineation of the lesion is done using 3–5% acetic acid and Lugol's iodine. The thermal probe is heated upto 100 °C

and placed on the cervix on the transformation zone ensuring good contact with the epi-

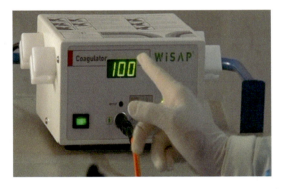

Fig. 9.3 Themal ablator

thelium, for 20–40 s. 1–5 overlapping applications of 20–40 s each can be used to cover the entire lesion (Fig. 9.4). At all times it is ensured that vaginal walls do not come in contact with the heated probe. After use, the probe is sterilized after cleaning, drying by reheating for 45 s at 120 °C.

Side effects are mild crampy pain, blood stained watery discharge (17%), vasovagal reactions (fainting, giddiness, mild cramps etc.), vag-

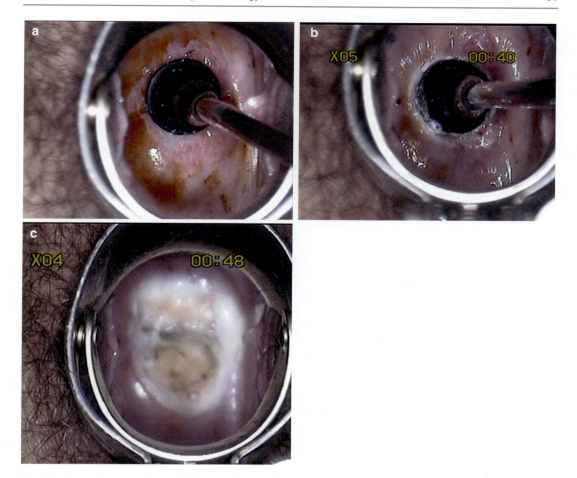

Fig. 9.4 (a) Application of thermal ablation probe. (b) Thermal damage at the point of probe application and surrounding tissue. (c) Post treatment

inal burns and rarely bleeding. Patients should be counseled about watery discharge that can present until 2–3 weeks post procedure. Long term consequences are rare and include pelvic inflammatory disease and cervical stenosis.

The patient is asked to report back if suffering fever for >2 days, foul smelling purulent discharge for >3 days, severe lower abdominal pain/cramps, bleeding for >2 days within 4 weeks of treatment.

The cure rate with thermal ablation is 96% [95% confidence interval (CI) 92–99%] and 95% (92–98%) for CIN1 and CIN2–3 disease, respectively [10].

The advantages and disadvantages of the cryotherapy and thermal ablation are summarized in Table 9.3.

9.4 Excisional Methods

An excisional biopsy is recommended when most of the ectocervix is replaced with high-grade abnormality, when low-grade colposcopic change is associated with high-grade dyskaryosis (severe) or worse, when a lesion extends into the canal in type 3 transformation zone. Common excisional methods include Large

Table 9.3 Advantages and disadvantages of ablative techniques

	Cryotherapy	Thermal ablation/cold coagulation
Advantages	1. Effective 2. Does not require anesthesia 3. Can be performed by trained nursing staff 4. Few side effects/complications	1. Effective 2. Does not require anesthesia 3. Easy portability 4. Can be performed by trained nursing staff 5. Multiple applications to cover large lesions 6. Less treatment time 7. Easy sterilization of probe 8. Few side effects/complications
Disadvantages	1. Logistic issues with gas cylinders as these are bulky, difficult to transport, expensive and not freely available. 2. Longer time to treat compared to thermal ablation 3. Single application only, hence not suitable for lesions occupying >75% of TZ	1. Expensive equipment 2. Requires electricity although battery operated devices have also been made recently

loop excision of transformation zone (LLETZ), straight wire excision of transformation zone (SWETZ), cold knife conisation (CKC) and laser excision.

The length of excised specimen depends on the transformation zone type, desire to preserve fertility and location of the lesion. The length of specimen varies from 8 mm to 1.5–2 cm for type 1 and type 3 TZ respectively. In a Cochrane meta-analysis, there was no difference in persistent disease at follow up with all three methods; LLETZ was associated with least morbidity [11]. Compared to destructive methods, the main advantage of excisional methods is that the tissue is available for histopathology, assessment of margins and depth of excision can be made.

9.4.1 Large Loop Excision of the Transformation Zone

Large loop excision of the transformation zone (LLETZ), also known as loop electrosurgical excision procedure (LEEP), is an excisional technique using a thin tungsten wire loop powered by an electrosurgical unit. It is the most common excisional method, performed in women with high-grade CIN (moderate and severe dyskaryosis). LLETZ and has a cure rate exceeding 90% for the treatment of CIN 2/CIN 3 lesions [12].

9.4.1.1 Preparation
Usually the procedure is carried out in the colposcopy clinic, under local anaesthesia after a informed consent as a day care procedure. If there is a large cervical lesion, the patient cannot tolerate the procedure under local anaesthesia, or there are contraindications to it, LLETZ can also be performed under general anaesthesia.

9.4.1.2 Procedure
The patient is positioned in lithotomy. If the procedure is performed under local anaesthetic, a dental syringe with needle and prefilled cartridges of local anaesthetic and vasoconstrictor are used. A four quadrant or circumferential superficial infiltration is performed in the cervix just outside the transformation zone.

Treatment is ideally conducted with the whole of the transformation zone visible within one field of view with low-magnification colposcopy. The transformation zone has a variable anatomy and the loop chosen should take this into account so that adequate excision may take place (Fig. 9.5).

Using a blend current with 70/30 or 80/20 cutting and coagulation settings for the excision, the loop is traversed across slowly from side to side or bottom to top to cause a fulguration effect. If the loop is pushed or hurried, desiccation will occur with a greater thermal damage to the excised specimen. The specimen should be retrieved ideally as a single piece but sometimes due to a large TZ or

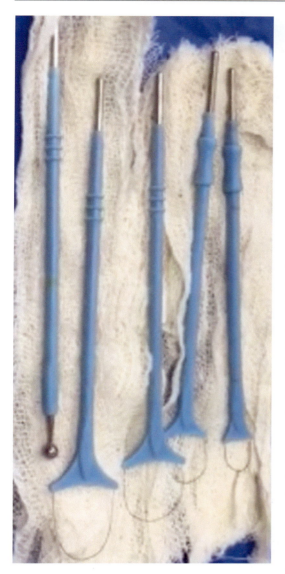

Fig. 9.5 Loops available in different sizes, roller ball for hemostasis

IFCPC has classified the excision types into types 1, 2, 3 depending on the type of transformation zone. The dimensions of the specimen according to IFCPC are standardized as length (distance from the distal or external margin to the proximal or internal margin), thickness (distance from the stromal margin to the surface of the excised specimen) and circumference (perimeter of the excised specimen) [3].

Post procedure patient may experience pain, bleeding and vaginal discharge which may last from few days up to 4 weeks. The patient should avoid tampons or menstrual cups, vaginal intercourse for 4 weeks. Complications are seen in 7–10% cases most commonly haemorrhage. Other complications include purulent vaginal discharge and pelvic pain. Long term morbidity includes cervical incompetence and preterm births, and cervical stenosis; especially, if the depth of excision (>1 cm) or repeat loops are performed. A meta-analysis estimated that the relative risk of delivery at <37 weeks after LLETZ was 1.56 (1.36–1.79) [13]. Cervical stenosis may lead to hematometra, infertility, and difficulties during subsequent colposcopy.

Straight wire excision is similar to LLETZ where instead of a loop, a straight tungsten wire is used to excise the cone tissue. In a randomised controlled trial, the risk of compromised or damaged endocervical margin in LLETZ-cone were significantly higher compared to SWETZ (RR 1.72, 95% CI: 1.14–2.6), and SWETZ specimens showed less fragmentation (ARR = 19.8%, 95% CI: 10.3–29.3%). There was no difference in the complication rate of the two procedures and SWETZ took a longer time compared to LLETZ [14].

9.4.2 Cold Knife Conisation

It is an excisional method using a scalpel and is reserved for type 3 transformation zone with suspicion of glandular disease. Conization is done for treatment of adenocarcinoma in situ and microinvasive disease [6]. The advantage of CKC is that the excision is in single piece with no thermal artifacts and desired depth of excised tissue

need of deep loop from endocervix more than one pass is required (Fig. 9.6a–d).

In case of bleeding, haemostasis can be ensured by using the diathermy ball in coagulative mode, using dessication or fulguration. Cotton tip buds and swabs are used to remove the excess blood. Other haemostatic techniques are using surgical oxycel, silver nitrate, ferric subsulphate (Monsel's solution or paste) or packing of the wound with gauze.

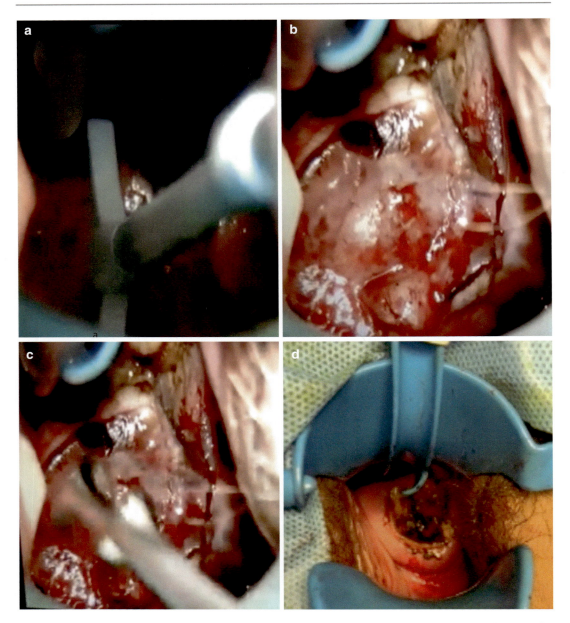

Fig. 9.6 (a) Activated loop is taken across the transformation zone from left to right. (b) LLETZ specimen seen after complete excision. (c) LLETZ Specimen retrieved from the cervix. (d) Post LLETZ view of cervix after hemostasis is obtained using ball cautrey

is obtained. However, compared to LLETZ, treatment related morbidity like haemorrhage and pregnancy complications are higher and it is always done under anaesthesia.

Laser conisation is similar except that ND Yag laser is used to excise and take out the conical tissue. This is much more expensive and requires good infrastructure.

9.4.2.1 Procedure

The lesion is outlined using 3–5% acetic acid and Lugol's iodine. Cervical infiltration with epinephrine (1:10,000), is done to reduce blood loss at surgery. One or two tenaculums are used to grasp the anterior lip of the cervix, away from the anticipated line of excision. A Beaver® blade is preferably used because it has two sharp edges which can be used to cut in either direction; an inward curve of the blade ensures that inadvertent injury to surrounding organs like the bladder or rectum is minimized.

The cone should be commenced from the 6 o'clock and curve upward; this prevents blood trickling down from obscuring the line of excision. As the cone is cut, it is pulled to the opposite side with a skin hook to provide visibility at the base of the incision. Every attempt should be made to remove the cone as a single piece, which should be symmetrically centred around the endocervical canal with the apex in the canal. After removal, the cone should be marked with a suture at the 12 o'clock position so that the histologist can orientate any positive margins or foci of invasive disease.

Methods to control post procedure bleeding are shown in Table 9.4. Post procedure advise is similar to that of loop excision.

The major long term risk is of cervical incompetence, preterm labour, premature rupture of membranes and perinatal mortality. The risk of preterm birth depends on depth of excision; with a depth ≥20 mm, the risk is 10.2% vs. 3.4% when less than 1 cm deep tissue is excised [12].

9.5 Endometrial Biopsy, Dilatation and Curettage

Indications for endometrial biopsy includes persistent or recurrent post menopausal bleeding, symptomatic patients on tamoxifen, endometrial thickness is ≥4 mm in asymptomatic post menopausal women, abnormal uterine bleeding (AUB) in age >45 years, and AUB in women who are obese, have PCOS, or not responding to medical treatment [15]. In a meta analysis, the weighted sensitivity of endometrial sampling with D&C as a reference for the diagnosis of endometrial cancer was 100% (range 100–100%) and 92% (71–100) for the diagnosis of atypical hyperplasia [16].

Endometrial biopsy is usually performed in the outpatient clinic by taking a Pipelle biopsy. Sometimes a Pipelle biopsy is not possible due to patient not tolerating the examination, body habitus, or cervical stenosis. In these circumstances, a dilatation and curettage with or without hysteroscopy is required. Hysteroscopy is also indicated if bleeding persists after negative office biopsy or where an inadequate specimen is obtained.

9.6 Hysteroscopy

Hysteroscopy improves diagnostic accuracy for evaluation of abnormal bleeding. In a recent meta analysis the diagnostic accuracy of hysteroscopy for endometrial cancer was high with sensitivity of 82.6% (95% CR 66.9–91.8%) and specificity of 99.7% (95% CR 98.1–99.9%) [17].

The procedure is contraindicated in the presence of pelvic infection and pregnancy should be ruled out if there is preceding amenorrhea.

The equipment consists of: video camera and monitor, light source and light lead, hysteroscope and sheath, irrigation system for fluid distension or CO_2 hysteroflator for gas distension (Table 9.5) [18]. The hysteroscope can be rigid or flexible, straight (0°) or oblique (12° and 30°). Usually a 30° optic is used for diagnostic hysteroscopy so that if the tip of the scope is 1–1.5 cm from the fundus, a view of the whole cavity and tubal ostia is obtained by rotating the instrument on its axis. On withdrawing the hysteroscope into the cervix, a panoramic view is obtained. The operator needs to understand the angulations of the optics of the hysteroscopy to achieve a safe insertion into the uterine cavity [19].

Table 9.4 Methods to control bleeding after cold knife conization

1. Ball diathermy
2. Cone bed is left open to granulate
3. Surgicel soaked in Monsel's solution (or paste)
4. Vaginal packing
5. Tranexamic acid (i.v)
6. Purse string cervical sutures in case of excessive bleeding

Table 9.5 Distention media used in hysteroscopy

Medium	Advantages	Disadvantages
Normal saline	• Low cost • For operative hysteroscopy in bipolar electrosurgical operative hysteroscopy • Lavage in the presence of bleeding	• Images not as clear as with CO_2 • Overload or excessive absorption can occur leading to pulmonary oedema and congestive cardiac failure
1.5% glycine	• Electrolyte-free and non-conductive • In monopolar electrosurgical operative hysteroscopy • Clear visibility	• Overload or excessive absorption causes hyponatremia. • Severe overload can lead to pulmonary oedema, congestive cadiac failure, haemolysis, seizures, coma and death
CO_2	• Well-tolerated, convenient and easy to use • Good visibility, it can be distorted in the presence of bleeding	• Bubble formation reduces visibility • Serious disadvantage of gas embolism • Shoulder tip pain • Bleeding reduces visibility in operative hysteroscopy as there isn't continuous irrigation as with fluid distension

Office hysteroscopy in outpatient settings as a One Stop approach includes diagnostic and operative hysteroscopic procedures like polypectomy which are done without general anaesthesia or dilatation of the cervix. It uses a non-touch vaginoscopic approach which cause less pain, and normal saline is used as distension media. Difficulties are encountered in nulliparous, postmenopausal women, cervical stenosis, severe patient anxiety, pre-existing pelvic pain and extreme retroversion.

9.7 Pyometra Drainage

Pyometra or collection of pus in the uterine cavity occurs when there is a stenosed cervical canal due to uterine or cervical malignancy or post radiotherapy cervical stenosis [20]. Pyometra has an incidence of 0.01–0.5%. It is more common in elderly and postmenopausal women, usually with concurrent medical conditions.

It may be asymptomatic and is found as an incidental finding on imaging. However, symptoms and signs of pyometra include blood-stained purulent vaginal discharge, symmetrical uterine enlargement and lower abdominal pain. Rare presentations include pyrexia or acute abdomen and pyoperitoneum due to perforation [21].

Treatment is pyometra drainage using graduated cervical dilatation with Hegar's dilator and the surgeon should be careful as the uterus is soft and may easily perforate. Occasionally, a false passage may be created in post radiotherapy cases. Antibiotics are only necessary if there is evidence of invasive infection, in the form of generalised malaise, pyrexia, or altered laboratory parameters. If antibiotics have to be used, seek advice from a microbiologist, and broad spectrum preparations covering both aerobic and anaerobic bacteria should be used.

9.8 Vulval Biopsy

Indications for vulval biopsy include presence of non-healing vulval ulcers, persistent eroded and indurated areas not responding to treatment, vulval melanosis, hypopigmented areas increasing in size or development of new areas, vulval growth and to confirm recurrence after treatment of vulval cancer [22].

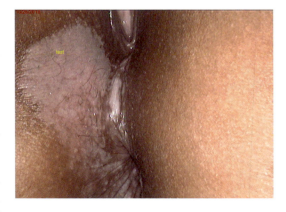

Fig. 9.7 Vulvoscopy showing dense acteowhitening after application of 5% acetic acid; histopathology: VIN 3

Biopsy from the lesion can be taken naked eye under good lighting or under vulvoscopic guidance. Vulvoscopy is performed using a gauze soaked in 5% acetic acid for 5 min or toluidine blue (Fig. 9.7). Before taking the biopsy, vulva, is cleaned with an antiseptic solution and 1–3 ml of 1% lidocaine (preferably with adrenaline) is administered for local anaesthesia. In the situation that larger excisional or multiple biopsies are required, general anaesthesia may be required.

Biopsy is taken using Keyes punch forceps which is available in 2–5 mm sizes (Fig. 9.8). The instrument is applied perpendicularly to the skin and rotated clockwise until the end of the metal blade to ensure full skin thickness specimen. The biopsy should be taken from the edge of the lesion or growth in order to avoid necrosis and include some normal tissue for appreciating the depth of invasion. The specimen is then excised with a scalpel blade. A representative site for the abnormality is selected, avoiding areas with inflammation, ulceration and necrosis. Multiple biopsies should be taken from multifocal lesions or if the lesion is large.

Post procedure bleeding can be controlled using Silver nitrate or ferric subsulfate (Monsel's solution). Larger lesions may require skin closure with interrupted absorbable sutures (i.e. Vicryl Rapide). An excisional biopsy should be avoided for larger lesions as it may be an under-treatment if the final histology shows cancer or vulval intraepithelial neoplasia.

9.9 Tru Cut Biopsy

Tru cut biopsy provides a tissue sample with preserved tissue architecture for histology and immunohistochemistry [23]. Biopsy is taken for histological verification, either under ultrasound or CT guidance, for advanced abdominal and pelvic tumors where diagnosis is uncertain in order to plan treatment. Other indications are to confirm metastasis, recurrence and residual tumours. Biopsy can be taken from the tumor mass, parietal nodules, omental cake, pelvic lymph nodes and recurrent masses [24].

The biopsy needles come in several sizes and the most common ones used are 18 G/25 cm long needles (Fig. 9.9). The 'Tru-Cut' needle consists

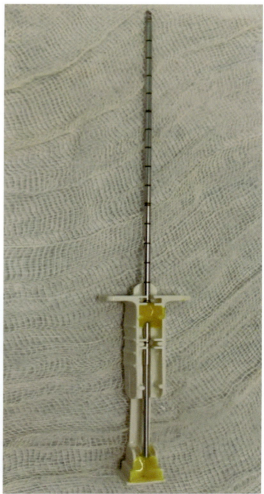

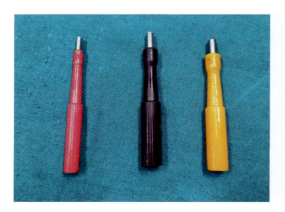

Fig. 9.8 Keyes punch biopsy forceps (Available in different sizes)

Fig. 9.9 Tru Cut biopsy needle

of an—inner solid needle—the obturator. It has a pointed end for tissue penetration and immediately behind this, there is a notch for the biopsy specimen—outer hollow needle—the cannula. It serves as a cutting sheath.

The skin in the area of the biopsy field is disinfected prior to the procedure, and local anaesthetic is administered. The skin is incised with a scalpel because the needle is not designed to puncture the skin. With the obturator fully retracted and held firm, the needle is inserted into the tissue being biopsied, the cannula is retracted (to expose the specimen notch) and then advanced (to cut the tissue which has prolapsed into the specimen notch), and the assembly withdrawn.

Under ultrasound guidance 1–3 tissue pieces 1–2 cm long are taken. Transvaginal tru cut biopsy can be obtained from pelvic masses and do not require local anaesthesia. To ensure safety, the tip of the needle should always be visualized during the entire procedure and always check for bleeding from the biopsy site. CT guided percutaneous biopsy is efficient and safe procedure for retroperitoneal and abdominal masses especially retroperitoneal nodal masses.

9.10 Fine Needle Aspiration Biopsy of Superficial Groin Lymph

Ultrasound guided fine needle aspiration (US-FNAC) is usually an outpatient procedure.

Ultrasound scan of the groin is initially performed with a high-frequency linear transducer (7–14 MHz). The criteria of suspicious nodes include increased size (short axis diameter >15 mm), altered shape (round or irregular rather than ovoid), loss of the fatty hilum, and perinodal irregularity. The presence of necrosis or abnormal blood flow pattern is also suspicious.

The groin is then cleaned with betadine. Local anaesthetic (1% lidocaine) is administered to the skin and subcutaneous tissues. Patient should be counselled regarding risk of bleeding and post operative mild pain. A 21- or 25-gauge needle is introduced into the selected node(s) under ultrasound guidance.

Two methods of specimen collection may be used depending on operator choice:

Non-Aspiration Capillary-Action Technique The needle is vigorously manipulated in a to-and-fro motion through the lymph node until a small amount of cellular material is seen in the needle well.

Suction Aspiration Technique A 10-ml syringe is applied to the hub of the needle and a similar to-and-fro manipulation is performed with minimal suction (1–2 ml) to aspirate a cellular specimen.

After each biopsy pass, the needle is withdrawn and the sample smeared onto a glass slide and fixed in alcohol. Multiple passes may be made into the same node to increase the detection rate for a cellular specimen. The specimen is then analysed at cytopathology. The main limitation of FNAC is small sample size and often disrupted tissue architecture.

9.11 Paracentesis

Ascitic tap can be both therapeutic and diagnostic, the former being done in massive ascites with marked abdominal distention. Contraindications include presence of an overlying infection. Caution must be exercised in cases of coagulopathy (INR > 2.0), pregnancy, presence of organomegaly, obstruction/ileus, distended bladder and abdominal adhesions. In cases with coagulopathy, the INR should be corrected to <1.5 and platelets count >50,000.

A consent should be obtained explaining the benefits (diagnostic purposes, relief of symptoms), as well as risks: infection, bleeding, pain, failure, damage to surrounding structures (especially bowel perforation—rare) and leakage.

Clinical examination should be performed to confirm ascites, followed by ultrasound (US) marking for the area of insertion to identify the deepest pool of fluid and to ensure that there are no vital organs beneath the drainage site. If US is not available for marking an appropriate point on the abdominal wall in the right or left lower quadrant, lateral to the rectus sheath is found with palpation and percussion. The landmark for needle insertion is one third—one half of the way between the anterior superior iliac spine and the umbilicus avoiding vessels and scars.

9.11.1 Procedure

After positioning, cleaning and draping, local anaesthesia is given in the skin and fascia upto the peritoneum up to a maximum of 10 ml of lidocaine. For a diagnostic tap, a 20 ml syringe is attached to a 19 gauge green needle for aspiration.

In therapeutic paracentesis, various catheters are available and can be left in situ for a longer period of time uptil 24 h. The procedure is described in Figs. 9.10, 9.11, 9.12, 9.13, and 9.14. At all times aseptic technique should be ensured and the catheter tip should not be touched. In cases of refractory ascites indwelling catheters may be placed for several days but these always carry risks of infection and blockage [25].

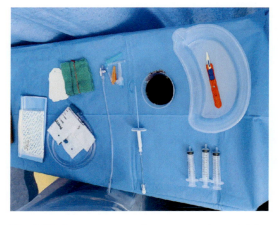

Fig. 9.10 Instrument tray for paracentesis containing Scalpel knife, paracentesis needle and catheter, iodine, swabs and syringes

9.12 Management of Wound Dehiscence

Wound dehiscence is most frequent between days 7 and 14 post surgery, when staples or sutures are removed. Dehiscence is most often preceded by a discharging wound.

The risk factors for wound dehiscence can be classified in three categories as shown in Table 9.6.

9.12.1 Superficial Dehiscence

Wound dehiscence is superficial when it does not involve the fascia. After careful inspection, gentle probation with a sterile cotton-tipped applicator is done to exclude fascial defect and a wound swab is taken for culture and sensitivity.

If there is no evidence of infection or subcutaneous collection, adhesive strips can be used to approximate the skin edges. Re-suturing is an alternative mainly in women with a raised BMI, under local or general anaesthesia. Wound review is done after 7 days.

If infection is suspected the wound should be cleaned and packed with gauze or covered with a sterile occlusive and a broad-spectrum antibiotic is commenced. Healing will take place by secondary intention. Also, delayed re-suturing can be considered.

9.12.2 Full-Thickness Wound Dehiscence

This type of wound involves fascia, muscles, rectus sheath or peritoneum and may be part of a complex clinical scenario associated with worsening of patient's condition. A thorough assessment of the patient is required, the patient may need to be stabilised (i.e. intravenous fluids, blood transfusion, nasogastric tube if ileus and vomiting). Antibiotics should be considered as part of the initial treatment, after sending a swab to microbiology.

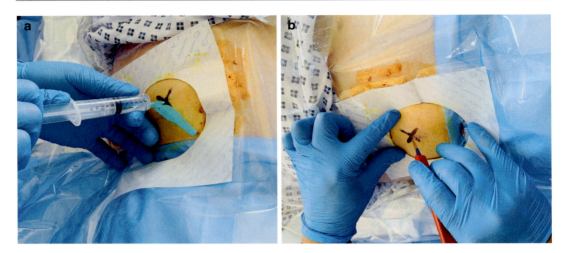

Fig. 9.11 (**a**) Local infilatration at the site marked on ultrasound. (**b**) No. 11 scalpel blade to make a small nick in the skin to allow easier passage of the catheter

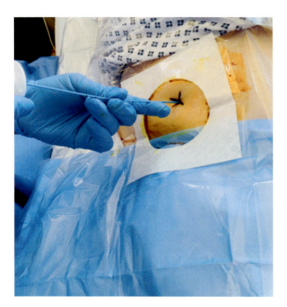

Fig. 9.12 The needle is inserted directly perpendicular to the selected skin entry point slowly

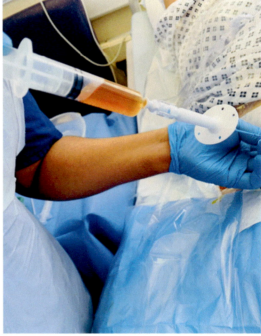

Fig. 9.13 Negative pressure is applied to the syringe as the needle is advanced and upon entry into the peritoneal cavity, loss of resistance is felt and ascitic fluid is filled in the syringe

The viability of surrounding tissues should be assessed and necrotizing fasciitis is excluded. Non-viable tissue should be removed.

The wound closure can be by immediate re-suturing, or sterile wound packing with healing by secondary intention. Resuturing may be partial (some layers closed) or full (all abdominal wall layers closed). In the case of full resuturing, mass closure should take place using a heavy, loop PDS suture. Deep retention sutures are used, to reinforce the wound closure by minimizing tension on the skin edges especially in obese patients. Particular attention is required to identify any

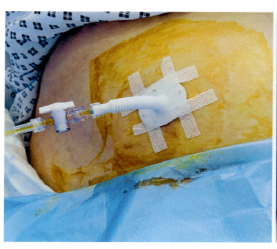
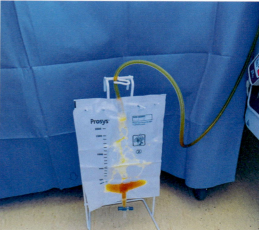

Fig. 9.14 Stopcock is held as the catheter is advanced and needle withdrawn; bag is attached for drainage

Table 9.6 Risk factors for wound dehiscence

Preoperative
– Age over 45 years
– Smoking
– Obesity
– Pulmonary disease
– Renal disease
– Liver disease (ascites, jaundice)
– Anaemia
– Malnutrition
Perioperative
– Emergency surgery
– Midline incision
– Prolonged surgery over 2.5 h
– Method of wound closure
Postoperative
– Raised intra-abdominal pressure (incl. postoperative coughing)
– Wound infection
– Trauma to the wound
– radiation

bowel loops in the wound. "Through-and-through" technique with each suture placed 2 cm apart, and at least 2 cm from the skin edges is recommended. The sutures should be left in situ for 3 weeks.

Superficial wound drains in subcutaneous tissue may be considered to reduce wound infections as prevent seroma collection which otherwise promote sepsis. Vacuum dressing, which is negative pressure wound therapy, involves the controlled application of subatmospheric pressure to the local wound environment using a sealed wound dressing connected to a vacuum pump [26]. The healing takes place by gradually decreasing the wound defect, encouraging granulation tissue formation, increasing local blood perfusion, reducing bacterial colonization, and removing interstitial fluid.

9.13 Cystoscopy

The indications of cystoscopy include suspected involvement of bladder in cervical and vaginal cancers, in suspected cases with post radiation/surgerical lower urinary tract fistula, diagnose cause of unexplained hematuria and intraoperatively to rule out surgical bladder injury or for ureteric stent insertion. Bladder biopsy may be taken from suspicious areas when indicated.

The patient s placed in dorsal lithotomy position, bladder is emptied and urine sent for cytology in cervical/vaginal cancers to exclude bladder involvement. Urethral orifice is cleaned and sometimes urethral dilation is required before inserting the assembled cystoscope. Hydrodistention of bladder is done using approximately 250–400 ml of saline. Trigone is identified and interureteric bridge is identified followed by identification of the two ureteric orifices. Air bubble orients the cystoscopy image towards the dome of the bladder. Biopsy of the bladder lesion maybe taken where required. Intra-procedure antibiotic is administered which is usually a single shot of Gentamicin 3–5 mg/kg if patient does not have any underlying renal compromise.

9.14 Chest Tube Drainage

Chest tube is inserted for pleurocentesis in stage 4 ovarian cancer for symptomatic relief and for cytological assessment of pleural cavity involvement as this influences the type of chemotherapy regimen patient receives.

Intraoperatively pleural drains are inserted in selected cases where major diaphragmatic resection has been performed and adequate water-tight closure of the diaphragm has not been achieved or in cases where extensive pleural disease is detected and not completely removed, to prevent build-up of pleural fluid and occasionally where any lung tissue has been dissected of from pleural disease so as to prevent any surgically induced pneumothorax. There is still debate about a routine intraoperative insertion of a chest tube drainage after every case of diaphragm resection. Chest drain is not mandatory after diaphragm resection and closure, however, it becomes important if there is suspected pneumothorax with injury or infiltration of lung from pleural deposits.

It is usually inserted through the 6th intercostal space in the anterior axillary line and kept in situ for 3–5 days (Fig. 9.15). A silk purse string suture is tied outside the chest drain fixation suture which is tied when the drain is removed postoperatively to prevent iatrogenic pneumothorax during removal of the chest drain.

9.14.1 PleurX Drain

PleurX drain is for intermittent drainage of ascites or pleural fluid which avoids multiple drainage insertions, allows drainage to be carried out in a domiciliary setting once the pleural drain has been inserted. PleurX drain has one-way valve allowing exit drainage and pre-

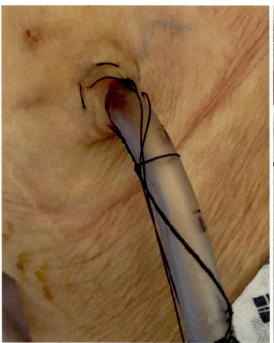
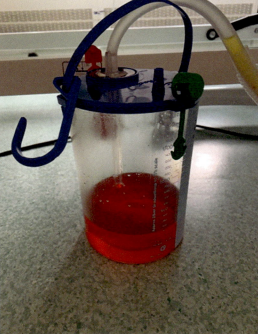

Fig. 9.15 Chest tube and drain

venting any entry of air/contamination from outside.

Drainage system is tunneled under the skin so requires two small incisions on skin for point of entry into pleural/peritoneal cavity and second entry in the skin for tunneling the pleurX drain kit in subcutaneous tissue. Insertion is done under sedation with local anaesthetic. Patient is trained to drain the fluid at home intermittently whenever experiences symptoms of fluid build up.

A PleurX drainage catheter is a thin, flexible tube placed in patient's chest/peritoneal cavity to drain pleural/ascitic fluid. It can stay in situ from few weeks up to several months, until the fluid stops draining.

It has three main parts:

- a catheter—one end of the catheter is inserted in the pleural/peritoneal space, the other one comes outside the body.
- A 1-way valve—on the end of the catheter outside the body. It lets pleural/ascitic fluid out but does not let air in.
- A valve cap—it protects the valve and keeps it clean.

The PleurX is inserted under sedation. The skin at the site of insertion is disinfected, and local anaesthetic is administered. Two small skin incisions are required, one into the pleural/peritoneal space, the other a few inches away through the skin. A tunnel is created under the skin between the two incisions. The PleurX catheter is inserted through the tunnel into the pleural/peritoneal space. Tunneling the catheter makes it more comfortable and helps it stay in place. Once the catheter is in place, the incision into the pleural/peritoneal space is closed, and a dressing is applied over the exit site. The end of the PleurX catheter is covered with a valve cap after the procedure. When fluid needs to be drained, the catheter is connected to a collection unit.

Key Points
1. Minor procedures include both diagnostic and therapeutic procedures and are usually carried out under local anaesthesia
2. Colposcopy is done in cases with abnormal screening tests or clinical presentation and examination suggestive of cervical malignancy. The findings are recorded in a standard format, according to the International Federation of Colposcopy and Cervical Pathology (IFCPC) criteria
3. Treatment of premalignant lesion can be done using ablative techniques like cryotherapy or thermal ablation and excisional methods like LLETZ, SWETZ or conisation
4. Endometrial biopsy with or without hysteroscopy is an important diagnostic procedure for postmenopausal or abnormal uterine bleeding to rule out endometrial cancer and is usually performed in the outpatient clinic by taking a Pipelle biopsy
5. Pyometra drainage is done using graduated cervical dilatation with Hegar's dilator and its very important to exclude malignancy in these cases
6. Vulval biopsy is taken using Keyes punch forceps from the edge of the lesion or growth
7. Ascitic tap can be both therapeutic and diagnostic and specialised catheters are inserted under aseptic precautions to be kept in situ for a longer time.
8. Chest tube is inserted prophylactically to reduce the morbidity due to pleural effusion in diaphragmatic surgery in ovarian cancer debulking. PleurX drainage catheter can be left in situ in refractory and recurrent malignant pleural effusions.

The procedure to place a PleurX drainage catheter usually takes about 45–90 min, and the patient goes home the same day, only constraint is, of course, the high cost compared to the conventional single time drainage system [27].

9.15 Conclusion

To conclude, this chapter summarizes the common minor procedures done in gynaecologic oncology. Although the number of complications associated are few compared to major surgery, a thorough knowledge regarding indications and procedure may minimize further morbidity.

References

1. Shafi M, Nazeer S. Colposcopy: a practical guide. 2nd ed. Cambridge: Cambridge University Press; 2018.
2. Comprehensive cervical cancer control: a guide to essential practice. 2nd ed. Geneva: World Health Organization; 2014. Annex 13, How to make Monsel's paste. Available from: https://www.ncbi.nlm.nih.gov/books/NBK269598/. Accessed 5 Aug 2021.
3. Bornstein J, Bentley J, Bösze P, Girardi F, Haefner H, Menton M, et al. colposcopic terminology of the International Federation for Cervical Pathology and Colposcopy. Obstet Gynecol. 2011;2012(120):166–72.
4. NHSCSP 20 Colposcopy and Programme management. 3rd ed. Available at https://www.bsccp.org.uk/assets/file/uploads/resources/NHSCSP_20_Colposcopy_and_Programme_Management_(3rd_Edition)_(2).pdf. Accessed 24 July 2021.
5. Wentzensen N, Walker JL, Gold MA, Smith KM, Zuna RE, Mathews C, et al. Multiple biopsies and detection of cervical cancer precursors at colposcopy. J Clin Oncol. 2015;33(1):83–9.
6. Basu P, Taghavi K, Hu SY, Mogri S, Joshi S. Management of cervical premalignant lesions. Curr Probl Cancer. 2018;42(2):129–36.
7. World Health Organization. WHO guidelines for screening and treatment of precancerous lesions for cervical cancer prevention. Geneva: World Health Organization. 2013. Available at: https://www.who.int/reproductivehealth/publications/cancers/screening_and_treatment_of_precancerous_lesions/en/. Accessed 12 Aug 2021.
8. Luciani S, Gonzales M, Munoz S, Jeronimo J, Robles S. Effectiveness of cryotherapy treatment for cervical intraepithelial neoplasia. Int J Gynaecol Obstet. 2008;101(2):172–7.
9. Chirenje ZM, Rusakaniko S, Akino V, Mlingo M. A randomised clinical trial of loop electrosurgical excision procedure (LEEP) versus cryotherapy in the treatment of cervical intraepithelial neoplasia. J Obstet Gynaecol. 2001;21(6):617–21.
10. Dolman L, Sauvaget C, Muwonge R, Sankaranarayanan R. Meta-analysis of the efficacy of cold coagulation as a treatment method for cervical intraepithelial neoplasia: a systematic review. BJOG. 2014;121(8):929–42.
11. Martin-Hirsch PP, Paraskevaidis E, Bryant A, Dickinson HO. Surgery for cervical intraepithelial neoplasia. Cochrane Database Syst Rev. 2013;(12):CD001318.
12. Santesso N, Mustafa RA, Wiercioch W, Kehar R, Gandhi S, Chen Y, et al. Systematic reviews and meta-analyses of benefits and harms of cryotherapy, LEEP, and cold knife conization to treat cervical intraepithelial neoplasia. Int J Gynaecol Obstet. 2016;132(3):266–71.
13. Kyrgiou M, Athanasiou A, Paraskevaidi M, Mitra A, Kalliala I, Martin-Hirsch P, et al. Adverse obstetric outcomes after local treatment for cervical preinvasive and early invasive disease according to cone depth: systematic review and meta-analysis. BMJ. 2016;28(354):i3633.
14. Russomano F, Tristao MA, Côrtes R, de Camargo MJ. A comparison between type 3 excision of the transformation zone by straight wire excision of the transformation zone (SWETZ) and large loop excision of the transformation zone (LLETZ): a randomized study. BMC Womens Health. 2015;15:12.
15. American College of Obstetricians and Gynecologists. ACOG Committee Opinion No. 426: the role of transvaginal ultrasonography in the evaluation of postmenopausal bleeding. Obstet Gynecol. 2009;113(2 Pt 1):462–4.
16. van Hanegem N, Prins MM, Bongers MY, Opmeer BC, Sahota DS, Mol BW, Timmermans A. The accuracy of endometrial sampling in women with postmenopausal bleeding: a systematic review and meta-analysis. Eur J Obstet Gynecol Reprod Biol. 2016;197:147–55.
17. Gkrozou F, Dimakopoulos G, Vrekoussis T, Lavasidis L, Koutlas A, Navrozoglou I. Hysteroscopy in women with abnormal uterine bleeding: a meta-analysis on four major endometrial pathologies. Arch Gynecol Obstet. 2015;291(6):1347–54.
18. Moore JF, Carugno J. Hysteroscopy. In: StatPearls. Treasure Island, FL: StatPearls Publishing; 2021.
19. Coomarasamy A, Shafi M, Willy DG. Gynecologic and obstetric surgery, challenges and management options. In: Conforti A, Magos A, editors. Hysteroscopy: endometrial resection and ablation

in the abnormal uterine cavity. Philadelphia: Wiley Blackwell; 2016. p. 197–8.
20. Kerimoglu OS, Pekin A, Yilmaz SA, Bakbak BB, Celik C. Pyometra in elderly post-menopausal women: a sign of malignity. Eur J Gynaecol Oncol. 2015;36(1):59–61.
21. Yousefi Z, Sharifi N, Morshedy M. Spontaneous uterine perforation caused by pyometra: a case report. Iran Red Crescent Med J. 2014;16(9):e14491.
22. American College of Obstetricians and Gynecologists' Committee on Practice Bulletins-Gynecology. Diagnosis and management of vulvar skin disorders: ACOG practice Bulletin, number 224. Obstet Gynecol. 2020;136(1):1–14.
23. Fischerova D, Cibula D, Dundr P, Zikan M, Calda P, Freitag P, Slama J. Ultrasound-guided tru-cut biopsy in the management of advanced abdomino-pelvic tumors. Int J Gynecol Cancer. 2008;18(4):833–7.
24. Zikan M, Fischerova D, Pinkavova I, Dundr P, Cibula D. Ultrasound-guided tru-cut biopsy of abdominal and pelvic tumors in gynecology. Ultrasound Obstet Gynecol. 2010;36(6):767–72.
25. Management of ascites in ovarian cancer patients. Royal College of Obstetricians and Gynaecologists. Available at: https://www.rcog.org.uk/globalassets/documents/guidelines/scientific-impact-papers/sip45ascites.pdf. Accessed 6 Aug 2021.
26. Coomarasamy A, Shafi M, Willy Davila G. Gynecologic and obstetric surgery, challenges and management options. In: Latte P, Gray J, editors. Wound Infection. Clark J, editor. Wound Dehiscence. Philadelphia: Wiley Blackwell; 2016. p. 142–149.
27. Burgers JA, Olijve A, Baas P. Chronic indwelling pleural catheter for malignant pleural effusion in 25 patients [in Dutch]. Ned Tijdschr Geneeskd. 2006;150(29):1618–23.

Management of Complications: Chemotherapy Related Complications, Acute Bowel Obstruction, Symptomatic Ascites and Pleural Effusion, Pulmonary Embolism, Deep Vein Thrombosis, Severe Pain, Chylous Ascites

10

Anastasios Tranoulis, Howard Joy, and Bindiya Gupta

10.1 Introduction

Women with gynaecological cancer often experience a significant burden of physical and emotional symptoms from the time of their diagnosis, through treatment, recurrences and end-of-life. Common complications amongst gynaecological oncology patients include pain, deep vein thrombosis/pulmonary embolism, haemorrhage, ascites/pleural effusion, chylous ascites, bowel obstruction and chemotherapy-related side effects. As with most other types of cancer, pain is a cardinal issue and can require multiple treatment modalities. Venous thromboembolism is a recognized adverse sequel amongst women with gynaecological cancer and represents one of the leading causes of morbidity and mortality in these patients. Women with epithelial ovarian cancer, often present with ascites, chylous ascites or malignant pleural effusion, which require tailored multidisciplinary management. Bowel obstruction remains a common problem resulting from progressive gynaecological cancer. Palliative surgery may be offered in carefully selected women. Chemotherapy-related side-effects are common. It is important to be able to prevent, recognize and manage chemotherapy-related side effects, as they can interfere with optimal and timely treatment and significantly affect the quality-of-life. This chapter focuses on the management of common complications in women with gynaecological malignancies.

A. Tranoulis (✉)
The Pan-Birmingham Gynaecological Cancer Centre, City Hospital, Birmingham, UK
e-mail: anastasios.tranoulis1@nhs.net

H. Joy
Sandwell and West Birmingham Hospitals NHS Trust, Birmingham, UK
e-mail: howard.joy@nhs.net

B. Gupta
Department of Obstetrics & Gynecology, University College of Medical Sciences & Guru Teg Bahadur Hospital, Delhi, India

10.2 Chemotherapy-Related Complications

To date, chemotherapy represents the cornerstone of neo-adjuvant and adjuvant treatment for most gynaecological malignancies. The most commonly used chemotherapeutic agents are platinum-based regimes (carboplatin/cisplatin) and taxanes (paclitaxel). Moreover, other cytotoxic agents are also used in recurrent or metastatic disease, such as topoisomerase inhibitors, doxorubicin, docetaxel, gemcitabine and ifosfamide. Recently, targeted therapy drugs, including bevacizumab and polyadenosine diphosphate ribose polymerase (PARP) inhibitors have emerged as novel treatment modalities amongst women with primary or recurrent gynaecological malignancies. Chemotherapeutic agents are usually used in doses causing some degree of toxicity to normal tissues. The most common side effects of the commonly used chemotherapeutic agents are listed in Table 10.1.

10.2.1 Management of Haematologic Toxicities

Anaemia Anaemia is one of the most common side effects of chemotherapy. Chemotherapeutic agents can suppress bone marrow and impair the synthesis of red blood precursors, leading to anaemia. Moreover, several chemotherapeutic agents (e.g. cisplatin) can cause nephrotoxicity, leading to a reduced renal production of erythropoietin and, thus, anaemia [1]. Treatment includes transfusion of packed red blood cells or administration of erythropoiesis-stimulating agents with or without iron supplementation [1].

Thrombocytopenia Women with sustained thrombocytopenia (platelets < 10,000/mm^3) carry a significantly higher risk of spontaneous bleeding. The management of chemotherapy-induced thrombocytopenia includes treating any underlying causes of thrombocytopenia, reducing the dose of chemotherapeutic agent or administering platelet transfusion [2]. Platelet transfusion is usually indicated when the patient is actively bleeding or about to undergo an urgent surgical procedure [2].

Neutropenia The severity of chemotherapy-induced neutropenia is usually graded using the scale of Common Toxicity Criteria of the National Cancer Institute based upon the absolute neutrophil count (ANC) [3]:

- Grade 1: ANC $\geq 1.5 \times 10^9/l$ & $<2 \times 10^9/l$
- Grade 2: ANC $\geq 1 \times 10^9/l$ & $<1.5 \times 10^9/l$
- Grade 3: ANC $\geq 0.5 \times 10^9/l$ & $<1 \times 10^9/l$
- Grade 4: ANC $<0.5 \times 10^9/l$.

Women with a neutrophils count <500/mm^3 for 5 days or longer are at high risk of febrile neutropenia (FN) [3]. FN is defined as an oral temperature > 38.5 °C or two consecutive temperatures > 38°C for 2 h and an ANC < $0.5 \times 10^9/l$. It is associated with increased mortality, prolonged hospitalisation and treatment delays [3]. Neutropenia can be managed by using Granulocyte-colony Stimulating Factor (G-CSF) [3], whilst FN requires fluid and electrolyte replacement, bowel rest, parenteral nutrition, administration of blood products and broad spectrum antibiotics. The most commonly used antibiotics consist of 3rd and 4th generation cephalosporins, meropenem, imipenem, aminoglycosides and metronidazole [3]. Empirical anti-fungal treatment can also be considered. Low-risk patient can be treated in the outpatient setting, whilst high-risk patients require hospitalisation for administration of IV broad spectrum antibiotics [3].

10.2.2 Management of Gastrointestinal Toxicities

Nausea/Vomiting The best combination for the management of chemotherapy-induced vomiting consists of a serotonin receptor antagonist (5-HT3) plus dexamethasone plus aprepitant [4]. In case of severe vomiting a combination of 5-HT3 receptor antagonist and neurokinin-1 (NK-1) receptor antagonist can be used which have got anxiolytic, antidepressant and anti-emetic properties and have receptors in the brain and peripherally in the gastrointestinal tract. If breakthrough treatment is required, an agent from a different drug class can be added [4].

Diarrhoea Loperamide is the recommended first-line treatment for the management of chemotherapy-induced diarrhoea [5]. Women with grade 1–2 diarrhoea, who have improve-

Table 10.1 The most common side effects of the most commonly used chemotherapeutic agents in gynaecological oncology

Drug	Route of administration	Common toxicities	Gynaecological malignancies
Alkylating-like agents			
Carboplatin	IV	Nausea and vomiting Myelossupression Neuropathy Ototoxicity Peripheral neuropathy	Ovarian cancer Endometrial cancer Cervical cancer
Cisplatin	IV	Nausea and vomiting Myelosuppresision Nephrotoxicity Peripheral neuropathy Tinnitus Heariing loss	Ovarian cancer Endometrial cancer Cervical cancer Germ cell ovarian tumours
Dacarbazine	IV	Nausea and vomiting Myelosuppression Hepatotoxicity Flu-like syndrome	Uterine sarcomas
Plant Alkaloids			
Paclitaxel	IV	Myelosuppression Cardiac arrhythmias Alopecia Allergic reactions	Ovarian cancer
Docetaxel	IV	Myelosuppression Peripheral oedema Alopecia Hypersensitivity reactions	Ovarian cancer
Vincristine	IV	Myelosuppression Neurotoxicity Gastrointestinal toxicity Cranial nerve palsies	Cervical cancer Sarcomas Germ cell ovarian tumours
Alkylating agents			
Ifosmamide	IV	Myelosuppression Nephrotoxicity Bladder dysfunction Central nervous system dysfunction	Cervical cancer Ovarian cancer Carcinosarcomas
Cyclophosmamide	PO, IV	Myelosuppression Bladder dysfunction Alopecia Hepatitis Amenorrhoea	Ovarian cancer Sarcomas
Antitumour antibiotics			
Bleomycin	IM, IV	Pulmonary toxicity Anaphylactic reactions Fever Dermatologic reactions	Germ cell ovarian tumours
Doxorubicin	IV	Nausea and vomiting Myelosuppression Cardiotoxicity Alopecia Mucosal ulcerations	Ovarian cancer Endometrial cancer

(continued)

Table 10.1 (continued)

Drug	Route of administration	Common toxicities	Gynaecological malignancies
Liposomal doxorubicin	IV	Myelosuppression Stomatitis	Ovarian cancer Endometrial cancer
Actinomycin-D	IV	Nausea and vomiting Myelossupression Skin necrosis Mucosal ulcerations	Germ cell ovarian tumours Gestational trophoblastic neoplasia Sarcomas
Antimetabolites			
Methotrexate	PO, IV	Myelosuppression Hepatotoxicity Mucosal ulceration Allergic pneumonitis	Gestational trophoblastic neoplasia
Gemcitabine	IV	Myelosuppression Fever	Ovarian cancer Sarcomas
5-fluoracil	IV	Nausea and vomiting Myelossupression Alopecia	Cervical cancer
Topioisomerase 1 Inhibitors			
Topetecan	IV	Myelosuppression	Ovarian cancer
Irinotecan	IV	Myelosuppression Diarhhoea	Ovarian cancer Cervical cancer
Anti-angiogenesis agents			
Bevacizumab	IV	Hypertension Proteinuria Bowel perforation	Ovarian cancer Cervical cancer
Polyadenosine diphosphate ribose polymerase inhibitors (PARPi)	PO	Nausea and vomiting Myelossupression Fatigue Diarrhoea Constipation Urinary tract infection Upper respiratory tract infection Abdominal pain	Ovarian cancer

ment or resolution of diarrhoea do not usually require any other intervention. On the other hand, high-risk women with ≥grade 3 diarrhoea require inpatient management [5]. Octreotide, dudesonide and atropine can also be used in cases of refractory diarrhoea [5]. Fluid and electrolyte replacement is usually required. Stool captures should be performed. If signs of peritonitis are present a CT scan is required. Necrotising enterocolitis includes a spectrum of severe diarrhoea, which is associated with increased mortality amongst women with neutropenia. IV broad spectrum antibiotics should be commenced in combination with bowel rest and parenteral nutrition [5].

- **Mangement of Neurologic Toxicities**: Several pharmacological treatment options are available for the management of chemotherapy-induced neurotoxicity with various efficacies: anticonvulsant drugs (gabapentin, pregabalin), tricyclic antidepressant drugs (amitriptyline), and duloxetine [6]. The non-pharmacological interventions consist of cognitive and behavioural treatments [6].
- **Management of Cardiac Toxicities**: Left ventricular dysfunction and overt heart failure are the most common manifestations of chemotherapy-induced cardiotoxicity. Carvedilol or dexrazoxane can be used for the prevention of cardiological adverse sequelae amongst patients receiving

anthracycline-based chemotherapy. Angiotensin-converting enzyme inhibitors can be used for the management of left ventricular dysfunction [7].

10.3 Acute Bowel Obstruction

The term bowel obstruction (BO) typically refers to a mechanical blockage of the bowel. BO is a rare presentation in women with gynaecological malignancy. It is most commonly associated with ovarian cancer. BO is often a clinical manifestation of recurrent disease and is associated with a poor prognosis [8]. BO bowel is usually associated with one or more of the following factors: widespread carcinomatosis causing intestinal motility dysfunction, intra-abdominal and/ or loco-regional recurrences causing extrinsic or extra-luminal occlusion, retroperitoneal disease with involvement of myenteric plexuses and adhesions [9]. In epithelial ovarian cancer, BO is linked with a number of factors, whilst more than one anatomical disease site usually contributes to the obstruction [10].

The most common symptoms of BO consist of [11]:

- Abdominal pain—colicky or cramping in nature
- Vomiting—occurring early in proximal obstructions and late in distal obstructions
- Abdominal distension
- Absolute constipation—occurring early in distal obstruction and late in proximal obstruction

All patients with suspected BO require routine urgent bloods, whilst a venous blood gas can be useful to evaluate the signs of ischaemia and metabolic derangements [11]. A CT scan with IV contrast of the abdomen and pelvis represents the gold standard imaging modality amongst women with suspected BO, whilst a plain abdominal x-ray can also be used in some settings as the initial investigation [11].

The management of BO is dependent upon the aetiology and whether it has been complicated by bowel ischaemia, perforation, and/or peritonism [11].

10.3.1 Conservative Management

Conservative management is recommended in the absence of signs of ischaemia or strangulation and consists of fasting, intravenous fluids and often insertion of a nasogastric tube (NGT). Fluid balance is crucial owing to fluid and electrolyte depletion [11]. Fluid management is not always easy, bearing in mind that women with epithelial ovarian cancer are also presented with severe ascites and hypoalbuminemia [11]. The insertion of a Foley catheter is usually recommended. The management of cardinal symptoms, including pain, nausea, vomiting and constipation should be individualized and involves the use of strong opioids, antiemetics, anticholinergics, somatostatin analogues and laxatives [11]. Antibiotics should be commenced at the confirmation of diagnosis of intestinal obstruction, especially in case of pyrexia and leucocytosis. The rationale of the use of antibiotics is based upon the control and treatment of intestinal overgrowth of bacteria and their translocation across the bowel wall [12]. Given that women with BO usually present with severe vomiting, drugs are usually administered by alternative routes, e.g. subcutaneously, trans-dermally, rectally or sublingually, whenever possible [11]. The use of intravenous steroids may also be considered [11]. Steroids carry an anti-emetic effect and can also reduce the bowel wall oedema, that characterises BO. A recent Cochrane review demonstrated that IV steroids are rather effective in resolving BO and controlling BO-related symptoms [12]. Adhesional small BO resulting from previous surgery can be treated conservatively with a water soluble contrast study (e.g. gastrografin) with a success rate of 80% [11]. Depending on the clinical situation, total parenteral nutrition (TPN) can also be considered. TPN should be used for a defined period, which typically is limited to a few weeks in the UK [11]. If conservative management does not relieve the symptoms, then surgery should be considered.

10.3.2 Surgical Management

There is currently no consensus on the definition of successful surgical palliation. The decision for palliative surgery amongst women with BO on the background of gynaecological malignancy is rather difficult owing to the increased mortality associated with such procedures, the uncertainty as to whether palliative goals would be achieved and the lack of quality-of-life data [11]. Palliative surgery should always be individualized and the following factors should be considered prior to any intervention:

- Previous surgical and non-surgical treatments
- Performance status and co-morbidities
- Nutritional status
- Location/site of bowel obstruction
- Presence of peritonitis
- Disease distribution
- Treatment-free survival

The possible surgical procedures should be individualized and include the following:

- "Open and close"
- Adhesiolysis
- Bowel resection with anastomosis and/or stoma formation
- Bypass procedures
- Decompression of an isolated obstructed segment of the bowel

Abdominal adhesiolysis via laparotomy has been the standard therapy for small bowel obstruction associated with adhesions; though laparoscopic adhesiolysis can be performed in selected patients [13]. Small bowel obstruction caused by tumour can be treated with resection and anastomosis or ileostomy formation based upon the extent of small bowel involvement, the general condition of the patient and the presence of peritonitis [14, 15].

Resection and stoma formation are the best options for malignant large bowel obstruction [16–18]. The reported rate of anastomotic leak following resection and anastomosis for malignant large BO ranges between 2 and 12%, which is comparable to the 2–8% rate after elective surgical procedures [16–18]; hence, resection and primary anastomosis may be offered in selected patients in the absence of significant risk factors or perforations. In women with single-site malignant BO, complete resection of the cancer is usually feasible [11, 16–18]. Nonetheless, most commonly, multiple sites of primary or recurrent disease typically cause the obstruction. In such cases, a palliative bypass procedure or a formation of a diverting stoma is usually opted, and the cancer sites causing the obstruction are often not resected [11, 16–18]. However, in such cases, it can be argued that women who are palliated surgically have the option to receive neo-adjuvant, adjuvant or second-line chemotherapy.

10.3.3 Alternative Treatment Options

Alternative treatment options should be considered for those women most likely not to benefit from surgical management, such as those with a poor performance and nutritional status or extensive carcinomatosis with multiple bowel obstruction sites and ascites [11].

1. **Stents**: radiologic or endoscopic placement of flexible, self-expanding metallic stents has recently emerged as an alternative, more conservative treatment modality amongst patients with BO. For palliation of obstructing left colon cancer, self-expanding metallic stents are preferred to colostomy because they are associated with similar mortality/morbidity rates but a shorter hospital stay [19]. Nonetheless, the main limitation of self-expanding stents, is the fact that they are recommended for single-site pelvic obstructions, in which a small segment of narrowed bowel is present or the pelvic anatomy is not notably distorted [11, 19].
2. **Palliative gastrostomy tubes**: palliative gastrostomy tubes can be offered in women with repeated vomiting. They can be placed endoscopically, radiologically or surgically via a small upper abdominal incision minimal mor-

bidity [11]. As an adequate decompression can be achieved, approximately 90% of women are able to tolerate oral intake, including a soft diet in 25% [20].

10.4 Symptomatic Ascites and Pleural Effusion

10.4.1 Ascites

Malignant ascites represents the accumulation of fluid within the abdominal cavity caused by underlying cancer. Ascites is most commonly associated with ovarian cancer which, together with tumours originating in the breast, bowel, pancreas, and endometrium, account for 80% of cases of malignant ascites in women [21]. It is probably caused by a combination of several factors, including obstruction of lymphatic drainage preventing absorption of intra-abdominal fluid and protein, disease producing a high volume of fluid with a high protein content, hypoproteinaemia and occasionally portal hypertension secondary to hepatic cancer [21]. In patients with ovarian or uterine cancer, liver metastases are less common; therefore, an exudative ascites is expected. In malignant disease, ascites may be present at diagnosis and also when the disease recurs [21]. Recurrent malignant ascites causes burdensome symptoms that significantly reduce the quality of life [22]. The accumulation and volume of fluid are difficult to predict; hence, women often need to be admitted to hospital as an emergency with a variety of symptoms, such as abdominal distension, anorexia, discomfort, nausea, constipation, and shortness of breath [22]. There is currently a paucity of reliable evidence regarding the optimum method of managing malignant ascites either at initial presentation, during treatment or palliation. Generally, the management of symptomatic malignant ascites consists of both mechanical interventions that aim to drain the ascites from the peritoneal cavity, and pharmacological interventions that prevent and diminish the development of ascites [23]. The treatment modalities for symptomatic ascites consist of the following:

10.4.1.1 Drainage of Ascites

Women with significant ascites under tension usually warrant percutaneous drainage. It is a common practice to perform image-guided paracentesis to identify the deepest pool of fluid and to avoid injuring vital organs beneath the drainage site. Drainage catheters are usually inserted following an ultrasound scan to mark an appropriate area, either at the same time as the scan or afterwards on the ward [24].

10.4.1.2 Indwelling Peritoneal Catheters

Indwelling catheters are usually used for women with recurrent or refractory ovarian cancers, whose ascites accumulates rapidly. In such cases, it is difficult to remove the drainage catheter due to excessive fluid production and may be a need to discharge patients with the drainage catheter in situ. Nonetheless, this practice comes with an increased risk of infection and blockage [25].

10.4.1.3 Diuretic Therapy

There is limited data, mainly deriving from small case series, supporting the role for PO to IV diuretics, such as spironolactone, amongst patients with malignant ascites [24, 26]. Diuretics are unlikely to shift ascitic fluid, whilst there is a high risk for patients to becoming dehydrated if not carefully supervised [24, 26]. Serum albumin ascitic gradient (SAAG) can be performed, should there be any doubt of non-malignant origin of the ascites. If the SAAG indicates a transudative mechanism, then a trial of diuretics may be considered, under close observation [24, 26].

10.4.1.4 Anti-neoplastic Therapy

The use of anti-neoplastic therapy may result in the prevention of ascitic fluid re-accumulation. Tumour necrosis factor (TNF) gave early promising results; yet, a randomized controlled trial demonstrated no effect against the re-accumulation of ascites [27]. Batimastat, an anti-angiogenesis drug, also yielded promising results; however, trials relating to this drug were closed early owing to the high incidence of bowel obstruction associated with its usage [28]. Catumaxomab, a monoclonal bispecific antibody, is seemingly an effective drug to alleviating ascites accumulation and significantly prolonging the interval between paracenteses [29]. The latter may have a benefit in decreasing the risk of infection, bowel perforation and adhesions. Further studies are warranted to draw firmer conclusions regarding its efficacy.

10.4.2 Pleural Effusion

A pleural effusion is an accumulation of extra fluid in the space between the lungs and the chest wall, which is called the pleural space. Malignant pleural effusion (MPE) is defined as pleural fluid containing malignant cells. It affects up to 15% of all patients with cancer and is the most common in lung, breast cancer, lymphoma, gynaecological malignancies and malignant mesothelioma [30]. MPE is with 33–53% the most common peritoneal manifestation of epithelial ovarian cancer, whilst in 15% of newly diagnosed women, MPE is the first clinical sign of disease [31]. Malignant cells infiltrate into the pleural space through haematogenous, direct or lymphatic spread [31]. Accumulation of fluid in the pleural space can be a consequence of tumour growth blocking the lymphatic drainage [30].

The treatment approach depends upon the physical status of the patient, the type of tumour itself and the expected overall survival [30]. Most patients develop dyspnoea at rest, whilst only a small proportion remains asymptomatic. Asymptomatic MPE, regardless of size, do not require specific interventions. On the other hand, in symptomatic patients, the main goal of treatment is to relieve dyspnoea in a minimally invasive manner. The treatment modalities for symptomatic MPE consist of the following:

10.4.2.1 Therapeutic Thoracentesis

Ultrasound scan-guided thoracentesis represents the first line intervention amongst women with symptomatic MPE. The advantages of ultrasound scan-guided thoracentesis include safety, ease of execution and reduced number of complications [32].

10.4.2.2 Pleurodesis

Pleurodesis leads to the obliteration of the pleural space and prevents the accumulation of MPE by merging the parietal and visceral pleura [33]. Various agents are used for pleurodesis, including talc, bleomycin, tetracycline, corynebacterium parvum and doxycycline [33].

10.4.2.3 Tunneled Pleural Catheter (TPC)

Tunneled Pleural Catheter (TPC)/PleurX drain is an alternative to pleurodesis for the treatment of recurrent MPE [15]. TPC is a silicone tube tunneled subcutaneously with a small cuff and inserted into the pleural cavity. The advantages of TPC consist of clinically significant improvement in dyspnoea, placement in the outpatient setting, and the ability of patient self-care at home [30, 34].

10.4.2.4 Pleurectomy

Radical total or subtotal pleurectomy, consisting of the resection of parietal and visceral pleura via removal of the fibrin pleural cortex can be used in patients with MPE, where pleurodesis is unsuccessful [30, 35]. It can be performed through a thoracoscopic approach and it is almost always effective in obliterating the pleural space [30, 35].

10.4.2.5 Intrapleural Application of Fibrinolytic

The use of fibrinolytic (urokinase) in patients with MPE has not been shown to be more effective compared to placebo in randomised control trials [30, 35]. Its use is not currently recommended as part of the standard clinical pathway [30, 35].

10.4.2.6 Anti-neoplastic Treatment

Anti-neoplastic therapy consists of chemotherapy, target therapy and immunotherapy [11, 17]. In most patients anti-neoplastic therapy is not considered more appropriate than standard interventions for symptom control related to MPE [30, 36].

10.5 Deep Vein Thrombosis and Pulmonary Embolism

10.5.1 Epidemiology and Aetiology

Venous thromboembolism (VTE) is a recognised adverse sequel amongst women with gynaecological cancer and represents the leading cause of morbidity and mortality in these patients [37]. Patients with malignancies and those undergoing pelvic surgery are known to be at higher risk of VTE, rendering gynaecological oncology patients a high-risk group. The reported incidence of VTE amongst women with gynaecological cancer ranges between 3 and 25%. This varied incidence is attributable to type of malignancy, stage and commencement of prophylactic treatment, as well as the marked heterogeneity of population groups and method of diagnosis [38].

Virchow triad, including hypercoagulability, venous stasis, and endothelial injury, represents the three general categories under which the most common risk factors for VTE in cancer will fall. Several patient's characteristics have been found to be significant risk factors of VTE including age > 60 years and BMI > 30 kg/m^2 [37]. Malignancy per se represents a well-known independent factor for development of VTE. Cancer growth is associated with the production of a hypercoagulable state, which is linked with three key mechanisms: (1) pro-coagulant, fibrinolytic and pro-aggregating activity; (2) release of pro-inflammatory and pro-angiogenic cytokines; (3) increased expression of adhesion molecules [39]. The main cells involved in these activities are endothelial cells, platelets and leukocytes. The activation of these pathway results in enhanced thrombin and fibrin production, which in turn, leads to a pro-thrombotic state [39]. Large pelvic tumours can also compress the pelvic veins leading to venous stasis via reduction of venous return, whilst invasion of parametria and/or side pelvic wall can damage endothelial cells [40]. Specific tumour parametres including type, size, grade and stage also contribute to the high-risk profile. Finally, pelvic surgery per se is a risk factor for VTE, while this risk increases with the addition of adjuvant or neo-adjuvant treatment [39]. Radiotherapy and chemotherapy can lead to thrombus formation via direct impediment of endothelial cells integrity [39]. A large study assessing the incidence of VTE amongst cancer patients undergoing chemotherapy demonstrated that overall 12.6% of the chemotherapy group patients developed VTE within 12 months of the treatment commencement compared to only 1.4% in the control group [41].

The development of VTE significantly increases mortality amongst gynaecological oncology patients. Pulmonary embolism remains the primary cause of mortality after gynaecological oncology procedure [37]. The type of malignancy is linked with risk of VTE, with ovarian cancer patients having the highest incidence amongst gynaecological malignancies [42]. Amongst ovarian and endometrial cancer patients, post-operative VTE is associated with a 2.3 and 1.5-fold higher mortality rate, respectively [42].

10.5.2 Clinical Presentation and Diagnosis

Leg oedema, erythema, warmth and pain are the most common presenting symptoms of deep vein thrombosis (DVT). Compression vein ultrasound with colour doppler is the most commonly used diagnostic test in the diagnosis of DVT [37]. Computed tomography (CT) or magnetic resonance venography can also be used, especially, when assessment of ilio-femoral DVT is required [37]. D-dimer levels are usually elevated in cases of VTE [1]. Nonetheless, D-dimer levels may also be elevated in cancer patients, even in the absence of VTE [1]. Although D-dimmers may guide diagnosis of VTE, with a sensitivity and specificity of 84% and 50% respectively, their use as a diagnostic tool in excluding isolated VTE, especially in women with levels <15 μg/ml, is limited [37].

With respect to the PE, common symptoms include dyspnoea, pleuritic chest pain, cough, haemoptysis and palpitations, whilst signs include hypoxia, tachypnoea and tachycardia [37]. Diagnosis is based upon these clinical findings in combination with laboratory tests and imaging studies. CT pulmonary angiography is commonly used diagnostic test, whilst chest x-ray may be useful in excluding other causes of deterioration [37]. ABG analysis may show hypoxia and hypocarbia. The most common ECG change, apart from sinus tachycardia, is T-wave inversion in the anterior leads. Echocardiopathy may be useful in the unstable women to investigate for right heart dysfunction [37].

10.5.3 Prophylaxis Strategies

10.5.3.1 Mechanical Prophylaxis

The aim of mechanical prophylaxis is to decrease venous stasis in the lower extremities, which is associated with decreased mean blood flow and pulsatile index within the capacitance veins of the calves and thus increased risk of VTE [37, 42]. Mechanical prophylaxis includes both passive and active methods [1, 6]. Active methods include devices such as intermittent pneumatic compression (IPC) devices, whilst passive methods include graduated compression stockings (GCS) [37, 42]. Both methods increase blood flow velocity and venous return within deep veins [37, 42]. Moreover, IPC devices can also trigger the production of tissue-type plasminogen activator and, in turn, activate endogenous fibrinolysis [37, 42].

Active mechanical prophylaxis when used intra-operatively or post-operatively after major gynaecological oncology procedures, can be as effective as pharmacological prophylaxis in preventing VTE [42]. In order to achieve their maximal efficacy, IPC devices should be used at least until ambulation and preferably throughout hospital stay or until the patient is completely mobile [42]. As IPC devices are not immediately available in moderate and low income countries, graduated compression stockings is an alternative option. Despite their low cost and easy use, their efficacy in preventing VTE is markedly lower compered to IPC devices [42]. Sole use of graduated compression stockings decreases the risk of VTE formation by only 50%; thus, they should be used in combination with pharmacological prophylaxis [42].

10.5.3.2 Pharmacological Prophylaxis

Pharmacological prophylaxis, including unfractionated heparin and low molecular weight heparin (LMWH), can also be used to minimise the risk of VTE. Pharmacological prophylaxis is usually used in combination with mechanical prophylaxis, as dual prophylaxis is superior to single mechanical or pharmacological prophylaxis in decreasing the risk of VTE [37, 42]. Given that some pharmacological prophylactic modalities increase the risk of bleeding, the option of type of prophylaxis should be tailored taking into account both benefits and risks.

Traditionally, unfractionated heparin was the pharmacological prophylaxis of choice. It prevents VTE by binding and accelerating the action of anti-thrombin [37, 42]. For women with gynaecological malignancy, 5000 units of unfractionated heparin administered subcutaneously 2 h before surgery and then every 8 h post-operatively is the recommended prophylactic protocol [37, 42]. The limitations of this prophylaxis include peri-operative risk of bleeding, three injections daily and risk of heparin-induced thrombocytopenia (HIT) [37, 42]. The reported risk of HIT amongst post-operative women receiving prophylactic dose of unfractionated heparin for more than 14 days is 1–5% [42].

Owing to the aforementioned limitations, LMWH has replaced unfractionated heparin in current clinical practice. Although LMWH has the same mechanism of action with unfractionated heparin, its benefits derive from the longer half-time. Moreover, in light of the lower anti-thrombin activity and higher anti-Xa levels, the risk of bleeding is lower compared to unfractionated heparin [42]. Disadvantages of LMWH include the higher cost and it is contraindicated in patients with impaired renal function [42]. 50% of VTE will occur within 24 h postoperatively, whilst an additional 25% within 24–72 h [42]. Mechanical prophylaxis does not increase the intra-operative risk of bleeding, thus, it should be used before and after surgery. On the other hand, the pre-operative use of LMWH is debatable. A study from the Memorial Sloan Kettering group, demonstrated a significant reduction in the incidence of VTE when LMWH was added to mechanical prophylaxis pre-operatively without significant increase of peri-operative bleeding sequelae or blood transfusion [43]. These findings were further supported by other smaller studies [42]. Therefore, the dual pre-operative prophylaxis is seemingly safe and decreases the incidence of VTE without increasing the risk of bleeding. The optimal post-operative time to initiate LMWH administration also remains to date a field of contention. Administration of LMWH < 6 h post-operatively is linked with increased risk of bleeding, whilst administration > 12 h is associated with increased risk of VTE [44]. In light of this evidence, it appears prudent to commence LMWH between 6 and 12 h post-operatively, until more robust data become available. It is recommended that an extended 28-day post-operative course of LMWH should be given to women with gynaecological malignancy undergoing abdo-pelvic surgery [42]. For morbid obese women (BMI > 40 and weight >99 kg) an increased dose of either unfractionated heparin or LMWH should be administered. Protamine sulphate can be used to reverse the effect of unfractionated heparin in case of excessive bleeding [42].

10.5.4 Treatment

Treatment with LMWH is the treatment of choice for VTE amongst women with gynaecological malignancy [37, 42]. According to the National Institute of Health and Care Excellence guidelines in United Kingdom, treatment dose of LMWH should be commenced amongst women with gynaecological cancer with confirmed VTE and continued for 6 months [37, 42]. Warfarin, a vitamin K antagonist, is an alternative option in case LMWH is contraindicated, notwithstanding, in long-term treatment setting, LMWH is seemingly more effective [37, 42]. Moreover, in light of the shorter half-life and more predictable pharmacokinetic profile, LMWH is a safer option compared to warfarin [37, 42]. Finally, new generation anticoagulants such as direct thrombin inhibitors (dabigatran) and factor Xa inhibitors (rivaroxaban, apixaban) is an alternative treatment option; yet, current evidence does not support any superiority over the LMWH or warfarin [37, 42].

Insertion of inferior vena cava (IVC) filters can be considered for women who already developed PE and are haemodynamically unstable and for women with VTE and absolute contraindication to pharmacological treatment, including haemorrhage, stroke and active bleeding [42]. Women who have an IVC filter inserted are at risk of immediate and later complications such as bleeding, infection, filter migration, IVC perforation and thrombosis [42]. It is recommended that IVC filters should be inserted and removed within 25–50 days [42].

10.6 Severe Pain

Cancer pain has a great impact on quality of life, and also leads to a number of psychological and social problems. The overall prevalence of cancer pain for all cancer sites is 39.3% after curative treatment; 55.0% during anticancer treatment; and 66.4% in advanced, metastatic, or terminal disease; 38% being moderate to severe pain [45, 46].

10.6.1 Mechanism of Pain

Pain can be somatic, visceral or neuropathic pain. Visceral pain is also associated with autonomic symptoms like nausea, vomiting, perspiration etc. and can be referred to peripheral structures. Mechanisms of pain are local tissue destruction, release of pain mediators like cytokines and proteases that enhance tissue destruction, increase inflammatory infiltration and production of neuro modulators that activate afferent neurons and overexpress nociceptive mediators [45, 46].

10.6.2 General Principles

Management of pain is a multidisciplinary team effort of the treating doctor, pain specialists, anesthesiologist, nurses, palliative care specialists, psychologists and counselors. The treating doctor should be empathetic in approach and should give some extra time in consultation. A detailed history includes questions on severity, location, radiation of pain, aggravating and relieving factors and temporal aspects. Associated co morbidities, treatment details, previous investigations should be seen and a detailed physical examination should be done [45, 46].

10.6.3 Analgesics

World Health organization (WHO) introduced the **analgesic ladder** for treatment of cancer pain. The WHO ladder consists of three steps; the first step includes non-opioid analgesics like aspirin, acetaminophen and Non-steroidal anti-inflammatory drugs (NSAIDs). In case the pain persists despite treatments, the second step should be implemented. This includes weak opioid analgesics like codeine, hydrocodone, Oxycodon. In case the patient doesn't respond to the second ladder constitution, higher doses of opioids can be given or one can resort to stronger opioid analgesics like morphine, dihydro-morphine, oxycodone or TTS -fentanyl patch. These drugs should be given round the clock. In addition to routine analgesics, adjuvant analgesics can be added at any step in the WHO ladder for pain relief. These include drugs like Amitriptyline, Paroxetine, Venlafaxine, Gabapentin, steroids, benzodiazepines etc. Tricyclic antidepressants besides providing pain relief, also act as mood elevators.

NSAID are the first line treatment for mild pain and are also used in combination with opioids in moderate to severe pain and thus help reducing the dose required for the latter. Relative contradiction includes peptic ulcer disease, thrombocytopenia and renal impairment. Cox 2 inhibitors and non-acetylated salicylate are safe and do not alter bleeding time.

The full agonists; morphine and codeine are the most commonly used drugs and are mainstay in management of cancer pain. The dose of morphine is 30 mg oral or 10 mg IM every 4 h while codeine is used as 130 mg IM or 200 mg oral every 4 h. Injectable steroids can also be administered in the form of patient controlled and analgesia (PCA). In this there is a special device or a pump which administers the drug intravenously subcutaneously or by epidural and the device is set at a basal infusion rate. Whenever the patient's experience increased pain they can administer boluses according to their requirements. The most common side effects are constipation and sedation. The other side effects include confusion, nausea, vomiting, dry mouth, urinary complaints, altered cognition, dysphoria and psychological dependence.

10.6.4 Interventions

Various neuronal blockade interventions have been developed that block the pain pathways and cause signaling interruptions of the neuronal innervations. These interventions are usually administered once the patient does not respond to medical management and is a second line approach for pain management in cancer patients. These are usually performed by specialized pain management team or by anesthetists under fluoroscopic or CT guidance. Commonly given blocks include celiac plexus, Lumbar sympathetic chain, superior hypogastric plexus or Ganglion impar (ganglion of Walther) blockade. Superior hypogastric plexus and ganglion of Walther blockade is especially useful in gynaecological cancers [45, 46].

10.6.5 Physical Modalities and Psychotherapy

Physical modalities are used in conjunction with drugs and together they help reduce pain and suffering. These interventions help to activate indigenous pain modulating pathways. Examples include hot fomentation, counter stimulation like transcutaneous electrical nerve stimulation

(TENS) therapy or acupuncture. Physical exercise also is useful for chronic pain, as is it helps to reduce stiffness restore balance and provide patient comfort.

Besides medical management several alternative remedies like psychological and cognitive behavioral treatments are available for management of cancer pain. This includes education (with coping skills training), hypnosis, yoga, cognitive behavioral approaches, and relaxation techniques including meditation. Cognitive behavioral treatments include learning skills like reinforcement of positive thoughts, adaptive coping skills and usually include both the patient and care giver [45, 46].

10.7 Chylous Ascites

Leakage and accumulation of lipid—rich milky and cloudy lymph into the peritoneal cavity is called chylous ascites. Lymph is the excess fluid from interstitial spaces that is not reabsorbed by postcapillary venules and consists of cells, particles, proteins and chylomicrons. The lymphatic system then collects this fluid or lymph and returns it back to the venous system. Destruction or obstruction of the lymphatics leads to leakage of the lipids in lacteals in the peritoneal cavity resulting in chylous ascites.

Common causes in gynaeoncology include complex surgical procedures, systematic lymphadenectomy, recurrent malignancy and radiation therapy. On ascitic tap, milky fluid is obtained (Fig. 10.1) and fluid analysis reveals elevated triglycerides (>110 mg/dl or >1.2 mmol/l). Investigation is usually not necessary but lymphangiography or lymphangioscintigraphy may demonstrate the site of leakage from the cisterna or the retroperitoneal lymphatics.

10.7.1 Management

It may take a longer time around 4–6 weeks to regress. Paracentesis provides symptom relief and may be required multiple times in a week. This can also be resolved by inserting long standing drains like Pleurex drains and it may gradually resolve spontaneously. Alteration in diet with high intake of protein and low fat diet with medium chain triglyceride supplementation is recommended. The basis is to decrease the intestinal lymphatic flow as dietary restriction of long chain fatty acids prevents their conversion into monoglycerides and free fatty acids (FFA), which are transported as chylomicrons to the intestinal lymph ducts, hence, preventing lymph and triglyceride accumulation. In contrast, medium chain triglycerides are absorbed

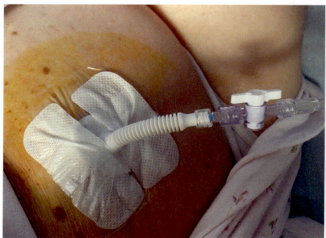
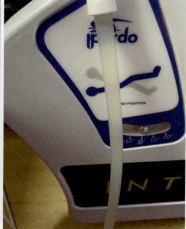

Fig. 10.1 Abdominal drain for chylous ascites (milky ascitic fluid)

directly into intestinal cells and transported as FFA and glycerol directly to the liver via the portal vein [47].

Other treatments that have been tried is cessation of oral intake and total parenteral nutrition for 2–3 weeks, somatostatin analogues to reduce splanchnic blood flow and decrease production of lymph and concomitant chemotherapy [48]. In refractory cases, surgical options include Trans juglar Intrahepatic Porto Systemic Shunt (TIPS), angiography and peritoneo-venous shunts [47–49].

This complication can be prevented by meticulous dissection techniques and ligation or clipping of major lymphatics during primary surgery. Use of hemostatic sponges like Tacosil over the aortic bed after systematic lymphadenectomy markedly reduces chylous leakage.

10.8 Summary

Management of common complications and symptoms by the gynaecological oncologists is integral to providing high-quality patient care. A multidisciplinary approach is associated with better symptom control, improved health-related quality-of-life and high patient satisfaction. The gynaecological oncologists with basic facility in symptom management will serve as an important team member in the interdisciplinary collaborations including doctors, nurses, pharmacists, social workers, psychologists, nutritionists, chaplains, patients and family members that can provide the most comprehensive approach to symptom management.

Key Points

- Chemotherapeutic agents are usually used in doses causing some degree of toxicity to normal tissues.
- BO is often a clinical manifestation of recurrent disease and is associated with a poor prognosis.
- The management of symptomatic malignant ascites or pleural effusion consists of both mechanical interventions that aim to drain the ascitic or pleural fluid, and pharmacological interventions that prevent the re-accumulation.
- Patients with malignancies and those undergoing pelvic surgery are known to be at higher risk of venous thromboembolism, rendering gynaecological oncology patients a high-risk group
- Management of chylous ascites includes long standing intrabdominal drains, dietary modification and occasionally total parenteral nutrition, somatostatin analogues, TIPS and peritoneo venous shunts.
- First line treatment of cancer pain is NSAID's but mainstay are opioids.

References

1. Rodgers GM 3rd, Becker PS, Blinder M, Cella D, Chanan-Khan A, Cleeland C, et al. Cancer- and chemotherapy- induced anemia. J Natl Compr Cancer Netw. 2012;10:628–53.
2. Kuter DJ. Managing thrombocytopenia associated with cancer chemotherapy. Oncology (Willis-ton Park). 2015;29:282–94.
3. de Naurois J, Novitzky-Basso I, Gill JM, Marti F, Cullen MH, Roila F. Management of febrile neutropenia: ESMO Clinical Practice Guidelines. Ann Oncol. 2010;21(supplement 5):v252–6.
4. National Comprehensive Care Network I. NCCN Clinical Practice Guidlines for Oncology (NCCN Guidlines); Antiemesis. 2015.
5. Andreyev J, Ross P, Donnellan C, Lennan E, Leonard P, Waters C, et al. Guidance on the management of diarrhoea during cancer chemotherapy. Lancet Oncol. 2014;15:e447–60.
6. Brewer JR, Morrison G, Dolan ME, Fleming GF. Chemotherpay-induced peripheral neuropathy. Current status and progress. Gynecol Oncol. 2015;140(1):176–83.
7. Curigliano G, Cardinale D, Super T, Plataniotis G, de Azambuja E, Sandri MT, Criscitiello C, et al. On behalf of the ESMO Guidelines Working Group, Cardiovascular toxicity induced by chemo-therapy, targeted agents and radiotherapy: clinical practice guidelines. Ann Oncol. 2012;23(Supplement 7):vii155–66.
8. Ripamonti C. Management of bowel obstruction in advanced cancer. Curr Opin Oncol. 1994;6:351–7.

9. Ripamonti C, Bruera E. Palliative management of malignant bowel obstruction. Int J Gynecol Cancer. 2002;12:135–43.
10. Dvoretsky PM, Richards KA, Angel C, et al. Distribution of disease at autopsy in 100 women with ovarian cancer. Human Pathol. 1988;19:57–83.
11. Kolomainen DF, Riley J, Wood J, Barton DPJ. Surgical management of bowel obstruction in gynaecological cancer. Obstet Gynaecol. 2017;19:63–70.
12. Feuer DJ, Broadley KE. Corticosteroids for the resolution of malignant bowel obstruction in advanced gynaecological and gastrointestinal cancer. Cochrane Database Syst Rev. 2000;2000(1):CD001219.
13. Ten Broek RPG, Krielen P, Di Saverio S, et al. Bologna guidelines for diagnosis and management of adhesive small bowel obstruction (ASBO): 2017 update of the evidence-based guidelines from the world society of emergency surgery ASBO working group. World J Emerg Surg. 2018;19(13):24.
14. Catena F, Ansaloni L, Gazzotti F, et al. Small bowel tumours in emergency surgery: specificity of clinical presentation. ANZ J Surg. 2005;75(11):997–9.
15. Vallicelli C, Coccolini F, Catena F, et al. Small bowel emergency surgery: literature's review. World J Emerg Surg. 2011;6(1):1.
16. Yeo HL, Lee SW. Colorectal emergencies: review and controversies in the management of large bowel obstruction. J Gastrointest Surg. 2013;17(11):2007–12.
17. Pisano M, Zorcolo L, Merli C, et al. 2017 WSES guidelines on colon and rectal cancer emergencies: obstruction and perforation. World J Emerg Surg. 2018;13(13):36.
18. Catena F, Pasqualini E, Tonini V, Avanzolini A, Campione O. Emergency surgery for patients with colorectal cancer over 90 years of age. Hepatogastroenterology. 2002;49(48):1538–9.
19. Takahashi H, Okabayashi K, Tsuruta M, Hasegawa H, Yahagi M, Kitagawa Y. Self-expanding metallic stents versus surgical intervention as palliative therapy for obstructive colorectal cancer: a meta-analysis. World J Surg. 2015;39(8):2037–44.
20. Rath K, Loseth D, Muscarella P, Phillips G, Fowler J, Mall D, et al. Outcomes following percutaneous upper gastrointestinal decompressive tube placement for malignant bowel obstruction in ovarian cancer. Gynecol Oncol. 2013;129:103–6.
21. Tamsma J. The pathogenesis of malignant ascites. Cancer Treat Res. 2007;134:109–18.
22. Meyer L, Suidan R, Sun C, Westin S, Coleman RL, Mills GB. The management of malignant ascites and impact on quality of life outcomes in women with ovarian cancer. Expert Rev Qual Life Cancer Care. 2016;1(3):231–8.
23. Hodge C, Badgwell BD. Palliation of malignant ascites. J Surg Oncol. 2019;120(1):67–73.
24. Macdonald R, Kirwan J, Roberts S, Gray D, Allsopp L, Green J. Ovarian cancer and ascites: a questionnaire on current management in the United Kingdom. J Palliat Med. 2006;9:1264–70.
25. O'Neill MJ, Weissleder R, Gervais DA, Hahn PF, Mueller PR. Tunneled peritoneal catheter placement under sonographic and fluoroscopic guidance in the palliative treatment of malignant ascites. AJR Am J Roentgenol. 2001;177:615–8.
26. Pockros PJ, Esrason KT, Nguyen C, Duque J, Woods S. Mobilization of malignant ascites with diuretics is dependent on ascitic fluid characteristics. Gastroenterology. 1992;103:1302–6.
27. Hirte HW, Miller D, Tonkin K, Findlay B, Capstick V, Murphy J, et al. A randomized trial of paracentesis plus intraperitoneal tumor necrosis factor-α versus paracentesis alone in patients with symptomatic ascites from recurrent ovarian carcinoma. Gynecol Oncol. 1997;64:80–7.
28. Kipps E, Tan DS, Kaye SB. Meeting the challenge of ascites in ovarian cancer: new avenues for therapy and research. Nat Rev Cancer. 2013;13:273–82.
29. Seimetz D, Lindhofer H, Bokemeyer C. Development and approval of the trifunctional antibody catumaxomab (anti-EpCAM × anti-CD3) as a targeted cancer immunotherapy. Cancer Treat Rev. 2010;36:458–67.
30. Skok K, Hladnik G, Grm A, Crnjac A. Malignant pleural effusion and its current management: a review. Medicina (Kaunas). 2019;55(8):490.
31. Porcel JM, Diaz JP, Chi DS. Clinical implications of pleural effusions in ovarian cancer. Respirology. 2012;17:1060–7.
32. Ataseven B, Chiva LM, Harter P, Gonzalez-Martin A, du Bois A. FIGO stage IV epithelial ovarian, fallopian tube and peritoneal cancer revisited. Gynecol Oncol. 2016;142:597–607.
33. Desai NR, Lee HJ. Diagnosis and management of malignant pleural effusions: state of the art in 2017. J Thorac Dis. 2017;9:S1111–22.
34. Li P, Graver A, Hosseini S, Mulpuru S, Cake L, Kachuik L, Zhang T, Amjadi K. Clinical predictors of successful and earlier pleurodesis with a tunnelled pleural catheter in malignant pleural effusion: a cohort study. CMAJ Open. 2018;6:E235–40.
35. Sterman DH, DeCamp MM, Feller-Kopman DJ, Maskell NA, Wahidi MM, Lee YCG, Gould MK, Rahman NM, Lewis SZ, Henry T, et al. Management of malignant pleural effusions. An official ATS/STS/STR clinical practice guideline. Am J Respir Crit Care Med. 2018;198:839–49.
36. Bibby AC, Dorn P, Psallidas I, Porcel JM, Janssen J, Froudarakis M, Subotic D, Astoul P, Licht P, Schmid R, et al. ERS/EACTS statement on the management of malignant pleural effusions. Eur J Cardiothorac Surg. 2019;55:116–32.
37. Cohen A, Lim CS, Davies AH. Venous thromboembolism in gynecological malignancy. Int J Gynecol Cancer. 2017;27:1970–8.
38. Satoh T, Matsumoto K, Tanaka YO, et al. Incidence of venous thromboembolism before treatment in cervical cancer and the impact of management on venous thromboembolism after commencement of treatment. Thromb Res. 2013;131:e127Ye132.

39. Piccioli A, Falanga A, Baccaglini U, et al. Cancer and venous thromboembolism. Semin Thromb Hemost. 2006;32:694Y699.
40. Barbera L, Thomas G. Venous thromboembolism in cervical cancer. Lancet Oncol. 2008;9:54Y60.
41. Khorana AA, Dalal M, Lin J, et al. Incidence and predictors of venous thromboembolism (VTE) among ambulatory high-risk cancer patients undergoing chemotherapy in the United States. Cancer. 2013;119:648Y655.
42. Barber EL, Clarke-Pearson DL. Prevention of venous thromboembolism in gynecologic oncology surgery. Gynecol Oncol. 2017;144:420–7.
43. Selby LV, Sovel M, Sjoberg DD, McSweeney M, Douglas D, Jones DR, et al. Pre-operative chemoprophylaxis is safe major oncology operations and effective at preventing venous thromboembolism. J Am Coll Surg. 2016;222:129–37.
44. Raskob GE, Hirsh J. Controversies in timing of the first dose of anticoagulant prophylaxis against venous thromboembolism after major orthopedic surgery. Chest. 2003;124:379–85.
45. van den Beuken-van Everdingen MH, Hochstenbach LM, Joosten EA, Tjan-Heijnen VC, Janssen DJ. Update on prevalence of pain in patients with cancer: systematic review and meta-analysis. J Pain Symptom Manage. 2016;51(6):1070–1090.e9.
46. Syrjala KL, Jensen MP, Mendoza ME, Yi JC, Fisher HM, Keefe FJ. Psychological and behavioral approaches to cancer pain management. J Clin Oncol. 2014;32(16):1703–11. https://doi.org/10.1200/JCO.2013.54.4825.
47. Manolitas TP, Abdessalam S, Fowler JM. Chylous ascites following treatment for gynecologic malignancies. Gynecol Oncol. 2002;86:370–3.
48. Al-Busafi SA, Ghali P, Deschênes M, Wong P. Chylous ascites: evaluation and management. International Scholarly Research Notices. 2014; Article ID 240473. https://doi.org/10.1155/2014/240473
49. Baiocchi G, Faloppa CC, Araujo RLC, et al. Chylous ascites in gynecologic malignancies: cases report and literature review. Arch Gynecol Obstet. 2010;281:677–81.

Chemotherapy in Gynaecological Cancers and Newer Developments

11

Michael Tilby, Sarah Williams, and Jennifer Pascoe

11.1 Introduction

Systemic anti-cancer treatment (SACT) including chemotherapy, immunotherapy, and targeted therapy form a key part of the multimodality management of patients with gynaecological cancers. Surgery and radiotherapy can be used for local control and debulking of gynaecological cancers and can be curative alone for early-stage cancers. SACT is required for the treatment of metastatic and micro-metastatic disease with a variety of mechanisms of action.

The hallmarks of cancer were first described by Hanahan and Weinberg in 2000 and updated in 2011 [1]. They describe the characteristics of cancer and can be therapeutic SACT targets. In this chapter we aim to summarise the underlying biology, pharmacology, and data for SACT in gynaecological cancers with a focus on ovarian and endometrial cancer. Newer developments including the role for PARP inhibitors and immunotherapy will be discussed (Fig. 11.1).

11.1.1 Systemic Anti-cancer Treatment Principles

SACT including chemotherapy aims to stop the unregulated growth of cancer cells and metastasis from their site of origin. Chemotherapy can be cytotoxic, that is killing cells including cancer cells, or cytostatic, stopping cancer cell growth and spread. However, chemotherapy is indiscriminate and will have an effect on all actively dividing cells. The aim is to have a therapeutic effect with the least possible toxicity on normal tissues. Traditionally cytotoxic chemotherapy dose is limited by bone marrow toxicity or toxicity to other rapidly dividing tissues, for example, mucous membranes in the GI tract, although newer targeted agents and immunotherapy have their own toxicity profiles. The pharmacological principle of therapeutic index is used in drug development to identify the maximal tolerated dose. The difficulty with anticancer agents is their narrow therapeutic index and it is the responsibility of a medical oncologist is to distinguish between activity and toxicity in drug development trials, and to balance clinical activity and toxicity in clinical practice. Following preclinical drug development active agents are included in phase 1 trials, establishing safety and

M. Tilby · S. Williams · J. Pascoe (✉)
Oncology Department, Queen Elizabeth Hospital, University Hospital Birmingham NHS Foundation Trust, Birmingham, UK
e-mail: michaeltilby@nhs.net; sarah.williams10@nhs.net; jenniferpascoe@nhs.net

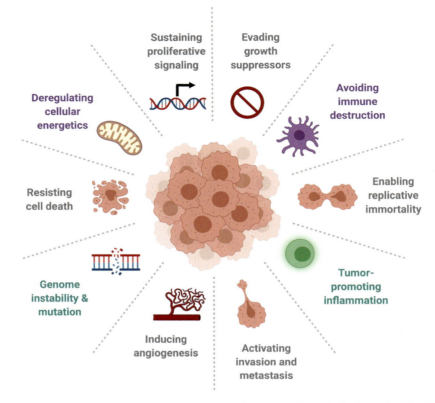

Fig. 11.1 Hallmarks of cancer described and updated with emerging hallmarks in 2011. The figure features capabilities involved tumour pathogenesis, metastasis, and cancer cell survival. Created with BioRender.com (Adapted from Hanahan and Weinberg [1])

a maximal tolerated dose to use in a phase 2 trial. Phase 2 trials aim to establish efficacy before evaluation against a current treatment or placebo in a phase 3 trials (summarised in Table 11.1).

SACT aims to kill cancer cells or stop their growth through their action on the cell cycle and interaction with DNA, RNA and cellular proteins. Different chemotherapeutic drugs may have activity at different stages of the cell cycle, or action on cellular signalling pathways. There are checkpoints between each phase of the cell cycle (Fig. 11.2) which must be met to proceed to the next phase, if not met, apoptosis, or programmed cell death is triggered. A key part of the cell cycle checkpoints is the need to ensure DNA integrity is maintained through homologous recombination repair, base excision repair and mismatch repair pathways. Cellular growth signalling pathways are driven by cell surface receptors linked to intracellular kinase, for example the mitogen-activated protein kinase (MAPK) pathway and nuclear receptors, for example the oestrogen receptor pathway. These pathways have been exploited in the newer therapeutics of targeted agents and immunotherapy which will be discussed later.

Chemotherapy agents can be classified according to their mechanism of action and those with activity in gynaecological cancers include platinum derivatives, taxanes and anthracyclines (Table 11.2). Unfortunately, drug resistance develops in cancer cells through upregulation of alternative pathways, for example through increasing cellular drug efflux pumps or a failure of apoptosis following DNA damage. This leads to growth of a genetically resistant clone of cells, leading to a loss of clinical effectiveness and requires a change in treatment where available.

Table 11.1 Clinical trials

	Number of people (approximately)	Aim	Cancer type	Randomised?	Timescale
Phase 0	10	First in human, establish safety at a low dose	Often any	No	Months
Phase 1	10–100	Establish safety and dose	Often any	No	Months
Phase 2	>100	Establish efficacy and safety	Usually one or two	Sometimes	Several months to years
Phase 3	>100–>1000	Compare new treatment to a current standard of care	Usually one	Usually	Years
Phase 4	Variable	Post licensing surveillance to establish long term efficacy and safety		No	Years

Chemotherapy dosing and scheduling differs depending on the pharmacokinetics of each drug and method of administration established during clinical trials. The most common regime for intravenous cytotoxic agents is to be administered intravenously every 3 weeks to allow recovery of toxicity before the next administration. Dosing can be uniform or calculated either by body surface area [2], body weight or in the case of carboplatin using the Calvert formula using estimated or actual glomerular filtration rate by area under the curve (AUC) [3]. Prior to each SACT treatment cycle patients are evaluated for signs of toxicity. Alterations can then be made in supportive medications, for example, additional anti-emetics or in the dosing of chemotherapy. Toxicity assessment and identification of adverse events can use the grading criteria set out by the National Institutes of Health Common Terminology Criteria for Adverse Events (CTCAE) [4]. Further guidance on management and monitoring is available from licensing authorities and in the UK in the summary of product characteristics available from the electronic medicine compendium [5].

Response assessment is an integral part of non-surgical cancer management and can use clinical, biochemical and radiological methods. Clinical assessment of response will depend on patient's symptoms and signs but may be clear, for example, the frequency of abdominal paracentesis required in patients with malignant ascites. Biochemical response assessment will depend on the primary site of gynaecological cancer. Serous ovarian cancers may secrete CA-125 which can be used to assess response to chemotherapy. The Gynaecologic Cancer Intergroup GCIG CA-125 response criteria were defined and used in clinical trials as a validated marker of biochemical progression during first line treatment and response in relapsed disease [6]. Other biochemical markers include AFP and HCG in germ cell tumours and include inhibin for granulosa cell tumours [7]. The role of circulating tumour cells and/or circulating tumour DNA (ctDNA) is under evaluation and may enter

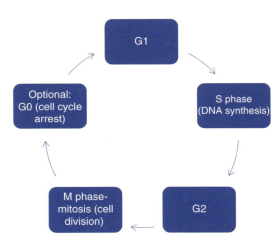

Fig. 11.2 Cell cycle. Phases of cell cycle: *G1* Growth, *S* DNA synthesis, *G2* growth and preparation for mitosis, *M* mitosis

Table 11.2 Different classes of chemotherapy drugs

Class	Mechanism of action	Active in gynaecological cancers
Platinum agents	Direct DNA damage Radiosensitiser	Cisplatin, carboplatin, oxaliplatin
Taxanes	Interferes with microtubule formation preventing mitosis	Paclitaxel, nab-paclitaxel, docetaxel
Anti-metabolites	Interfere with DNA and RNA synthesis	Gemcitabine, fluorouracil, capecitabine, pemetrexed, methotrexate
Anthracyclines	Effect DNA stability and DNA damage, cellular damage through generation of free radicals	Doxorubicin, liposomal doxorubicin, epirubicin
Topoisomerase inhibitors	Interfere with DNA stability and repair pathways	Topotecan, irinotecan
Alkylating agents	Direct DNA damage	Cyclophosphamide, ifosfamide, dacarbazine
Epipodophyllotoxins	DNA damage	Etoposide
Miscellaneous	Interfere with transcription and DNA repair	Trabectedin, eribulin

clinical practice in the future as both a diagnostic and response assessment tool [8]. Radiological response can be assessed through cross sectional imaging, most commonly CT and MRI, although PET-CT has an important role in cervical cancer and is increasingly being used in the management of other gynaecological malignancies [9]. Radiological response in clinical trials is assessed using the RECIST criteria [10] with a similar reporting format advocated in clinical practice outside of clinical trials.

Personalised medicine and the role for targeted cancer treatments is an increasing possibility in cancer medicine. Personalised medicine aims to use a management strategy for an individual patient taking into account the patient's tumour biology and likelihood of response to particular therapy whilst reducing potential toxicity. In gynaecological cancer this has been through the introduction of PARP inhibitors, initially in those patients with a germline BRCA mutation and later for all patients. These targeted agents have a different side effect profile compared to traditional cytotoxic chemotherapy and specific mechanisms of action linked to cancer biology. For example, NTRK (neurotrophic tyrosine kinase) fusion positive solid tumours, for example in uterine sarcoma, can be targeted with drugs such as larotrectinib and entrectinib [11]. There are other targeted anti-cancer treatments used in gynaecological cancer and these are summarised in Table 11.3.

Anti-angiogenic agents are used in the treatment of ovarian and cervical cancer, in particular the monoclonal antibody bevacizumab in combination with chemotherapy and as a maintenance agent post induction chemotherapy. Hormonal agents also have a role in those cancers with an underlying hormonal driver such as endometroid endometrial cancer.

SACT can be used in gynaecological cancers in the adjuvant, neo-adjuvant and metastatic setting. Adjuvant treatment aims to increase survival by reducing the risk of relapse and is used after definitive local control to target a much smaller group of cancer cells

Table 11.3 Targeted agents used in gynaecological cancer

Class	Mechanism of action	Drug	Cancer type
Poly-ADP ribose polymerase (PARP) inhibitor	Inhibition of DNA repair pathway	Olaparib Niraparib Rucaparib	High grade serous ovarian cancer
Anti-angiogenic inhibitor antibody/tyrosine kinase inhibitor (TKI)	Target VEGF signalling, prevent angiogenesis, immunomodulatory	Bevacizumab Cediranib (in clinical trials) Lenvatinib	High grade serous ovarian cancer Cervical cancer
Anti-PD-L1/Anti-PD1	Immunotherapy	Pembrolizumab Nivolumab Dostarlimab Cemiplimab Avelumab	Endometrial cancer Cervical cancer Trials in ovarian cancer
MEK inhibitor	Inhibition of MEK in MAPK pathway	Trametinib Binimetinib	Low grade serous ovarian cancer
NTRK inhibitor	Oncogene driven NTRK gene fusion-positive cancers	Larotrectinib Entrectinib	Any NTRK gene-fusion positive cancer
Anti-oestrogens—aromatase inhibitors, oestrogen receptor antagonists (SERM)	Inhibition of endogenous oestrogen synthesis in post-menopausal women	Letrozole Anastrozole Exemestane Tamoxifen (SERM)	Endometrial cancer Ovarian cancer Granulosa cell tumours Low grade endometrial stromal sarcoma
Progestins	Reduce LH secretion and oestrogen levels	Megestrol acetate	Endometrial cancer

once the bulk has been improved through surgery. Neo-adjuvant treatment aims to control symptomatic or bulky disease and may facilitate less morbid surgery. It can also give an indication of the underlying disease biology at post-surgery pathological assessment and likelihood of achieving long term cancer cure [12]. Neo(adjuvant) treatment also has oncological advantages in that it treats cancer when cancer cells are most susceptible to chemotherapy. SACT in the advanced, incurable cancer setting has two main aims, to alter the disease course and in doing so improve survival, and to improve symptoms (palliation).

11.1.2 Systemic Anti-cancer Therapy in Ovarian, Fallopian Tube and Primary Peritoneal Cancer

SACT is an integral part of the treatment of patients with ovarian, fallopian tube and primary peritoneal cancer at early and advanced stages.

11.1.2.1 Early Stage Disease (FIGO I–II)

Platinum based chemotherapy in early-stage disease (FIGO I-II) has been shown to reduce the risk of recurrence and improve overall survival. The ICON 1 (International Collaborative Ovarian Neoplasm) trial and ACTION trials demonstrated a significant improvement in relapse free survival and overall survival [13, 14]. This benefit was confirmed in a meta-analysis by the Cochrane group including an analysis of five prospective clinical trials showing that adjuvant chemotherapy has a survival advantage over observation following surgery. Chemotherapy options include single agent carboplatin, at a dose of AUC 5 or 6, or carboplatin and paclitaxel for 6 cycles scheduled every 3 weeks [15]. ESMO, NCCN and UK guidelines recommend adjuvant chemotherapy [16–18]. There is evidence of benefit across risk groups and the ESMO recommendations are summarised in Table 11.4. Response rates to non-serous epithelial ovarian cancer histology is poorer than serous and there is little data to guide recommendations in these subtypes.

Table 11.4 Recommendations for adjuvant chemotherapy by histology

Histology	Recommendations
Serous	High grade any stage ≥1A
	Low grade >Stage 1B/IC1
Mucinous	Infiltrative >Stage 1B/IC1
	Optional infiltrative stage 1A
	Expansile grade 1–2 >Stage 1B/IC1
Clear cell	Optional stage 1A and 1B/1C1
	>Stage 1C2–IC3
Endometrioid	High grade (grade 3) any stage >1A
	Grade 1–2 optional stage >IB/IC1
	Grade 1–2 Recommended Stage 2A

11.1.2.2 Advanced Disease (FIGO III–IV)

Primary debulking surgery is the standard of care where complete cytoreduction is probable and the patient's fitness and burden of disease makes surgery possible. However neoadjuvant chemotherapy followed by interval debulking surgery has been shown to be non-inferior to primary surgery followed by adjuvant chemotherapy [19]. For advanced disease the standard of current standard chemotherapy is intravenous carboplatin AUC 5/6 and paclitaxel 175mg/m^2 every 3 weeks for 6 cycles. There is potentially a role for intraperitoneal chemotherapy and HIPEC (hyperthermic intraperitoneal chemotherapy) but is currently confined to centres where the technical ability is possible and clinical trials [18, 20]. There is no survival benefit from adding in a third chemotherapy drug [18, 21]. Anti-angiogenics have been trialled as a maintenance treatment post adjuvant chemotherapy in advanced disease and bevacizumab is funded in the UK currently for any patients with stage 4 or incompletely resected Stage 3C disease (>1 cm residual disease). Maintenance bevacizumab has a progression free survival advantage in this group when given for 18 cycles (12 months) following surgery or where surgery is not feasible [22, 23]. Bevacizumab is given intravenously every 3 weeks and has side effects including hypertension, proteinuria, venous and arterial thromboembolic events, and gastrointestinal toxicity including rarely perforation [22, 23]. There is a role for PARP inhibitors as a maintenance treatment post adjuvant chemotherapy which will be discussed later in this chapter.

11.1.2.3 Relapsed Disease: Focus on High Grade Serous Ovarian Cancer

Patients need a rigorous surveillance routine post first line treatment as relapse rates are high and further surgery and systemic treatment may be feasible. Secondary debulking surgery should be considered in appropriate patients and followed by further systemic therapy. The decision to offer further systemic therapy on relapse is based on symptoms, performance status and radiological findings. There is no survival benefit in starting systemic therapy based on rising CA125 alone [24]. In those patients suitable for further chemotherapy with a longer treatment free interval (TFI) combination treatment with platinum rechallenge is recommended. For those patients with short TFI (less than 6 months) or progressing on first line therapy an alternative single agent chemotherapy is equally effective and less toxic [16]. The choice of further chemotherapy depends on patient factors including patient choice, performance status, toxicity from previous treatment and any hypersensitivity reactions, and the treatment and platinum free interval. Response rates to platinum chemotherapy fall on a continuum from around 50–60% to less than 20% depending upon platinum free interval. Resistance to platinum chemotherapy can be intrinsic to the tumour and progression may occur early, or develop later after first or subsequent line of platinum chemotherapy. GCIG categories are summarised in Table 11.5 and definitions based on the probability of responding to further platinum chemotherapy [25].

Combination platinum chemotherapy options for recurrent disease include carboplatin and pegylated liposomal doxorubicin (PLD), gemcitabine or paclitaxel [26–30]. Different schedules are possible but in general patients are offered six cycles of platinum based chemotherapy with imaging response assessment halfway through. Each regime has shown a progressive free survival benefit of between 9 and 12 months. Bevacizumab in combination with platinum based therapy and continued as maintenance treatment has also shown a benefit in progression free survival and increased response rates in the recurrent ovarian cancer setting but availability in clinical practice will depend on local funding arrangements [30].

Table 11.5 Classification based on platinum free interval

Classification	Definition
Platinum sensitive	Progression >12 months after completion of platinum chemotherapy
Partially platinum sensitive	Progression 6–12 months after completion of chemotherapy
Platinum resistant	Progression less than 6 months after completion of chemotherapy
Platinum refractory	Progression during or within 1 month after completion of chemotherapy

Patients with a short platinum free interval are conventionally treated with single agent chemotherapy and the most efficacious options include weekly paclitaxel, PLD and gemcitabine. Response rates to these agents have been shown to be increased with the addition of bevacizumab [31] However, response rates are generally low, in the region of 20% and further dose dense platinum chemotherapy can have a role for some patients. For example, cisplatin in a dose dense schedule has shown evidence of high response rates [32]. There is also a role for hormonal therapy in relapsed ovarian cancer especially in later lines of therapy. Hormonal therapy with tamoxifen or AI has shown modest overall response rates and evidence of disease control. Data is largely from retrospective case series with response rates of 15% [33], and in the Paragon phase 2 trial anastrozole showed evidence of clinical benefit in 35% of patients [34] although the ESGO-ESMO consensus guideline statement highlights the uncertain benefit [16]. Hormonal therapy does have a role in non-epithelial ovarian tumours such as granulosa cell tumours and is recommended by ESMO [35].

11.1.3 PARP Inhibitors in Ovarian Cancer

PARP inhibitors have changed the treatment landscape in advanced high-grade platinum sensitive ovarian cancer. There are multiple pathways involved in DNA repair that can be affected in cancer and exploited through SACT (Fig. 11.3a).

Approximately 50% of patients with high grade serous ovarian cancer have defects in DNA repair via homologous recombination (HR) due to germline or somatic mutations, summarised in Fig. 11.4 [36]. Defective DNA repair is an important target both through platinum-based chemotherapy inducing crosslinking and DNA damage and can be exploited through PARP inhibitors. PARP inhibitors use the concept of synthetic lethality in ovarian cancer whereby a defect in one gene, for example BRCA1 has little effect but when combined with another deficit leads to cell death [37]. PARP is a DNA repair pathway enzyme required to repair single strand breaks in DNA through the base excision repair pathway. PARP inhibitors stop this process and lead to double stranded DNA breaks. In patients with germline or somatic deficiencies in this pathway, through BRCA 1 or 2 mutation or loss of other proteins involved in homologous DNA repair, DNA repair cannot continue leading to cell death (summarised in Fig. 11.3b).

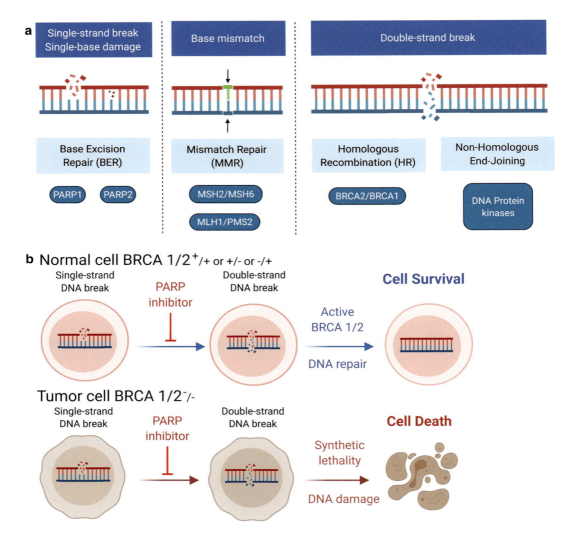

Fig. 11.3 (a) DNA repair pathways including relevant proteins in gynaecological cancers. *PARP* Poly (ADP-ribose) polymerase, *BRCA* Breast cancer gene. (b) Effect of PARP inhibitors on ovarian cancer cells with BRCA mutations. (Created with BioRender.com)

11 Chemotherapy in Gynaecological Cancers and Newer Developments

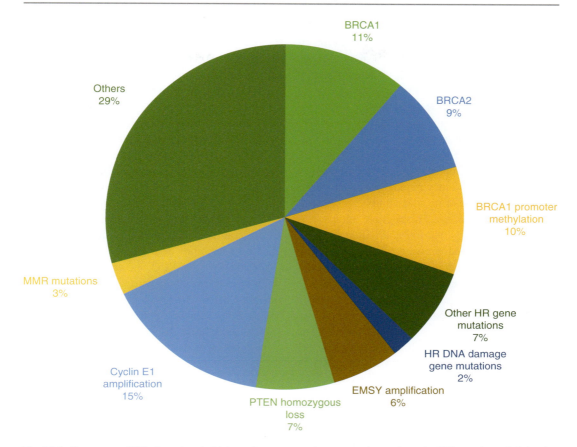

Fig. 11.4 Frequency of HR alterations in high grade serous ovarian cancer. Approximately 50% may have deficiencies in HRD. (Adapted from Konstantinopoulos et al. [40])

Patients can be tested for BRCA1 and BRCA2 germline and tumour mutations to guide both future cancer risk and individual cancer management. There are other mutations in DNA repair pathways that lead to homologous recombination deficiency (HRD). There are different methods of assessing for HRD. This can be by tumour next generation sequencing or proprietary assays. For example, the Myriad Genetics myChoice assay was used in the PAOLA-1 trial to guide maintenance therapy post first line chemotherapy [38] and Foundation Medicine next generation sequencing can assess for mutations in homologous recombination pathway genes and LOH (loss of heterozygosity) [39].

PARP inhibitors were first introduced as a maintenance treatment following platinum based chemotherapy for patients with recurrent ovarian cancer and have subsequently been shown to improve outcomes following first line treatment for patients with stage 3 or 4 high grade ovarian serous ovarian, fallopian tube or primary peritoneal cancer. Efficacy is more pronounced in patients with a BRCA mutation or homologous repair deficiency (HRD) but clinical benefit is also seen in patients without HRD. Olaparib was the first agent used in clinical trials and has a shown a very significant relapse free and overall survival benefit in patients with a germline or somatic BRCA mutation in the first line setting and following treatment for a platinum sensitive relapse [41–43]. Niraparib is licensed as a maintenance treatment post first or subsequent platinum sensitive relapse following platinum-based chemotherapy irrespective of BRCA or HRD status [44]. Rucaparib is licensed as a maintenance treatment post chemotherapy in a platinum sensitive relapse irrespective of BRCA or HRD status [45]. More recently the combination of Olaparib and bevacizumab as a maintenance treatment post platinum-based chemotherapy has shown evidence of efficacy compared to PARP inhibitor alone and has been approved in the UK for patients that are HRD positive [46].

PARP inhibitors do have adverse events associated with their use. Haematological toxicity including anaemia, neutropenia and thrombocytopenia can be common and may require dose alternations [42–44]. There are some specific toxicities associated with certain drugs. For example, niraparib is associated with hypertension and requires regular monitoring of blood pressure when starting and rucaparib can cause deranged liver function. PARPi can also be associated with systemic symptoms including fatigue, nausea, and anorexia although often this is short lived. Patients also need to be counselled regarding rare but serious toxicity of an increased risk of myelodysplasia and acute myeloid leukaemia (MDS/AML) with PARPi treatment. A systematic review published in 2020 of over 5000 patients treated with PARPi reported a significantly increased risk of MDS/AML, OR 2.63 (0.73% vs. 0.41% in normal controls) [47] and in long term data from the SOLO2 trial, use of PARPi in platinum pre-treated BRCA mutant patients increased the rate of MDS/AML from 4 to 8% [48].

11.1.4 Targeted Treatment in Low Grade Serous Ovarian Cancer

Low grade serous ovarian cancer (LGSOC) is a rare subtype of ovarian cancer which often presents at a younger age with a different molecular pathogenesis with alternations in the RAS and MAPK (mitogen-activated protein kinase) signalling pathways, described in Fig. 11.5. Treatment is centred on surgery and optimal cytoreduction as often there is a much lower response to platinum-based chemotherapy, less than 25% compared to 60–70% in high grade serous cancers [49]. Hormonal therapy can form part of the first line treatment with a survival benefit shown in a retrospective series following adjuvant chemotherapy [50]. In relapsed disease response rates for platinum based and other chemotherapy is poor.

MEK inhibitors have been developed and trialled in this setting. The first, ENGOTov11/MILO study using binimetinib compared to chemotherapy showed no significant benefit [51]. However more recently the LOGS trial using trametinib compared to physician's choice of chemotherapy or hormonal therapy showed a statistically significant benefit for progression free and overall survival compared to standard of care. There was also a much-improved overall response rate, around 26% compared to only 6% in the control group [52]. In particular further chemotherapy showed a response rate of 9% for paclitaxel, 3% for PLD and 0% for topotecan. Hormonal therapy with letrozole had a response rate of 13.6%. However, there is toxicity with MEKi most commonly diarrhoea, nausea, skin rashes, and change in heart function. Further trials including in combination with other treatments are ongoing.

11.1.5 Systemic Anti-cancer in Endometrial Cancer

SACT and radiotherapy form a key part of the management of patients with early and advanced uterine cancer. Currently risk stratification is based on pathological findings including histology type, grade, and presence or absence of lymphovascular space invasion (LVSI). Although currently not routinely available in clinical practice in the future it may be feasible to refine this further using molecular pathology, to assess for POLE and p53 mutation status and presence of mismatch repair deficiency [53]. Risk groups have been defined in the 2020 ESGO/ESTRO/ESP guidelines and summarised in Table 11.6.

Patients in the high-intermediate risk groups with or without complete nodal staging may be considered for chemotherapy especially in high grade disease with significant LVSI. Patients in the advanced, metastatic, and high-risk groups should be counselled regarding the benefits of adjuvant chemotherapy.

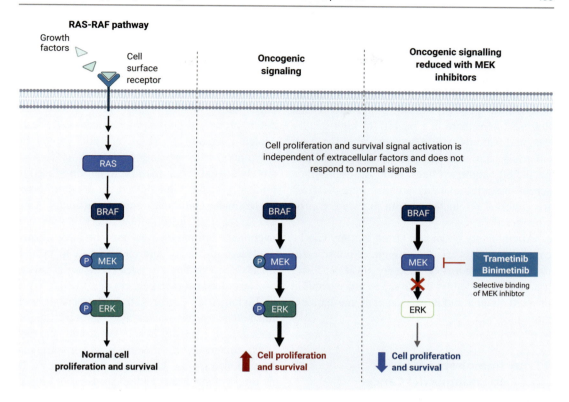

Fig. 11.5 RAS-MAPK signalling pathway (Created with BioRender.com)

Table 11.6 ESGO-ESMO prognostic risk groups

Risk group	Pathological classification
High-intermediate	• Stage 1 endometroid + substantial LVSI regardless of grade and depth of invasion • Stage 1B endometroid high-grade regardless of LVSI status • Stage 2
High	• Stage 3–4A with no residual disease • Stage 1–4A non-endometroid (serous, clear cell, undifferentiated carcinoma, carcinosarcoma, mixed) with myometrial invasion, and with no residual disease
Advanced metastatic	• Stage 3–4A with residual disease • Stage 4B

Adapted from Concin et al. [53]

The PORTEC-3 trial studied patients with high-risk features comparing radiotherapy to concurrent chemoradiotherapy and four cycles of adjuvant carboplatin and paclitaxel. The trial demonstrated an overall survival benefit for chemotherapy over radiotherapy alone which was most pronounced in patients with serous histology and stage 3 disease [54]. Studies are ongoing to define molecular subtypes with a risk of relapse and how adjuvant treatment can be tailored to risk. For example, the benefit of adjuvant chemotherapy in stage 1 and 2 clear cell cancers has not been consistently demonstrated across clinical trials [53]. In practice in the UK if chemotherapy is recommended to patients would be 4–6 cycles of carboplatin AUC5/6 and paclitaxel 175 mg/m^2 every 3 weeks followed by external beam radiotherapy and vaginal brachytherapy where indicated.

For advanced endometrial cancer maximal cytoreduction followed by chemotherapy should be considered after specialist MDT assessment. Patients with oligometastatic disease should be considered for local control including surgery, radiotherapy including stereotactic radiotherapy or other ablative techniques. In patients with unresectable disease SACT can have a role in improving patient's symptoms and improving overall survival [55]. Systemic treatment options including platinum-based chemotherapy with the combination of carboplatin and paclitaxel. This was shown to be non-inferior and less toxic than the previously used regime of cisplatin, doxorubicin plus paclitaxel [56]. Beyond first line treatment there is a paucity of high-quality data and patients should be considered for clinical trials. Active chemotherapy agents include paclitaxel, anthracyclines and for high grade serous endometrial cancers with a long platinum free interval re-challenge with platinum can be considered.

Alternatively hormonal based therapy can be considered. This can have high response rates especially for hormone receptor positive, lower grade cancers. This is discussed in more detail in the next chapter and is advocated in international guidelines [53, 57].

11.1.6 Immunotherapy in Endometrial Cancer

Immunotherapy has revolutionised the treatment of malignancy and clinical trials have been ongoing in the role for immunotherapy in gynaecological cancer. Immunotherapy has been reviewed in detail by Waldman [58]. In summary immunotherapy or checkpoint inhibition aims to use the patient's immune system to target cancer. Summarised by Chen and Mellman in the cancer immunity cycle, cancer cells produce new antigens that are recognised by the immune system however tumours develop means of avoiding the immune system through upregulation of immune checkpoint pathways [59]. Programmed cell death protein (PD-1), programmed cell death protein ligand 1 (PDL-1) and cytotoxic T-lymphocyte-associated protein 4 (CTLA-4) targeted agents were the first to be introduced to clinical practice. Anti-PD1 drugs include: pembrolizumab, nivolumab and dostarlimab. Anti-PD-L1 agents: atezolizumab, durvalumab, and avelumab. Immunotherapy currently has shown evidence of efficacy and clinical benefit in mismatch repair deficit advanced endometrial cancer and advanced cervical cancer (Fig. 11.6).

Endometrial cancer can be associated with mismatch repair deficiency through germline deficiencies, in Lynch syndrome, or sporadic mutations in mismatch repair proteins. Immunotherapy has been studied in patients with recurrent or metastatic endometrial cancer following platinum-based chemotherapy. Dostarlimab, a PD-1 targeting agent, has shown evidence of high response rates and anti-tumour activity. Pembrolizumab and nivolumab have shown evidence in dMMR tumours and in the United States have been licensed by the Federal Drug Agency (FDA) as a pan-tumour indication for mismatch repair deficiency (dMMR) or microsatellite insta-

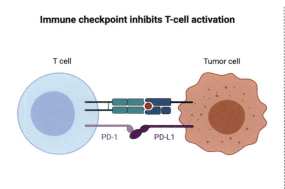
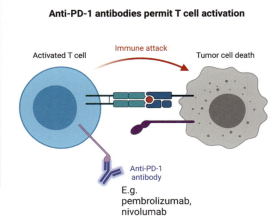

Fig. 11.6 Immune system regulation and role of checkpoint inhibitors. (Created with BioRender.com)

bility high (MSI-H) cancers or tumour with a high tumour mutational burden (TMB) [60].

Cancer treatment with immunotherapy is a rapidly evolving field and is under investigation in combination with targeted agents. In the LEAP-001 (NCT03884101) trial the combination of pembrolizumab and lenvatinib, a multi-kinase targeting TKI, is being investigated are used in combination for patients with mismatch repair proficient or deficient advanced endometrial cancer. In ovarian cancer immunotherapy is also being trialled in combination with PARP inhibitors in the ATHENA trial (NCT03522246) and dostarlimab and niraparib in combination (NCT04679064).

Immunotherapy has a very different toxicity profile to conventional chemotherapy due to its mechanism of action effecting the immune system. Checkpoint inhibitors targeting PD-1, PD-L1 and CTLA-4 can lead to a wide range of immune related adverse events effecting any organ. This can be mild requiring only symptomatic treatment through to life threatening organ dysfunction that can be fatal. Commonly this can lead to rashes, endocrinopathies, pneumonitis, colitis, and rarely fatal effects such as myocarditis [61]. Immune related side effects can happen at any time during or after treatment with immunotherapy and can have a significant impact on quality of life. Immune related side effects need specialist management from oncologists and medical specialists.

11.1.7 Cervical, Vulval and Rare Gynaecological Cancers

Systemic anti-cancer therapy also forms an integral role in the treatment of cervical, vulvar and other rarer gynaecological cancers such as non-epithelial ovarian cancer, germ cell tumours and gestational trophoblastic disease. Common regime used for germ cell tumor is the combination of Bleomycin, Etoposide and cisplatin for four cycles. For gestational trophoblastic neoplasia (GTN) Methotrexate is used for low risk disease while combination of Etoposide, Methotrexate and Dactinomycin- cyclophosphamide and vincristine (EMACO regime) is used for high risk GTN. Chemotherapy is also used a radiosensitiser in concurrent chemoradiation protocols used in the treatment of gynaecological cancers. Treatment is guided by national and international guidelines, for example ESMO and NCCN [62, 35].

11.2 Conclusions

Chemotherapy and other systemic anti-cancer treatment form a key part of the management of gynaecological cancers in combination with surgery and radiotherapy. Conventional chemotherapy using platinum based and taxanes have a significant role in the treatment of gynaecological cancers. There is an established role for targeted therapies including PARP inhibitors and other protein kinase inhibitors especially in ovarian cancer. Immunotherapy has revolutionised the treatment of cancers and has an evolving role in endometrial cancer with future work ongoing in combination with other agents. The trade-off is toxicity. This can be dose related but can also be unpredictable and life threatening. There is much to be done to refine SACT in patients' management and how improve the lives of patients living with and beyond cancer.

Key Points
- Chemotherapy in early and advanced stage disease should be considered where appropriate in a patient's cancer journey.
- Personalised cancer medicine is evolving and aims to maximise benefit whilst limited toxicity.
- PARP inhibitors have changed the prospects for patients with ovarian cancer and recommended for patients with platinum sensitive disease.
- Immunotherapy has an evolving role in gynaecological cancers and most applicable to patients with mismatch repair deficient endometrial cancer.

References

1. Hanahan D, Weinberg RA. Hallmarks of cancer: the next generation. Cell. 2011;144(5):646–74. https://doi.org/10.1016/j.cell.2011.02.013.
2. du Bois D, du Bois EF. Clinical calorimetry: tenth paper a formula to estimate the approximate surface area if height and weight be known. Arch Int Med. 1916;17((6_2):863–71. https://doi.org/10.1001/archinte.1916.00080130010002.
3. Calvert AH, Newell DR, Gumbrell LA, O'Reilly S, Burnell M, Boxall FE, Siddik ZH, Judson IR, Gore ME, Wiltshaw E. Carboplatin dosage: prospective evaluation of a simple formula based on renal function. J Clin Oncol. 1989;7(11):1748–56. https://doi.org/10.1200/JCO.1989.7.11.1748.
4. https://ctep.cancer.gov/protocolDevelopment/adverse_effects.htm
5. https://www.medicines.org.uk/emc/about-the-emc
6. Rustin GJS, Vergote I, Eisenhauer E, et al. Definitions for response and progression in ovarian cancer clinical trials incorporating RECIST 1.1 and CA 125 agreed by the gynecological cancer intergroup (GCIG). Int J Gynecol Cancer. 2011;21:419–23.
7. Lyubimova NV, Beyshembaev AM, Kushlinskiy DN, Zordania KI, Adamyan LV. Granulosa cell tumors of the ovary and inhibin B. Bull Exp Biol Med. 2011;150(5):635–8. https://doi.org/10.1007/s10517-011-1209-z.
8. Roncati L, Lusenti B. Liquid biopsy to monitor early relapse of gynaecological malignancies. Eur J Gynaecol Oncol. 2020;41(6):849–51. https://doi.org/10.31083/j.ejgo.2020.06.5430.
9. Narayanan P, Sahdev A. The role of 18F-FDG PET CT in common gynaecological malignancies. Br J Radiol. 2017;90(1079):20170283. https://doi.org/10.1259/bjr.20170283.
10. Schwartz LH, Litière S, de Vries E, et al. RECIST 1.1—Update and clarification: from the RECIST committee. Eur J Cancer. 2016;62:132–7. https://doi.org/10.1016/j.ejca.2016.03.081.
11. Drilon A, Laetsch TW, et al. Efficacy of larotrectinib in TRK fusion-positive cancers in adults and children. N Engl J Med. 2018;378:731–9.
12. Kerr DJ, et al. Oxford textbook of oncology. 3rd ed. Oxford: Oxford University Press; 2016.
13. Colombo N, Guthrie D, Chiari S, Parmar M, Qian W, Swart AM, Torri V, Williams C, Lissoni A, Bonazzi C. International collaborative ovarian neoplasm trial 1: a randomized trial of adjuvant chemotherapy in women with early-stage ovarian cancer. J Natl Cancer Inst. 2003;95(2):125–32. https://doi.org/10.1093/jnci/95.2.125.
14. Trimbos JB, Parmar M, Vergote I, Guthrie D, Bolis G, Colombo N, Vermorken JB, Torri V, Mangioni C, Pecorelli S. International collaborative ovarian neoplasm trial 1 and adjuvant chemotherapy in ovarian neoplasm trial: two parallel randomized phase III trials of adjuvant chemotherapy in patients with early-stage ovarian carcinoma. J Natl Cancer Inst. 2003;95(2):105–12. https://doi.org/10.1093/jnci/95.2.105.
15. Lawrie TA, Winter-Roach BA, Heus P, Kitchener HC. Adjuvant (post-surgery) chemotherapy for early stage epithelial ovarian cancer. Cochrane Database Syst Rev. 2015;2015(12):CD004706. https://doi.org/10.1002/14651858.CD004706.pub5.
16. Colombo N, Sessa C, du Bois A, et al. ESMO-ESGO consensus conference recommendations on ovarian cancer: pathology and molecular biology, early and advanced stages, borderline tumours and recurrent disease. Ann Oncol. 2019;30(5):672–705. https://doi.org/10.1093/annonc/mdz062.
17. Armstrong DK, et al. Ovarian cancer, version 2.2020, NCCN clinical practice guidelines in oncology. J Natl Compr Canc Netw. 2021;19(2):191–226.
18. Fotopoulou C, Hall M, Cruickshank D, et al. British Gynaecological Cancer Society (BGCS) epithelial ovarian/fallopian tube/primary peritoneal cancer guidelines: recommendations for practice. Eur J Obstet Gynecol Reprod Biol. 2017;213:123–39. https://doi.org/10.1016/j.ejogrb.2017.04.016.
19. Vergote I, Tropé CG, Amant F, et al. Neoadjuvant chemotherapy or primary surgery in stage IIIC or IV ovarian cancer. N Eng J Med. 2010;363(10):943–53. https://doi.org/10.1056/nejmoa0908806.
20. Jaaback K, Johnson N, Lawrie TA. Intraperitoneal chemotherapy for the initial management of primary epithelial ovarian cancer. Cochrane Database Syst Rev. 2016;2016(1):CD005340. https://doi.org/10.1002/14651858.CD005340.pub4.
21. du Bois A, Weber B, Rochon J, et al. Addition of epirubicin as a third drug to carboplatin-paclitaxel in first-line treatment of advanced ovarian cancer: a prospectively randomized gynecologic cancer intergroup trial by the Arbeitsgemeinschaft Gynaekologische Onkologie Ovarian Cancer Study Group and the Groupe d'Investigateurs Nationaux pour l'Etude des Cancers Ovariens. J Clin Oncol. 2006;24:1127–35.
22. Burger RA, Brady MF, Bookman MA, et al. Incorporation of bevacizumab in the primary treatment of ovarian cancer. N Eng J Med. 2011;365(26):2473–83. https://doi.org/10.1056/nejmoa1104390.
23. Perren TJ, Swart AM, Pfisterer J, et al. A phase 3 trial of bevacizumab in ovarian cancer. N Eng J Med. 2011;365(26):2484–96. https://doi.org/10.1056/nejmoa1103799.
24. Rustin GJS, van der Burg MEL, Griffin CL, et al. Early versus delayed treatment of relapsed ovarian cancer (MRC OV05/EORTC 55955): a randomised trial. Lancet. 2010;376(9747):1155–63. https://doi.org/10.1016/S0140-6736(10)61268-8.
25. Wilson M, et al. Fifth ovarian cancer consensus conference of the gynecologic cancer intergroup: recurrent disease. Ann Oncol. 2017;28:727–32.
26. Gladieff L, Ferrero A, de Rauglaudre G, et al. Carboplatin and pegylated liposomal doxorubicin versus carboplatin and paclitaxel in partially platinum-sensitive ovarian cancer patients: results from a subset analysis of the CALYPSO phase III trial. Ann Oncol. 2012;23(5):1185–9. https://doi.org/10.1093/annonc/mdr441.

27. Wagner U, Marth C, Largillier R, et al. Final overall survival results of phase III GCIG CALYPSO trial of pegylated liposomal doxorubicin and carboplatin vs paclitaxel and carboplatin in platinum-sensitive ovarian cancer patients. Br J Cancer. 2012;107(4):588–91. https://doi.org/10.1038/bjc.2012.307.
28. ICON and AGO Collaborators. Paclitaxel plus platinum based chemotherapy versus conventional platinum based chemotherapy in women with relapsed ovarian cancer: the ICON/ AGO-OVAR 2.2 trial. Lancet. 2003;361:2009–106.
29. Pfisterer J, et al. Gemcitabine plus carboplatin compared with carboplatin in patients with platinum-sensitive recurrent ovarian cancer: an intergroup trial of the AGO-OVAR, the NCIC CTG, and the EORTC GCG. J Clin Oncol. 2006;24(29):4699–707.
30. Aghajanian C, Blank SV, et al. OCEANS: a randomized, double-blind, placebo-controlled phase III trial of chemotherapy with or without bevacizumab in patients with platinum-sensitive recurrent epithelial ovarian, primary peritoneal, or fallopian tube cancer. J Clin Oncol. 2012;30:2039–45.
31. Pujade-Lauraine E, Hilpert F, Weber B, et al. Bevacizumab combined with chemotherapy for platinum-resistant recurrent ovarian cancer: the AURELIA open-label randomized phase III trial. J Clin Oncol. 2014;32:1302–8.
32. Van der Burg ME, de Wit R, Van Putton WL, et al. Weekly cisplatin and daily oral etoposide is highly effective in platinum pre-treated ovarian cancer. B J Cancer. 2002;7:19–25.
33. George A, et al. The role of hormonal therapy in patients with relapsed high-grade ovarian carcinoma: a retrospective series of tamoxifen and letrozole. BMC Cancer. 2017;17:456. https://doi.org/10.1186/s12885-017-3440-0.
34. Kok PS, Beale P, O'Connell RL, et al. PARAGON (ANZGOG-0903): a phase 2 study of anastrozole in asymptomatic patients with estrogen and progesterone receptor-positive recurrent ovarian cancer and CA125 progression. J Gynecol Oncol. 2019;30(5):e86. https://doi.org/10.3802/jgo.2019.30.e86.
35. Ray-Coquard I, Morice P, Lorusso D, Prat J, Oaknin A, Pautier P, Colombo N. Non-epithelial ovarian cancer: ESMO Clinical Practice Guidelines for diagnosis, treatment and follow-up. Ann Oncol. 2018;29(Suppl 4):iv1–iv18. https://doi.org/10.1093/annonc/mdy001.
36. Konstantinopoulos PA, Ceccaldi R, Shapiro GI, D'Andrea AD. Homologous recombination deficiency: exploiting the fundamental vulnerability of ovarian cancer. Cancer Discov. 2015;5(11):1137–54. https://doi.org/10.1158/2159-8290.CD-15-0714.
37. Ashworth A, Lord CJ. Synthetic lethal therapies for cancer: what's next after PARP inhibitors? Nat Rev Clin Oncol. 2018;15(9):564–76. https://doi.org/10.1038/s41571-018-0055-6.
38. https://medicines.astrazeneca.co.uk/home/oncology/hrd-tbrca-testing/hrd-testing.html
39. https://www.foundationmedicine.com/test/foundationone-cdx
40. Konstantinopoulos PA, Ceccaldi R, Shapiro GI, D'Andrea AD. Homologous Recombination Deficiency: Exploiting the Fundamental Vulnerability of Ovarian Cancer. Cancer Discov. 2015;5(11):1137–54. https://doi.org/10.1158/2159-8290.CD-15-0714. Epub 2015 Oct 13. PMID: 26463832; PMCID: PMC4631624.
41. Ledermann JA, Harter P, Gourley C, et al. Overall survival in patients with platinum-sensitive recurrent serous ovarian cancer receiving olaparib maintenance monotherapy: an updated analysis from a randomised, placebo-controlled, double-blind, phase 2 trial. Lancet Oncol. 2016;17(11):1579–89. https://doi.org/10.1016/S1470-2045(16)30376-X.
42. Moore K, Colombo N, Scambia G, et al. Maintenance olaparib in patients with newly diagnosed advanced ovarian cancer. N Eng J Med. 2018;379(26):2495–505. https://doi.org/10.1056/nejmoa1810858.
43. Poveda A, Floquet A, Ledermann JA, et al. Final overall survival (OS) results from SOLO2/ENGOT-ov21: a phase III trial assessing maintenance olaparib in patients (pts) with platinum-sensitive, relapsed ovarian cancer and a BRCA mutation. J Clin Oncol. 2020;22(5):620–31. https://doi.org/10.1200/jco.2020.38.15_suppl.6002.
44. Mirza MR, Monk BJ, Herrstedt J, et al. Niraparib maintenance therapy in platinum-sensitive, recurrent ovarian cancer. N Eng J Med. 2016;37(32)):2968–73. https://doi.org/10.1056/nejmoa1611310.
45. Coleman RL, Oza AM, Lorusso D, et al. Rucaparib maintenance treatment for recurrent ovarian carcinoma after response to platinum therapy (ARIEL3): a randomised, double-blind, placebo-controlled, phase 3 trial. Lancet. 2017;390(10106):1949–61. https://doi.org/10.1016/S0140-6736(17)32440-6.
46. Ray-Coquard I, Pautier P, Pignata S, et al. Olaparib plus bevacizumab as first-line maintenance in ovarian cancer. N Eng J Med. 2019;381(25):2416–28. https://doi.org/10.1056/nejmoa1911361.
47. Morice PM, Leary A, et al. Myelodysplastic syndromeand acute myeloid leukaemia in patients treated with PARP inhibitors: a safety meta-analysis of randomised controlled trials and a retrospective study of the WHO pharmacovigilance database. Lancet Haematol. 2021;8(2):e122–34.
48. Poveda A, Floquet A, et al. SOLO2/ENGOTOV21 investigators. Olaparib tablets as maintainance therapy in patients with platinum-sensitive relapsed ovarian cancer and a BRCA1/2 mutation: a final analysis of a double blind, randomised, placebo controlled phase 3 trial. Lancet Oncol. 2021;22(5):620–31. https://doi.org/10.1016/S1470-2045(21)00073-5.
49. Grabowski JP, Harter P, Heitz F, et al. Operability and chemotherapy responsiveness in advanced low-grade serous ovarian cancer. An analysis of the AGO Study Group metadatabase. Gynecol Oncol. 2016;140(3):457–62. https://doi.org/10.1016/j.ygyno.2016.01.022.
50. Gershenson DM, Bodurka DC, Coleman RL, Lu KH, Malpica A, Sun CC. Hormonal maintenance therapy

for women with low-grade serous cancer of the ovary or peritoneum. J Clin Oncol. 2017;35(10):1103. https://doi.org/10.1200/JCO.2016.71.0632.

51. Monk BJ, Grisham RN, Banerjee S, et al. MILO/ENGOT-ov11: binimetinib versus physician's choice chemotherapy in recurrent or persistent low-grade serous carcinomas of the ovary, fallopian tube, or primary peritoneum. J Clin Oncol. 2020;38(32):3753. https://doi.org/10.1200/JCO.20.01164.

52. Gershenson D. A randomised Phase II/III study to assess the efficacy of trametinib in patients with recurrent or progressive low grade serous or peritoneal cancer. Gynecol Oncol. 2020;159(Suppl 1):v897–8. https://doi.org/10.1016/j.ygyno.2020.06.045.

53. Concin N, Matias-Guiu X, Vergote I, et al. ESGO/ESTRO/ESP guidelines for the management of patients with endometrial carcinoma. Int J Gynecol Cancer. 2021;31(1):12–39. https://doi.org/10.1136/ijgc-2020-002230.

54. de Boer SM, Powell ME, Mileshkin L, et al. Adjuvant chemoradiotherapy versus radiotherapy alone in women with high-risk endometrial cancer (PORTEC-3): patterns of recurrence and post-hoc survival analysis of a randomised phase 3 trial. Lancet Oncol. 2019;20(9):1273–85. https://doi.org/10.1016/S1470-2045(19)30395-X.

55. Vale CL, Tierney J, Bull SJ, Symonds PR. Chemotherapy for advanced, recurrent or metastatic endometrial carcinoma. Cochrane Database Syst Rev. 2012;2012(8):CD003915. https://doi.org/10.1002/14651858.CD003915.pub4.

56. Miller D, Filiaci V, Fleming G, Mannel R, Cohn D, Matsumoto T, Tewari K, DiSilvestro P, Pearl M, Zaino R. Late-breaking abstract 1: randomized phase III noninferiority trial of first line chemotherapy for metastatic or recurrent endometrial carcinoma: a Gynecologic Oncology Group study. Gynecol Oncol. 2012;125(3):771. https://doi.org/10.1016/j.ygyno.2012.03.034.

57. Sundar S, Balega J, Crosbie E, et al. BGCS uterine cancer guidelines: recommendations for practice. Eur J Obstet Gynecol Reprod Biol. 2017;213:71–97. https://doi.org/10.1016/j.ejogrb.2017.04.015.

58. Waldman AD, Fritz JM, Lenardo MJ. A guide to cancer immunotherapy: from T cell basic science to clinical practice. Nat Rev Immunol. 2020;20(11):651–68. https://doi.org/10.1038/s41577-020-0306-5.

59. Chen DS, Mellman I. Oncology meets immunology: the cancer-immunity cycle. Immunity. 2013;39(1):1–10. https://doi.org/10.1016/j.immuni.2013.07.012.

60. Yoshino T, et al. JSCO-ESMO-ASCO-JSMO-TOS: international expert consensus recommendationfor tumour agnostic treatments in patients with solid tumours with microsatellite instability or NTRK fusions. Ann Oncol. 2020;31(7):861–72. https://doi.org/10.1016/j.annonc.2020.03.299.

61. Haanen JBAG, Carbonnel F, Robert C, Kerr KM, Peters S, Larkin J, Jordan K. Management of toxicities from immunotherapy: ESMO Clinical Practice Guidelines for diagnosis, treatment and follow-up. Ann Oncol. 2017;28(suppl_4):iv119–42. https://doi.org/10.1093/annonc/mdx225.

62. Marth C, Landoni F, Mahner S, McCormack M, Gonzalez-Martin A, Colombo N. Cervical cancer: ESMO Clinical Practice Guidelines for diagnosis, treatment and follow-up. Ann Oncol. 2017;28(suppl_4):iv72–83. https://doi.org/10.1093/annonc/mdx220.

Hormonal Treatment in Gynaecological Malignancies

12

Anastasios Tranoulis and Indrajit N. Fernando

12.1 Introduction

In this chapter, the role of hormonal therapy (HT) in gynaecological malignancies is discussed with an emphasis on endometrial cancer (EC), uterine sarcomas and ovarian cancer (OC). Most gynaecological cancers, including EC, OC, low grade endometrial stromal sarcomas (LG-ESS), uterine leiomyosarcomas (u-LMS) and granulosa cell tumours (GCT) express oestrogen (ER) and/or progesterone receptors (PR) to various extend [1]. To this end, HT has an established role in the management of selected patients with advanced or recurrent disease, including first-line treatment [1]. A variety of agents have been used for treatment of advanced or recurrent disease as well as amongst selective women with early-stage EC, who wish to preserve their fertility. Historically, progestin therapy has been the most widely applied HT and it is still the preferred choice as first line HT. Progesterone acts as an anti-oestrogen by reducing ER and increasing oestrodiol dehydrogenase; thus, leading to suppression of endometrial gland growth and stromal decidu-

alisation [2]. Currently used anti-oestrogenic drugs are selective oestrogen receptor modulators (SERM) or down-regulators (SERD) and aromatase inhibitors (AIs). SERMs and SERDs such as tamoxifen and fulvestrant have an anti-proliferative effect by blocking the oestrogen receptor (ER) through which oestrogen effects are mediated [3]. Aromatase inhibitors like anastrozole, letrozole, and exemestane, limit the oestrogen tumour exposure by aromatase in fat tissue, especially in postmenopausal women [3]. Finally, targeted therapies, including mTOR inhibitors, have recently emerged as a promising treatment option, especially in combination with HT [4]. In light of the recent advances in immunotherapy, the role of combined HT and mTOR inhibitors is also covered in this chapter.

12.2 Endometrial Cancer

Endometrial cancer (EC) is the most common malignancy of the gynaecological genital tract in the developed world. There are two pathological sub-types according to oestrogen dependence [5]. Type I (oestrogen related) represents the most common type of EC and it is usually associated with obesity and diabetes mellitus. The most common characteristics of type I EC are: (1) endometrioid histology; (2) lower grade; (3) high PR expression; (4) younger age; (5) less myometrial invasion; (6) genetic aberrations (microsatel-

A. Tranoulis (✉)
The Pan-Birmingham Gynaecological Cancer Centre, City Hospital, Birmingham, UK
e-mail: anastasios.tranoulis1@nhs.net

I. N. Fernando
University Hospitals Birmingham NHS Foundation Trust, Birmingham, UK
e-mail: indrajit.fernando@uhb.nhs.uk

© The Author(s), under exclusive license to Springer Nature Switzerland AG 2022
K. Singh, B. Gupta (eds.), *Gynecological Oncology*, https://doi.org/10.1007/978-3-030-94110-9_12

lite instability, DNA mismatch repair defects, K-ras/b-catenin/PI3K mutations) [5]. On the other hand, type II EC is characterised by: (1) non-endometrioid histology (serous, clear cell); (2) p53 mutations; (3) over expression of Her2/neu; (4) aneuploidy [5].

Unopposed oestrogen is the most significant risk factor for type I EC and its precursor, endometrial hyperplasia [5]. ER/PR expression is associated with grade of histological differentiation with 70%, 55% and 41% of grade 1, 2 and 3 EC expressing ER (+) and/or PR (+), respectively [5]. Of note, the recent analysis of the Cancer Genome Atlas Project (TCGA) confirmed the presence of a hormonal phenotype, characterised by marked expression of ER/PR correlated with endometrioid histology [6]. In view of this evidence, HT including progestins, SERMS/SERDS and AIs has been extensively investigated in EC with various responses. Interestingly, with the recent advances in immunotherapy, the combined HT with mTOR inhibitors has also emerged as an attractive option.

12.2.1 Hormonal Therapy as Treatment for Fertility Preservation in Early-Stage Endometrial Cancer (EC)

For EC patients at reproductive age and wishes to preserve fertility, fertility-sparing treatments may be considered. The criteria for conservative management in premenopausal EC patients are: (1) grade 1 well-differentiated endometrioid tumour; (2) FIGO stage IA tumour without invasion of myometrium on MRI; (3) absence of lymphovascular invasion on specimen; (4) no evidence of intra-abdominal disease or adnexal mass; (5) strong desire for pregnancy; (6) exclusion of infertility [7]. A meta-analysis of 28 studies enrolling 1038 women with early-stage EC or atypical complex hyperplasia (ACH) evaluated the oncologic and reproductive outcomes after fertility-sparing management with monotherapy or combined HT [8]. The study reported complete remission rate (CRR) of 71%, pregnancy rate of 34% and a live birth rate of 20% amongst women managed with oral progestins [8]. Correspondingly, the pooled CRR for women managed with levonorgestrel-releasing intrauterine device (LNG-IUD) was 76%, whilst the pooled pregnancy and live birth rate was 18% and 14% respectively [8]. Finally, the combined treatment with progestin plus LNG-IUD resulted in 87% CRR, with 40% and 35% pregnancy and live birth rate, respectively [8]. In light of these findings, systemic or local progestins can be safely used in selected young women with ACH or early-stage EC fulfilling the aforementioned fertility-sparing criteria. LNG-IUD appears to be effective and avoids side effects of systemic progestins. The combined treatment with oral progestins plus LNG-IUD is seemingly the most effective treatment modality; yet, further studies are warranted to confirm this notion.

Metformin has recently emerged as a potential treatment option in EC, as it prevents cancer recurrence and increases radiosensitivity [9]. Limited data has suggested that obese patients with type I endometrial cancer had less risk of cancer recurrence on metformin [9]. Mitsuhashi et al. reported the concurrent use of metformin inhibited disease relapse after fertility-sparing management with medroxyprogesterone acetate in women with ACH and early-EC [10]. Ongoing trials investigate the combination of progestins with dietary modifications or with metformin in this setting; however, this is still regarded as experimental.

12.2.2 Hormonal Therapy as Adjuvant Treatment Following Surgical Management in Endometrial Cancer (EC)

Standard therapy for EC consists of surgery followed by adjuvant radio- and/or chemotherapy depending upon final tumour characteristics [11]. It is currently recommended that progestins have no role in the adjuvant treatment of endometrial cancer [11, 12]. A Cochrane review enrolling nine randomised trials addressed the use of adjuvant vs. no adjuvant progestins therapy amongst women who had previously undergone surgery for apparent early-stage EC [12]. There was no overall survival benefit for women given adjuvant progestins therapy, whilst the main side effects included thromboembolic and cardiovascular events [12]. It is noteworthy that the majority of women in the included studies were high-risk EC, which are usually ER/PR negative. Therefore, future research should focus on women with low/intermediate-risk ER/PR positive EC to ascertain the prognostic role of HT in such tumours. This should include patients with endometroid cancers with stage 3 and 4 ER/PR positive tumours, who may or may not also be suitable for adjuvant chemotherapy.

12.2.3 Hormonal Therapy as Treatment in Advanced and Recurrent Endometrial Cancer (EC)

Progestin-based HT has long been used with a view to counter the hyperestrogenism associated with the advanced and recurrent EC. A Gynaecological Oncology Group (GOG) study demonstrated a 24% CRR; yet, this response was not sustained most likely owing to the downregulation of PR [13]. On the contrary, as tamoxifen was shown to increase PR expression, it was hypothesised that pre-treatment with tamoxifen could increase the response of tumours to progestins [14, 15]. As tamoxifen is linked with increased PR expression, two phase II trials have evaluated the combination of progesterone and tamoxifen [9, 10]. The reported CRR was 27% and 33%, respectively [14, 15]. Overall, the reported CRR amongst women managed with combined progestin/tamoxifen treatment ranged between 19% and 37% [16], whilst for those managed with tamoxifen monotherapy between 10% and 53%, respectively [16]. At present there is no level 3 evidence to support this as an alternative to progestins alone. The opposite strategy of reducing circulating oestrogen by inhibiting aromatase or by direct inhibition of ER has been less successful. AIs have shown minimal activity in advanced/recurrent EC [16]. The reported CRR varied between 9 and 31% [16]. The addition of progestin and tamoxifen to chemotherapy was evaluated by Ayoub et al., who reported a higher RR for the combination compared to chemotherapy alone [17]. The combination of tamoxifen and progestins can be considered as an option of treatment but there is still no level 3 evidence compared to progestins alone. Aromatase can be considered a second-line HT option in EC. However it should be noted that they are not formally licensed in EC. The effect of anti-oestrogens in advanced/recurrent EC needs further improvement. Currently, selection for HT is mainly based upon ER/PR status necessitating a shift in the focus of future research into incorporating additional biomarkers to improve selection of women that would benefit most from HT.

In an effort to improve the efficacy of HT combinations with agents targeting cross-talking signaling pathways and/or metformin have been investigated. In EC, oestradiol signaling is mediated via ERa and is capable of activating the mitogen activated protein kinase (MAPK) signaling pathway, which further triggers downstream molecules ERK and AKT (part of the PIEK/AKT/mTOR pathway). PR signaling also partially acts through the MAPK and PI3K/AKT/mTOR pathways [18]. Therefore, combinations of HT and mTOR inhibitors with or without metformin were tested. Fleming et al., carried out a randomised phase II trial of intravenous temsirolimus 25 mg weekly versus the combination of weekly temsirolimus with a regimen of megestrol acetate 80 mg BD for 3 weeks alternating with tamoxifen 20 mg BD for 3 weeks in women with recurrent or metastatic EC [19]. The authors reported that adding the combination of megestrol acetate and tamoxifen to temsirolimus therapy did not enhance activity, whilst the combination treatment was associated with an excess of venous thrombosis. Slomovitz et al. carried out a phase II trial of everolimus and letrozole in women with recurrent EC [20]. The reported RR was 32%. Soliman et al. evaluated the addition of metformin in treatment with evelolimus and letrozole, which resulted in 50% clinical benefit and 28% overall response [21]. A phase II trial assessing the efficacy of the combination of ribociclib and letrozole for treatment of relapsed ER-positive EC demonstrated a promising 55% 12-week PFS, whilst 45% of the patients with grade 1 or 2 endometrioid EC obtained substantial benefit with no evidence of progression for at least 24 weeks [22]. Few ongoing clinical trials are aiming to further investigate the role of targeted treatment and metformin in the management of advanced/recurrent EC. The ENGOT-EN3-NSGO/PALEO 1:1 randomised trial is designed to assess the efficacy of letrozole vs. letrozole/palbociclib in ER-positive advanced or recurrent EC, whilst the GOG 3007 trial the efficacy of everolimus plus letrozole vs. tamoxifen plus MPA. Finally, the MD Anderson Cancer Centre group is currently carrying out a single arm phase II trial (NCT01797523) to evaluate the therapeutic role of everolimus plus letrozole plus metformin in this setting. It is hoped that some of these new treatments may turn out to be beneficial once we have completed phase 3 trials.

12.3 Uterine Sarcomas

12.3.1 Uterine Leiomyosarcomas (u-LMS)

ER/PR have been found to be positive in 40–70% of u-LMS [23]. ER/PR appear to have a pivotal role in regulating the growth and remodeling of uterine smooth muscle, thus, their activation seemingly plays an important role in tumour development in uterine leiomyosarcomas (u-LMS). The Memorial Sloan Kettering Cancer group reported that ER/PR expression was found to be associated with survival outcomes in 43 women with high-grade uterine-limited LMS [23]. The role of HT has been minimally studied in two phase II trials [24, 25]. A single-arm phase II study investigated the prognostic role of letrozole at a dose of 2.5 mg daily in 27 patients with unresectable u-LMS with ER and/or PR expression confirmed by immunohistochemistry [24]. The 12-week PFS was 50%. Patients with the longest PFS rate were those, whose tumours strongly and diffusely expressed ER and PR (>90%). Moreover, a recent open-label, phase 2 study investigated the prognostic impact of letrozole 2.5 mg daily versus observation in completely resected u-LMS without any previous adjuvant treatment [25]. Nine patients were randomized. Four patients were in the letrozole arm and five patients were in the observation arm. The percent progression free at 12 and 24 months was 100% for patients receiving letrozole compared to 80% at 12 months and 40% at 24 months for patients in the observation arm. Although these findings are encouraging, robust conclusions cannot be made owing to early study closure and the small patient numbers. Similar findings were reported in few retrospective studies. Thanopoulou et al., reported a retrospective study of 16 women with ER/PR positive advanced u-LMS treated with first line letrozole and second line exemestane (83%) or letrozole (17%) [22]. Median PFS in 1st line was 14 months, and prolonged PFS was more likely to be observed in patients with low grade compared to high grade u-LMS (20 months vs. 11 months), and in moderately/strongly ER positive compared to weakly ER positive u-LMS (20 months vs. 12 months) [26].

Progestins were amongst the first hormonal modulators to be explored in the management of metastatic u-LMS; notwithstanding, AIs are currently the preferred hormonal agents for 1st line treatment, owing to their high therapeutic index [26]. Moreover, AIs have shown activity as 2nd line treatment in progestin-resistant u-LMS [26]. ER and PR expression appears to be a prognostic factor and AIs may play an active therapeutic role especially amongst u-LMS with strong (>90%) ER/PR expression. Nonetheless, despite this promising evidence, HT could not be routinely recommended as an adjuvant treatment until more robust data become available. HRT may be considered only in selected cases with negative ER/PR. Ovarian preservation is seemingly not associated with worse oncological outcomes, nevertheless most centers would not advise against this particularly in hormone sensitive LMS [26].

12.3.2 Low Grade Endometrial Stromal Sarcoma (LG-ESS)

Low grade endometrial stromal sarcomas (LG-ESS) are commonly ER and PR positive (approximately 70–80%) [27]. In light of this high expression, the use of HT with either progestins or AIs has been investigated in localised and mainly in advanced or recurrent LG-ESS with various responses. In the absence of randomised or prospectives studies, this evidence stems mainly from small cohort studies.

Progestins induce durable responses in women with LG-ESS and have been used after surgical management or in recurrent setting [28]. Responses to AIs have also been reported, even after progression on progestins [28]. Therefore, HT with progestin or AIs is considered as the front-line treatment of metastatic or recurrent LG-ESS. Six retrospective studies enrolling 40 women with advanced or recurrent LG-ESS treated with progestins reported an overall response of approximately 50% with about 15% of women experiencing disease progression as the best response [28]. Correspondingly, seven retrospective studies reported that approximately 90% of the 50 enrolled women patients treated with AIs experienced clinical benefit, including an objective response in about 2/3 of all cases [28]. In terms of localised LG-ESS, the existing evidence is conflicting and the responses can be durable, there are no robust data to support the regular implementation of adjuvant HT. According to the ESMO-EURACAN guidelines, although adjuvant HT is not a current standard in LG-ESS, it might represent an alternative in this setting and can be considered for ER/PR positive disease [29]. HRT and tamoxifen are both contraindicated in cases of LG-ESS [29]. Ovarian preservation is associated with higher recurrence rates, thus, it may be an option only in a well-informed patient population [29].

12.4 Ovarian Cancer (OC)

12.4.1 Epithelial Ovarian Cancer (EOC)

Targeting oestrogen signaling in epithelial ovarian cancer (EOC) is supported by the compelling evidence suggesting that the majority of ovarian tumours express ER/PR and oestogens trigger OC cell proliferation and migration [30]. The recent study by Sieh et al., enrolling approximately 3000 women with invasive EOC undergoing central hormone receptor assay, demonstrated that the expression of ER and PR was associated with subtype-specific survival, with highest positivity for endometrioid carcinoma and low-grade serous carcinoma, intermediate for high-grade serous carcinoma, and lowest for mucinous carcinoma and clear-cell carcinoma [31]. In view of this evidence, HT, particularly tamoxifen and AIs, may be an invaluable treatment option in metastatic/recurrent EOC. A number of phase II trials have reported moderate RR and prognostic benefit amongst women with recurrent/metastatic EOC; notwithstanding, with wide variation in reported RR depending upon the different treatment modalities used [32].

A recent meta-analysis by Peleari et al. evaluated the effect of HT on EOC outcome [32]. The overall clinical benefit rate (CBR) was 43%. In the sub-group analyses, the reported CBRs were: tamoxifen (43%), AIs (41%), progestins (39%), and tamoxifen plus progestins (40%) respectively [32]. Of note, there was no statistical significance after stratification for chemoresistance or ER/PR status [32]. Finally, comparing the survival outcomes amongst six randomised controlled trials, the authors demonstrated a significant reduced risk of death (OR = 0.69) [32]. This evidence suggests that HT may induce a small but modest clinical benefit amongst patients with metastatic/recurrent EOC. Similarly with EC, the patient's selection for HT is mainly based upon ER/PR. Nonetheless, in the absence of other robust predictive markers and with the wide spread of novel treatment modalities, including anti-angiogenic agents and PARP inhibitors, it is likely that the use of HT, especially in the sub-group of high-grade serous EOC, will be confined to patients who have reached the end of the road with standard systemic therapy and no alternatives are available. There are currently ongoing phase II trials evaluating the combination of HT with mTOR or CDK4/6 inhibitors. A study of letrozole and everolimus in women with platinum-resistant/refractory EOC is currently recruiting patients (NCT0218850), whilst another trial of letrozole plus ribociclib in women with relapsed ER (+) OC is underway (NCT02657928).

In light of the marked ER/PR expression and platinum resistance [31], low-grade serous EOC seemingly represents an EOC sub-group with a higher reported clinical response. A recent retrospective study from the MD Anderson Cancer Centre group enrolling 203 women with stage II–IV low-grade serous EOC, who received maintenance HT following primary treatment demonstrated a better PFS in HT compared to surveillance group (64.9 vs. 26.4 months); notwithstanding, no significant difference in OS was observed between groups (102.7 vs. 115.7 months) [32]. In another observational study, HT was administered instead of chemotherapy after debulking surgery amongst women with low-grade serous EOC. The reported 3-year PFS and OS were 79% and 92.6%, respectively [33]. Although large randomised trials are warranted to provide more robust data, the existing evidence has rendered HT as a relatively effective treatment modality, which is currently at the forefront of treatment for advanced/recurrent low-grade EOC in clinical practice.

12.4.2 Granulosa Cell Tumours

Classified as sex cord stromal tumours, granulosa cell tumours (GCT) in the vast majority of cases express ER/PR [34]. Abnormal secretion of sex hormones is associated with clinical symptoms of hyper-oestrogenism or vitrilisation, respectively [34]. Based on these considerations, different HT modalities have been used in recurrent GCT. Possible mechanisms of action have been proposed for how HT may inhibit tumour growth in GCTs: (1) indirect action on tumour through suppression of gonadotropins or endogenous steroids; (2) direct effect on the tumour; (3) combination of the first two mechanisms [35].

A recent meta-analysis assessed the clinical response to HT in women with adult type ovarian GCT [35]. HT was given after multiple treatments of recurrences (median 2, range 1–7). The overall clinical RR was 71%, whilst the complete and partial RR was 25.8% and 45.2%, respectively. Anastrozole and letrozole yielded most complete and partial responses. These AIs as well as medroxyprogesterone acetate or megestrol acetate alternating with tamoxifen and diethylstilbestrol had a 100% response rate. Megestrol acetate, leuprolide plus tamoxifen, goserelin and leuprolide had response rates of 66.7%, 50%, 50% and 30%, respectively. The rarity of this condition makes randomized control studies almost impossible to perform so data from such meta-analyses have to be used to guide treatment. However, the existing evidence, deriving from small cohort studies, points to modest level of activity for HT in GCT, whilst the best available data thus far support the use of AIs or GnRH-agonists in women with recurrent GCT.

12.5 Summary

HT is an attractive treatment option for selected women with recurrent or metastatic endometrial cancer. It is also the treatment of choice for selected women with early-stage endometrial carcinoma wishing to maintain their fertility. It is currently recommended that HT have no role in the adjuvant treatment of endometrial cancer; yet, a post hoc analysis of PORTEC 3 trial showed that a sub-group of patients with specific molecular profile may benefit from adjuvant HT. The ongoing PORTEC 4a trial remains to confirm the aforementioned notion. The role of HT in the treatment of uterine sarcomas and granulosa cell tumours remains controversial. In light of the rarity of many of the tumour types, this evidence derives from phase II studies and case series. Recently, HT has been supplemented with targeted therapies, including mTOR inhibitors, which is a welcome development of immunotherapy. The main challenge remains of how to best identify women who are most likely to respond to HT. The development of additional markers or signatures and a better understanding of ER/PR pathway biology are pivotal to improving responses of women with gynaecological cancers and designing new targeted treatments.

Key Points

- Hormonal therapy with oral progestins and/or with levonorgestrel-releasing intrauterine device (LNG-IUD) is the treatment of choice amongst selected women with early-stage endometrial cancer, who wish to maintain their fertility.
- Hormonal therapy is currently not routinely recommended as adjuvant treatment of endometrial cancer. However, it might be considered for selected patients with specific molecular profile.
- Hormonal therapy is an attractive treatment option for selected women with recurrent or metastatic endometrial cancer.
- HT as a relatively effective treatment modality for advanced/recurrent low-grade EOC.
- Its role in the treatment of uterine sarcomas and granulosa cell tumours remains controversial, as the response rates vary significantly amongst studies.
- Hormonal therapy has been recently supplemented with targeted therapies, including mTOR inhibitors.
- The development of additional markers or signatures and a better understanding of ER/PR pathway biology are pivotal to improving responses of women with gynaecological cancers and designing new targeted treatments.

References

1. Sommeijer DW, Sjoquist KM, Friedlander M. Hormonal treatment in recurrent and metastatic gynaecological cancers: a review of the current literature. Curr Oncol Rep. 2013;15:541–8.
2. Yu Song J, Fraser IS. Effects of progestagens on human endometrium. Obstet Gynecol Surv. 1995;50:385–94.
3. Carlson MJ, Thiel KW, Leslie KK. Past, present, and future of hormonal therapy in recurrent endometrial cancer. Int J Women's Health. 2014;6:429–35.
4. Jerzak KJ, Duska L, McKay HJ. Endocrine therapy in endometrial cancer: an old dog with new tricks. Gynecol Oncol. 2019;153:175–83.
5. Bokhman JV. Two pathogenetic types of endometrial carcinoma. Gynecol Oncol. 1983;15:10–7.
6. Cancer Genome Atlas Research, Kandoth NC, Schultz N, et al. Integrated genomic characterisation go endometrial carcinoma. Nature. 2013;497:67–73.
7. Rodolakis A, Biliatis I, Morice P, Reed N, Mangler M, Kesic V, Denschlag D. European Society of Gynecological Oncology Task Force for fertility preservation: clinical recommendations for fertility-sparing management in young endometrial cancer patients. Int J Gynecol Cancer. 2015;25(7):1258–65.
8. Wei J, Zhang W, Feng L, Gao W. Comparison of fertility-sparing treatments in patients with early endometrial cancer and atypical complex hyperplasia. A meta-analysis and systematic review. Medicine (Baltimore). 2017;96(37):e8034.
9. Hall C, Stone RL, Gehlot A, et al. Use of metformin in obese women with type I endometrial cancer is associated with a reduced incidence of cancer recurrence. Int J Gynecol Cancer. 2016;26:313–7.
10. Mitsuhashi A, Sato Y, Kiyokawa T, et al. Phase II study of medroxyprogesterone acetate plus metformin as a fertility-sparing treatment for atypical endometrial hyperplasia and endometrial cancer. Ann Oncol. 2016;27:262–6.
11. Colombo N, Creutzberg C, Amant F, Bosse T, Gonzalez-Martin A, Ledermann J, et al. ESMO-ESGO-ESTRO consensus conference on endometrial cancer: diagnosis, treatment and follow-up. Int J Gynecol Cancer. 2016;26:2–30.
12. Martin-Hirsch PL, Jarvis G, Kitchener H, et al. Progestagens for endometrial cancer. Cochrane Database Syst Rev. 1999;4:CD001040.
13. Lentz SS, Brady MF, Major FJ, et al. High-dose megestrol acetate in advanced or recurrent endometrial carcinoma: a Gynecologic Oncology Group Study. J Clin Oncol. 1996;14:357–61.
14. Whitney CW, Brunetto V, Zaino RJ, et al. Phase II study of medroxyprogesterone acetate plus tamoxifen in advanced endometrial carcinoma: a Gynecologic Oncology Group study. Gynecol Oncol. 2004;92:4–9.
15. Florica JV, Brunetto V, Hanjani P, et al. Phase II trial of alternating courses of megestrol acetate and tamoxifen in advanced endometrial carcinoma: a Gynecologic Oncology Group study. Gynecol Oncol. 2004;92:10–4.
16. van Weelden WJ, Massuger LFAG, Pijnenborg JMA, Romano A. Anti-estrogen treatment in endometrial cancer: a systematic review. Front Oncologia. 2019;9:359.
17. Ayoub J, Audet-Lapointe P, Methot Y, Hanley J, Beaulieu R, Chemaly R, et al. Efficacy of sequential cyclical hormonal therapy in endometrial cancer and its correlation with steroid hormone receptor status. Gynecol Oncol. 1988;31:327–37.
18. Zhang G, Cheng Y, Zhang Q, Li X, Zhou J, Wang J, et al. ATX-LPA axis facilitates oestrogen-induced endometrial cancer cell proliferation via MAPK/ERK singling pathway. Mol Med Rep. 2018;17:4245–52.

19. Fleming GF, Filiaci VL, Marzullo B, Zaino RJ, Davidson SA, Pearl M, et al. Temsirolimus with or without megestrol acetate and tamoxifen for endometrial cancer: a gynecologic oncology group study. Gynecol Oncol. 2014;132:585–92.
20. Slomovitz BM, Jiang Y, Yates MS, Soliman PT, Johnston T, Nowakowski M, et al. Phase II study of everolimus and letrozole in patients with recurrent endometrial carcinoma. J Clin Oncol. 2015;33:930–6.
21. Soliman PT, Westin SN, Iglesias DA, Fellman B, Yuan Y, Zhang Q, Yates M, et al. Everolimus, letrozole, and metformin in women with advanced or recurrent endometrioid endometrial cancer: a multicenter, single arm, phase II study. Clin Cancer Res. 2020;26:581–7.
22. Colon-Otero G, Zanfagnin V, Hou X, Foster NR, Asmus EJ, Hendrickson AW, Jatoi A, et al. Phase II trial of ribociclib and letrozole in patients with relapsed oestrogen receptor-positive ovarian or endometrial cancers. ESMO Open. 2020;5(5):e000926.
23. Leitao MM, Hensley ML, Barakat RR, Aghajanian C, Gardner CJ, Jewell EL, et al. Immunohistochemical expression of estrogen and progesterone receptors and outcomes in patients with newly diagnosed uterine leiomyosarcoma. Gynecol Oncol. 2012;124:558–62.
24. George S, Feng Y, Manola J, Nucci MR, Butrynski JE, Morgan JA, Ramaiya N, Quek R, Penson RT, Wagner AJ, Harmon D, Demetri GD, Krasner C. Phase 2 trial of aromatase inhibition with letrozole in patients with uterine leiomyosarcomas expressing estrogen and/or progesterone receptors. Cancer. 2014;120:738–43.
25. Slomovitz BM, Taub MC, Huang M, Levenback C, Coleman RL. A randomized phase II study of letrozole vs. observation in patients with newly diagnosed uterine leiomyosarcoma (uLMS) Gynecol. Oncol Rep. 2018;27:1–4.
26. Thanopoulou E, Thway K, Khabra K, Judson I. Treatment of hormone positive uterine leiomyosarcoma with aromatase inhibitors. Clin Sarcoma Res. 2014;26:4–5.
27. Yoon A, Park JY, Park JY, Lee YY, Kim TJ, Choi CH, et al. Prognostic factors and outcomes in endometrial stromal sarcoma with the 2009 FIGO staging system: a multicenter review of 114 cases. Gynecol Oncol. 2014;2014(132):70–5.
28. Zhang YY, Li Y, Qin M, Cai Y, Jin Y, Pan LY. High-grade endometrial stromal sarcoma: a retrospective study of factors influencing prognosis. Cancer Manag Res. 2019;11:831–7.
29. Casali PG, Abecassis N, Bauer S, Biagini R, Bielack S, Bonvalot S, Boukovinas I, et al. ESMO Guidelines Committee and EURACAN. Soft tissue and visceral sarcomas: ESMO-EURACAN Clinical Practice Guidelines for diagnosis, treatment and follow-up. Ann Oncol. 2018;29:iv51–67.
30. Andersen CL, Sikora MM, Boisen MM, et al. Active estrogen receptor-alpha signaling in ovarian cancer models and clinical specimens. Clin Cancer Res. 2017;23:3802–12.
31. Paleari L, Gandini S, Provinciali N, Puntoni M, Colombo N, DeCensi A. Clinical benefit and risk of death with endocrine therapy in ovarian cancer: a comprehensive review and meta-analysis. Gynecol Oncol. 2017;146:504–13.
32. Gershenson DM, Bodurka DC, Coleman RL, et al. Hormonal maintenance therapy for women with low grade serous carcinoma of the ovary or peritoneum. J Clin Oncol. 2017;35(10):1103–11.
33. Fader AN, Bergstrom J, Jernigan A, et al. Primary cytoreductive surgery and adjuvant hormonal mono therapy in women with advanced low-grade serous ovarian carcinoma: reducing over treatment without compromising survival? Gynecol Oncol. 2017;147:85–91.
34. Farinola MA, Gown AM, Judson K, et al. Estrogen receptor alpha and progesterone receptor expression in ovarian adult granulosa cell tumors and Sertoli-Leydig cell tumors. Int J Gynecol Pathol. 2007;26:375–82.
35. van Meurs HS, van Lonkhuijzen LRCW, Limpens J, van der Velden J, Buist MR. Hormone therapy in ovarian granulosa cell tumors: a systematic review. Gynecol Oncol. 2014;134:196–205.

13. Radiation Protocols Relevant for Gynaecological Oncology and Management of Complications

Beshar Allos, Indrajit N. Fernando, and Nawaz Walji

13.1 Introduction to Radiotherapy

Radiotherapy utilises ionising radiation mainly to treat invasive cancers; it can also be used to treat some pre-invasive tumours and benign conditions. The aim of radiotherapy treatment is to irradicate cancer by delivering a high radiation dose whilst minimising the impact on surrounding healthy tissues and organs which are referred to as organs at risk (OAR).

Gynaecological malignancies are commonly treated with external beam radiotherapy (EBRT) and brachytherapy. Concurrent chemoradiation (CCRT), where chemotherapy is given synchronously with EBRT, is a standard of care for the treatment of advanced cervical cancer. Advanced radiotherapy techniques such as Image Guided Radiotherapy (IGRT) together with Intensity-Modulated Radiotherapy (IMRT) or Volumetric Modulated Arc Therapy (VMAT) have largely replaced other techniques including conformal radiotherapy or virtual simulation and conventional radiotherapy. Intra-cavity (ICBT) and vaginal brachytherapy (VBT) are commonly used for the treatment of cervical, endometrial and vaginal cancers; interstitial brachytherapy (ISBT) is gaining increasing traction in the treatment of cervical cancer but can also be used to treat cancers of the vulva and vagina.

13.1.1 Radiation Physics

Radiation dose is measured in Grays (Gy) where 1 Gy equates to 1 J/kg. The majority of radiotherapy is delivered using megavoltage x-rays (photons) which form part of the electromagnetic spectrum. Photons are produced by colliding electrons with a heavy metal target (e.g. tungsten) inside a machine called a linear accelerator (see Fig. 13.1). The photons are subsequently directed as a beam towards the treatment target producing therapeutic tissue ionisation. Higher energy photons are associated with greater tissue penetration; typically pelvic EBRT requires photon energies between 6 and 10 megavolts (MV).

Therapeutic irradiation can also be delivered by particulates including electrons, protons and neutrons. Proton beam therapy (PBT) is delivered using a cyclotron. Its main advantage is that it can be used to treat deep-seated tumours with a rapid dose fall off that occurs once the beam has reached its peak (called the Bragg peak) thus reducing the dose to surrounding OAR. PBT is

---

B. Allos (✉) · I. N. Fernando
Cancer Centre, University Hospitals Birmingham NHS Foundation Trust, Birmingham, UK
e-mail: Beshar.allos@uhb.nhs.uk;
Indrajit.fernando@uhb.nhs.uk

N. Walji
Arden Cancer Centre, University Hospitals Coventry and Warwickshire NHS Trust, Coventry, UK
e-mail: Nawaz.walji@uhcw.nhs.uk

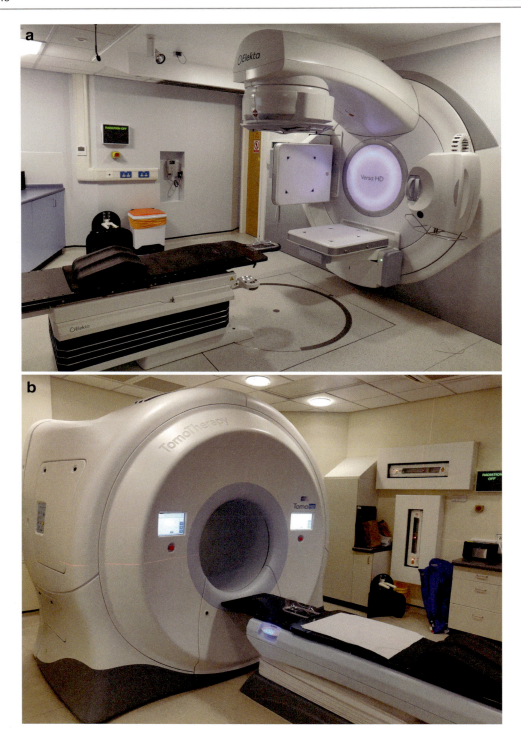

Fig. 13.1 A linear accelerator (**a**) and a tomotherapy unit (**b**) in a radiotherapy treatment room. Both deliver IMRT. The linear accelerator rotates 360° around the treatment couch, thus is able to deliver multiple beams in multiple directions, either via arcs or fixed positions. Tomotherapy uses a continuous 360° helical fan-beam technique to deliver ionising radiation

mainly utilised for the treatment of paediatric cancers, prostate cancer and cancers of the central nervous system in adults; future indications for treatment may expand, including its use in gynaecological cancers, with the greater availability of cyclotrons and as results from a number of trials looking at the benefit of PBT in other cancer sites become available.

High-energy electrons are produced in linear accelerators by removing the heavy metal target. Electrons are mainly used to treat superficial cancers (typically at a depth no more than 3 cm) as electron beams are rapidly attenuated by tissues. They are mainly used in the treatment of cancers of the vulva in the context of managing gynaecological malignancies.

Brachytherapy involves the placement of a sealed radioactive source either within close proximity of or directly into tumours to deliver a dose of radiation. It takes advantage of the inverse square law (radiation dose is inversely proportional to the square of the distance from the source) allowing delivery of a very high of dose of radiotherapy to the tumour with relative sparing of surrounding OAR. It involves treatment with gamma-rays which are produced from the decay of radioactive isotopes. Iridium-192 is commonly used to deliver high-dose-rate (HDR) brachytherapy treatment which has largely replaced low-dose-rate treatment for the management of gynaecological malignancies.

13.1.2 Radiobiology

Radiotherapy initiates cell death via irreparable deoxyribonucleic acid (DNA) damage leading to cessation of uncontrolled cell division which is the hallmark of invasive cancers. Such cell kill also affects normal cells which leads to the side effects caused by radiotherapy. The ability of ionising radiation to successfully kill cancer cells revolves around the five "Rs" of radiobiology: radiosensitivity, repair, repopulation, reoxygenation and redistribution (see Table 13.1).

Intrinsic tumour radiosensitivity is considered to be the most important factor, however, in order to get the best therapeutic outcome, all the five "Rs" need to be optimised. For example prolongation of overall treatment time beyond 56 days is associated with poorer outcomes (due to the impact of repopulation) in the treatment of cervical carcinoma, as is a haemoglobin concentration below 120 g/L during treatment (effect of reoxygenation) [1].

Normal cells have a greater ability than cancer cells to repair themselves following sublethal DNA damage provided the total radiation dose does not exceed the tolerance dose. Thus fractionated radiotherapy (the process of dividing a total dose of radiation into multiple small treatments called fractions) is advantageous as it allows normal cells to repopulate and repair in-between fractions but also allows for reoxygenation and redistribution of cancer cells into the active cell cycle, both of which improve the radiosensitivity of the cancer being treated with radiotherapy. Radiotherapy is normally delivered at a dose of 1.8–2 Gy per fraction.

Another concept to consider is the long-term health of OAR which is dependent on that tissue/organ's own tolerance range. A tolerance dose of any given OAR is the maximum dose that organ can receive before harm is done, potentially leading to functional damage. Tolerance doses are based on dose delivered using 2 Gy per fraction. Another parameter for assessing radiation side effects is the TD5/5 for a given organ. This is the estimated dose that gives a 5% chance of a late effect occurring in 5 years following radiotherapy. There are many factors to consider when assessing the probability of late effects to OAR including fraction size, volume of tissue treated, total dose, concurrent use of chemotherapy and pre-existing patient comorbidities (e.g. diabetes, connective tissue disorders, inflammatory bowel disease, presence of adhesions) [2]. In gynaecological radiotherapy, the tolerance doses of the bladder, rectum and small bowel must be respected when planning treatment in order to avoid long-term toxicity.

Table 13.1 The five "Rs" of radiobiology

Radiobiological Factor	Mechanism	Clinical relevance
Radiosensitivity	Tumour cells and normal cells have varying radiosensitivity	Responses can vary between histological types—squamous cell cancers and lymphomas are relatively more radiosensitive compared to melanomas or gliomas
Repair	Not all DNA damage caused is irreparable, late-responding tissue (usually non/low-proliferating cells) are effective at DNA repair	DNA damage can be repaired by some tumour cells leading to treatment failure
Repopulation	Once radiotherapy commences, surviving cells in acute responding tissues can regrow at a faster rate	Minimising overall treatment time and avoiding treatment gaps is beneficial in reducing this phenomenon
Reoxygenation	Tumour cells are generally hypoxic but surviving cells reoxygenate over time so improving radiosensitivity	Ensuring patients are not anaemic improves outcomes in radiotherapy. Overall treatment times should equally not be too short to allow for reoxygenation of cells
Redistribution	Cells redistribute between different phases of the cell cycle during radiotherapy. Cells in the resting phase are relatively radioresistant	During a course of radiotherapy, cells redistribute from resting phase to the active cell cycle, where they are more radiosensitive allowing for increased cell kill

13.2 Radiotherapy Toxicity

Pelvic radiotherapy, including EBRT and brachytherapy cause unwanted side effects, the extent of which is dependent upon both tumour-related and patient-related factors. This morbidity can leave long-term physical and psychological damage. Broadly speaking, radiotherapy related side effects are divided into early effects—occurring within 90 days of treatment—and late effects, which can develop months or years following completion of treatment. The main OAR are the bladder, rectum and small bowel (see Table 13.2).

13.2.1 Radiotherapy Dose-Fractionation

Standard radiation therapy is delivered using once daily treatment for 5 days a week, prescribing 1.8–2 Gy per fraction, typically over a period of 5–7 weeks. The dose prescription includes the total dose (in Gy), the number of fractions over which the dose will be delivered, and the total length of time required to deliver the treatment. The equivalent dose in 2 Gy fractions (EQD2) is quoted when prescribing radiotherapy using

Table 13.2 Early and late effects of radiotherapy on normal organs

Organ	Early effect	Late effect
Bladder and ureter	Radiation cystitis—frequency, urgency, dysuria	Bladder dysfunction Fistulae Haematuria
Rectum	Radiation proctitis—frequency, urgency, diarrhoea	Radiation proctitis Altered bowel habit Fistulae Stenosis
Small bowel	Nausea and sickness	Fistulae Stenosis Enteropathy
Bone		Insufficiency fractures Osteoradionecrosis
Lymph nodes		Lymphoedema
Skin	Erythema Desquamation	Telangiectasia Fibrosis
Vagina	Mucositis—bleeding, discharge	Fistulae Stenosis
Ovaries		Infertility Early menopause
Spinal cord		Myelopathy
Kidneys		Renal failure
General		Loss of libido Secondary cancers

more than 2 Gy per fraction. This EQD2 figure helps to rationalise different dose/fractionation schedules into a comparable standard.

The total dose prescribed varies depending on the purpose of treatment. Typically, a dose of 45–50.4 Gy over 23–28 fractions is prescribed for the adjuvant treatment of gynaecological cancers where the aim is to treat potential areas of microscopic disease to prevent disease recurrence. Conversely radical treatment delivered for tumour eradication requires doses exceeding 60 Gy. For advanced cervical cancers for instance, an EQD2 of 80–85 Gy is recommended [3].

Hypofractionated radiotherapy entails treatment using more than 2 Gy per fraction delivered over fewer fractions. The total dose prescribed is reduced in order to keep to an equivalent dose in 2 Gy per fraction (EQD2). Advanced radiotherapy techniques such as IGRT with IMRT or VMAT make it possible to deliver higher radiation doses to areas of macroscopic disease using hypofractionated radiotherapy without prolonging overall treatment duration times.

Palliative radiotherapy, for instance to control bleeding or treat pain, is typically delivered with hypofractionated radiotherapy over one, five or ten fractions which is more convenient for patients.

13.3 Radiotherapy Treatment Planning and Delivery

EBRT and brachytherapy are the two primary techniques used in gynaecological radiotherapy, with EBRT being the most commonly used modality. EBRT starts with the planning process. A planning CT scan of the pelvis (and abdomen if treating para-aortic lymph nodes), using 2–3 mm slices of the area being treated, is acquired with the patient in the treatment position. Intravenous contrast is administered to assist with delineation of lymph node basins. Tattoos laterally and anteriorly are required to maintain patient positioning and alignment for each subsequent treatment and patients must be immobilised comfortably throughout the course. A bladder filling protocol is initiated to reduce the amount of bowel in the treatment field. Enemas are used to minimise the impact of bowel distension on radiotherapy planning.

The planning CT scan is used to delineate the target volumes. The Gross Tumour Volume (GTV) is created by delineating the tumour on the planning CT scan. The diagnostic MRI scan, or an MRI scan taken in the RT planning position, can be fused with the planning CT scan to help with GTV delineation. Any enlarged lymph nodes suspicious for involvement by cancer are delineated as a separate GTV for treatment with simultaneous integrated boost (SIB). In postoperative radiotherapy the GTV doesn't exist.

The GTV is grown to include areas of potential microscopic disease to form the Clinical Target Volume (CTV). A margin may be added to the CTV to account for internal organ motion which can impact the shape or position of the CTV; this is called the Internal Target Volume (ITV). A margin is added to the ITV to account for day-to-day set up uncertainties to create the final Planning Target Volume (PTV); the PTV margin can also account for internal organ motion if the ITV is not created. The PTV is the target to which radiotherapy is planned to for delivery of the treatment dose taking into account the OAR, which are also delineated on the planning CT scan. The purpose of radiotherapy treatment is to deliver a dose of radiation which is sufficient to eradicate areas of macroscopic and microscopic disease without exceeding the dose tolerance constraints of the OAR within close proximity of the PTV.

IGRT combined with IMRT or VMAT allow for a higher dose conformity to the PTV by using multi-leaf collimators (MLC) within the beam head, whose positions can be varied in time as the gantry moves, to deliver beams of varying intensity and shaped to the PTV (see Fig. 13.2). This also enables multiple PTVs to be treated to different dose levels, including dose escalation (SIB) within a single plan, thus permitting treatment times to be maintained and removing the need for multiple phases of treatment. This more precise delivery of radiotherapy also leads to lower doses to OAR thus reducing the risk of both early and late effects from treatment [4, 5]. The downside to IMRT is that it leads to a larger volume of tissue overall receiving a low dose of radiation, the "low dose bath". Long-term consequences of this are unknown but such risks are outweighed by the perceived benefits of IMRT. We await the results of prospective long-term studies to confirm this is the case.

13.4 Brachytherapy

Brachytherapy is an integral component for the curative treatment of gynaecological cancers. Brachytherapy is the only demonstrated method of delivering doses >80 Gy for the treatment of

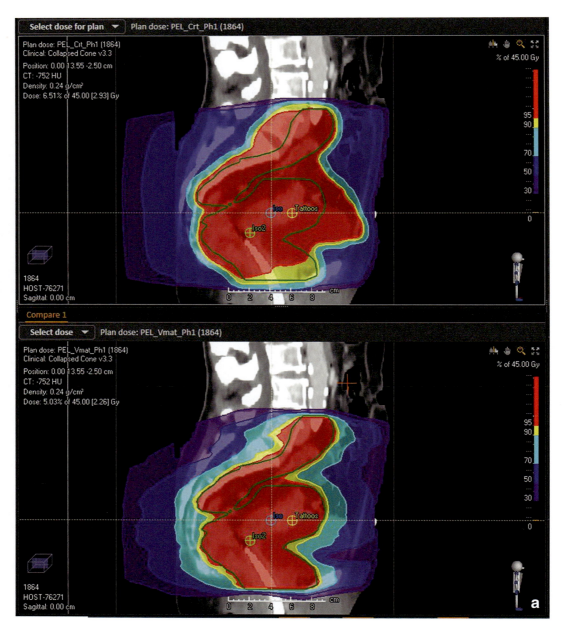

Fig. 13.2 An axial (**a**) and sagittal (**b**) CT slice from a radical cervical cancer radiotherapy plan aiming to treat the cervix, uterus, parametria and pelvic lymph nodes. The green volume outlines the PTV. The red zones demonstrate the high-dose area. The upper slices represent a standard 4-field conformal plan. The lower slices represent the same PTV planned with IMRT and demonstrates the benefit IMRT brings in reducing the amount of normal tissue exposed to higher doses of radiotherapy

13 Radiation Protocols Relevant for Gynaecological Oncology and Management of Complications 153

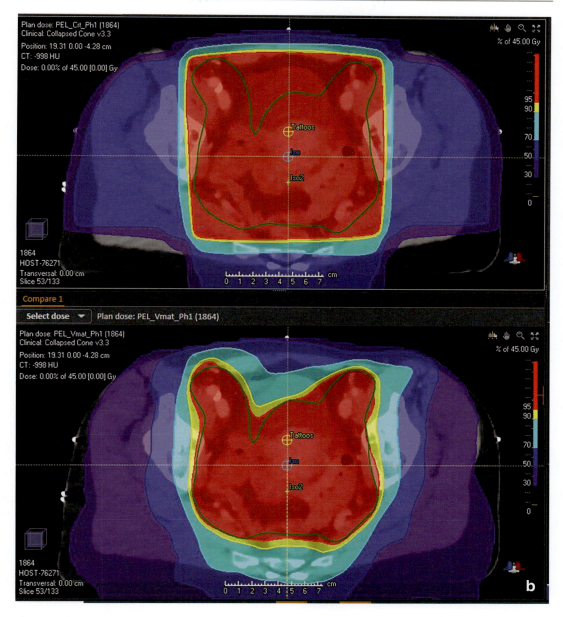

Fig. 13.2 (continued)

advanced cervical cancer whilst minimising the dose received by the OAR. Failure to deliver brachytherapy in cervical carcinoma is associated with poorer outcomes [6].

In the management of cervical cancer brachytherapy is commonly delivered following, or towards the end of, CCRT which allows for maximum tumour shrinkage and smaller brachytherapy treatment volumes [7]. Brachytherapy is performed using ICBT alone or in combination with ISBT. An MRI scan of the pelvis performed in the final week of CCRT is useful to assess treatment response and aid with brachytherapy planning, including assessing the need for ISBT.

ICBT is the most commonly practiced method of brachytherapy. The two commonly used applicator systems for ICBT include a tandem and ovoid or tandem and ring design. ISBT involves the placement of hollow catheters directly into tumour and is indicated where the residual disease following CCRT is not likely to be adequately covered with ICBT alone.

Prior to the insertion of applicators for brachytherapy patients must have bloodwork measured and receive appropriate treatment to correct anaemia or hypomagnesaemia resulting from CCRT. Patients who are neutropenic require antibiotic cover. The applicators are usually inserted in an operating theatre under general or spinal anaesthesia which may be given with light sedation. An examination is undertaken in the lithotomy position to assess tumour response following which a Foley catheter is inserted in the urinary bladder. Trans-abdominal or trans-rectal ultrasound may be used to guide insertion of the tandem into the endometrial cavity. Hollow catheters to deliver ISBT are inserted once the tandem and ovoid/ring applicator is in place (see Fig. 13.3).

Image guided brachytherapy (IGBT) is considered the standard of care for the delivery of brachytherapy treatment. Following insertion of the applicators an MRI is performed to reconstruct the applicators and delineate the residual tumour—referred to as the high-risk CTV (HR-CTV)—and the OAR. A CT scan may be required to delineate any catheters inserted for ISBT. Following delineation of the HR-CTV and OAR, a plan is produced to optimise treatment and the dose is prescribed is treat the HR-CTV (see Figs. 13.4 and 13.5). Alternatively, the dose may be prescribed to the ICRU reference point A if not treating with IGBT.

Patients are commonly treated with 3–5 fractions of IGBT. Where access to theatre proves challenging, applicators may be kept in-situ and patients may be treated with two or more fractions with a single insertion provided there is an inter-fraction gap of more than 6 h. In such instances caution must be exercised to ensure the applicators have not moved and a repeat CT scan prior to each treatment can help with determining the dose received by the OAR.

ISBT is also used in the treatment of primary vaginal cancer and vaginal metastases arising from endometrial or cervical cancers. Typically, this is done following EBRT or CCRT although in some instances ISBT may be used as the primary treatment modality. A perineal template is utilised to insert hollow catheters into the tumour typically under trans-rectal ultrasound guidance. An MRI and/or CT scan is undertaken following placement of the catheters to delineate the target volume and OAR and to assist with planning of treatment. Treatment is typically delivered with 4–6 fractions over 2–3 days with a minimum inter-fraction gap of 6 h. ISBT for treatment of vaginal cancers can also be undertaken by placing radioactive seeds directly into the tumour using a perineal template.

VBT is used in the adjuvant treatment of intermediate and intermediate-high risk endometrial cancer; it can also be used following EBRT to deliver an additional dose to the CTV in the treatment of endometrial and vaginal cancer. Treatment is delivered using a vaginal cylinder which is typically inserted in the brachytherapy treatment suite. The dose is prescribed at 5 mm from the surface of the applicator with treatment typically being delivered over 2–3 fractions depending on indication for treatment.

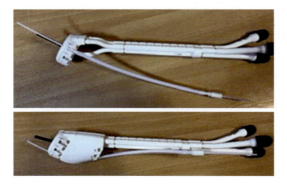

Fig. 13.3 The Venezia applicator used for ICBT and ISBT. The top image demonstrates the tandem and ovoid set-up with one interstitial needle placed. The bottom image is the same applicator but with an additional vaginal cap meaning upper vaginal disease can also be treated with ISBT

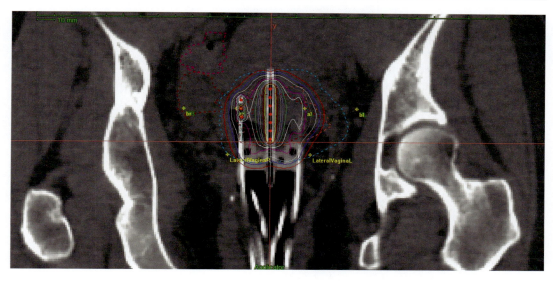

Fig. 13.4 A coronal CT slice from an ISBT plan utilising bilateral interstitial needles for ISBT to treat large residual disease post CCRT. HR-CTV is delineated as the light red dotted line

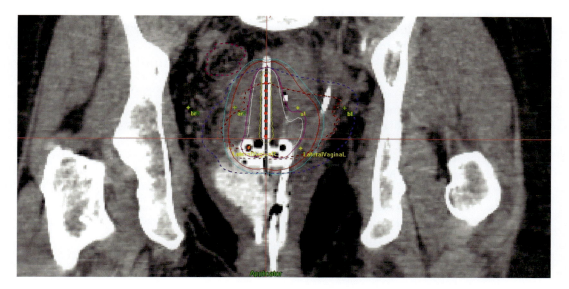

Fig. 13.5 A coronal CT slice from an ISBT plan utilising an oblique interstitial needle for ISBT to treat pelvic side wall disease. HR-CTV once again demonstrated by the light red dotted line

13.5 Radiotherapy in Endometrial Cancer

The majority of patients diagnosed with endometrial cancer present with organ confined disease thus proceed with surgery as the primary treatment modality. The main role of radiotherapy in the management of endometrial cancer is to reduce the risk of pelvic recurrence; treatment with adjuvant radiotherapy does not improve overall survival [8].

Following surgery patients can be categorised in to four risk groups based on parameters derived from the final histology assessment, which include tumour grade, FIGO stage, and presence of lymphovascular space invasion (LVSI) [9].

Table 13.3 summarises the different risk groups based on final histology and potential treatment options for each risk group.

Whilst effective in reducing the risk of disease recurrence, EBRT can be associated with an increased risk of late effects impacting on long-term bowel and bladder function. VBT provides an equally effective option for the treatment of intermediate risk disease and also for high-intermediate risk disease where lymph node dissection has been undertaken [10].

Adjuvant EBRT is recommended for the adjuvant treatment of high-intermediate risk disease where a lymph node dissection has not been performed, and for those with high-risk disease. A dose of 45–50.4 Gy in 25–28 fractions is prescribed; VBT at a dose of 6–12 Gy in 1–2 fractions can be used following EBRT in those with cervical involvement.

The PORTEC3 trial compared CCRT followed by adjuvant chemotherapy with radiotherapy only for the adjuvant treatment of high-risk endometrial cancer [11]. Patients in the experimental arm received a dose of 48.6 Gy in 27 fractions alongside two cycles of concurrent cisplatin chemotherapy followed by four cycles of adjuvant chemotherapy with paclitaxel and carboplatin. A statistically significant survival advantage of 5% was demonstrated in a post-hoc analysis at the expense of an increase in grade 3 adverse events. A statistically significant difference was demonstrated for serous cancers and those with stage 3 disease. As the experimental arm included the addition of concurrent and adjuvant chemotherapy, it remains uncertain whether the overall survival benefit was due to CCRT, adjuvant chemotherapy, or both. As a consequence, the practice of giving adjuvant chemotherapy followed by EBRT is accepted as a standard of care for patients with stage 3 disease and those with non-endometrioid histology.

The management of inoperable endometrial cancer, either due to disease stage or patient co-morbidities, presents a challenge. Some patients may be treated with downstaging chemotherapy in order to render the cancer operable. Where

Table 13.3 Risk stratification for endometrial cancer post-operative with possible adjuvant treatment options

Risk category	Histology features	Adjuvant treatment options
Low	• Low grade (grade 1 or 2), stage 1A, no or focal LVSI	• No adjuvant treatment
Intermediate	• Low grade (grade 1 or 2), stage 1B, no or focal LVSI • High grade (grade 3), stage 1A, no or focal LVSI • Non-endometrioid histology (serous, clear cell, undifferentiated, carcinosarcoma, mixed), stage 1A (no myometrial invasion)	• VBT • No adjuvant treatment
High-intermediate	• Stage 1 endometrioid with substantial LVSI regardless of grade and depth of invasion • Stage 1B, grade 3 endometrioid, regardless of LVSI status • Stage 2	• EBRT • VBT only (if lymph node dissection performed)
High risk	• Stage 3–4A, with no residual disease • Non-endometrioid histology (serous, clear cell, undifferentiated, carcinosarcoma, mixed), stage 1–4A with myometrial invasion, no residual disease	• CCRT and adjuvant chemotherapy • Adjuvant chemotherapy with sequential EBRT
Advanced/metastatic	• Stage 1–4A with residual disease • Stage 4B	• Adjuvant chemotherapy with sequential EBRT including SIB to macroscopic residual disease • Palliative treatment if disease cannot be encompassed with high dose EBRT treatment

such an approach is not feasible, definitive radical radiotherapy may provide a treatment option and can provide good disease control in early stages [12]. Treatment consists of EBRT to the pelvis treating with 45–50.4 Gy in 25–28 fractions followed by ICBT prescribing 21–28 Gy in 3–4 fractions. In selected patients where the disease is confined to the endometrium based on radiology brachytherapy alone can be considered, again with high local control rates, but such practice is rare [13].

13.6 Radiotherapy in Cervical Cancer

Patients with stage IA1-IB2 are treated with primary surgery; those with stage II-IVA disease are treated with primary chemoradiotherapy. Patients with stage IB3-IIA disease can be treated with surgery or CCRT with equivalent survival rates [14]. The decision to treat with surgery or radiotherapy is based on factors such as tumour size, histology (squamous cell cancer or adenocarcinoma) and patient co-morbidities.

Following surgery adjuvant CCRT is indicated (or radiotherapy alone if chemotherapy is contra-indicated) in the presence of high-risk features including node positive disease; parametrial spread; or a positive margin. Radiotherapy alone is considered if one or more of the following moderate risk factors are present: deep stromal invasion; lymphovascular space invasion is present; or tumour size is >4 cm, adenocarcinoma histological type. In such cases if the patient is fit with limited co-morbidities then concurrent chemotherapy can be added. Accepted dose schedules delivered to the pelvis and lymph nodes include 45–50.4 Gy in 25–28 fractions.

Primary CCRT involves EBRT to the primary tumour and lymph nodes followed by ICBT and ISBT (where indicated). Total treatment time for both phases should not exceed 56 days in total in order to not detrimentally effect local control or cure rates [15]. Typical dose ranges for EBRT, delivered via IMRT technique, are 45–50.4 Gy in 25–28 fractions over 5–5.5 weeks. Involved pelvic or para-aortic lymph nodes can be boosted to 55–57.5 Gy in 25–28 fractions via a simultaneous integrated boost (SIB) or sequential boost if considered more appropriate.

Concurrent chemotherapy is given with 5–6 cycles of weekly Cisplatin 40 mg/m^2 provided the patient has a WHO performance status of 0–1 and sufficient renal function. The addition of chemotherapy to EBRT has been shown to improve overall survival, progression-free survival and reduce local and distant relapse rates [16]. However, both early and some late toxicity is increased with the addition of chemotherapy. Radiotherapy alone is given if chemotherapy is contra-indicated.

13.7 Radiotherapy in Vulval Cancer

The cornerstone of management of vulval cancer is surgery. Surgery for advanced cancers may be associated with significant morbidity. EBRT, with or without chemotherapy, provides an alternate treatment option for the management of advanced disease in patients who are not fit for surgical management and in those with stage 4B disease confined to the involvement of pelvic lymph nodes only.

Adjuvant radiotherapy can be given following surgery to reduce the risk of local recurrence. Whilst there is a paucity of data, published evidence suggests that adjuvant EBRT reduces the risk of local recurrence in patients with close or positive resection margins [17]. The presence of two or more positive inguinal nodes or extracapsular spread, is another indication for adjuvant EBRT further. The GROINSS-V-II study is assessing the role of EBRT in sentinel node positive disease. Interim analysis suggests there may be a role for adjuvant treatment with EBRT in the presence of micrometastatic disease ($\leq$2 mm). In such patients, inguinal recurrence rate was 3.8% with minimal toxicity [18]. This practice has presently not been widely adopted yet.

The whole vulva, bilateral inguinal nodal chains and pelvic lymph nodes up to the level of common iliac vessels bifurcating should be treated. A recommended dose of 45–50 Gy in 25 fractions over 5 weeks is given. There is no evidence for adding concurrent chemotherapy in the adjuvant setting but practice varies with some centres treating with concurrent weekly cisplatin based on data extrapolated from the treatment of cervical cancer.

Patients with inoperable disease receiving EBRT as the definitive treatment require a higher treatment dose to the primary tumour and involved lymph nodes. Increasingly, this is delivered with IMRT using the SIB approach whereby potential areas of microscopic disease receive 45 Gy in 25 fractions and areas of macroscopic disease receiving a dose of 60 Gy in 25 fractions. Good response rates are garnered from EBRT often with both complete clinical and pathological responses seen.

CCRT improves relapse-free and overall survival for the definitive treatment of vulval cancers [19]. Patients with WHO PS 0–1 and adequate renal function are commonly treated with concurrent weekly cisplatin; alternative options include treatment with cisplatin and fluorouracil (5-FU) or mitomycin C and 5-FU.

Recurrent disease can often be removed with more radical surgery. However, in the EBRT-naïve patient, CCRT is an alternative to surgery and gives good long-term disease control [20].

13.8 Radiotherapy in Vaginal Cancer

Primary vaginal cancer is rare and as such there is a paucity of high quality published evidence to guide the management of vaginal cancer. Surgery may be considered for the treatment early stage I cancers. Treatment with radiotherapy is the mainstay of treatment otherwise.

In general terms, cancers arising in the upper third of the vagina are treated akin to cervical cancers and those arising in the lower third of the vagina are treated akin to vulval cancers. Definitive treatment is normally delivered with EBRT followed by brachytherapy (vaginal or interstitial). ISBT provides a better treatment option for bulky residual disease following EBRT. Small or superficial cancers not amenable to surgical resection can be treated with ISBT alone. Where it is not feasible to treat with brachytherapy, a radical dose of radiotherapy can be delivered either with SIB or using multiple treatment phases.

Concurrent chemotherapy with Cisplatin can be used alongside EBRT with the data taken from the cervical cancer experience. Therapy with this combination of treatment, utilising radiotherapy doses between 70 and 80 Gy EQD2 appear to confer a survival advantage [21].

13.9 Radiotherapy for Palliation

Palliative EBRT alone can be used to treat symptoms such as bleeding or pain in patients with metastatic disease, or localised disease otherwise not fit for surgery nor radical chemoradiotherapy. Typical doses used include 8 Gy in one fraction, 20 Gy in five fractions or 30 Gy in ten fractions. As the primary aim is symptom control with less emphasis on protecting OAR, simple radiotherapy plans can be delivered with conventional radiotherapy.

13.10 Summary

Radiotherapy is an important treatment in the management of gynaecological malignancies utilising different modalities including EBRT and brachytherapy. Radiotherapy as a primary treatment for cervical and vulval cancers gives good responses and outcomes, especially with the addition of concurrent chemotherapy, but this must be balanced against toxicity associated with treatment. It is, thus, a good alternative to surgery in such patients whom are inoperable or unfit for resection. Adjuvant radiotherapy reduces the risk of local recurrence and is widely used in endometrial cancer. Palliative radiotherapy in advanced malignancy gives good symptomatic relief from symptoms including bleeding and pain.

Key Points
1. Most radiotherapy is delivered using high-energy megavoltage x-rays created by a linear accelerator or through radioactive isotopes placed in applicators during brachytherapy. Both techniques are commonly used in gynaecological cancers.
2. Radiation doses are fractionated in order to allows normal cells to repopulate and repair in-between fractions but also to improve the radiosensitivity of the target tumour through reoxygenation and redistribution of cancer cells into the active cell cycle.
3. Advancements in therapeutic EBRT techniques has led to IMRT becoming the standard of care as it offers more precise delivery of radiotherapy to the target PTV whilst also lowering doses to OAR.
4. Early and late effects of radiation on OAR, including those on the bladder, gastrointestinal system and vagina, can have a substantial long-term impact on a patient's quality of life.
5. CCRT with cisplatin chemotherapy is widely accepted as gold standard management for cervical and vulval cancers when considering a radical non-surgical approach.
6. Brachytherapy can deliver high doses of radiation to localised areas by virtue of the principle of inverse square law, thus also minimising dose to surrounding OAR. It is an integral component in the radical management of cervical cancers.
7. IGBT is considered the standard of care for the delivery of brachytherapy treatment, utilising ICBT alone or in combination with ISBT.
8. The management of endometrial cancer in the adjuvant setting is based on postoperative risk-stratification and can range from surgical follow-up to adjuvant CCRT.
9. Palliative EBRT is an important and useful treatment to help with symptomatic relief of gynaecological cancers, particularly bleeding and apin, not suitable for radical management.

References

1. Winter WE 3rd, Maxwell GL, Tian C, et al. Association of hemoglobin level with survival in cervical carcinoma patients treated with concurrent cisplatin and radiotherapy: a Gynecologic Oncology Group study. Gynecol Oncol. 2004;94(2):495–501.
2. Fernandes DCR, Andreyev HJN. Gastrointestinal toxicity of pelvic radiotherapy: are we letting women down? Clin Oncol. 2021;S0936-6555(21):00166–7.
3. Mazeron R, Castelnau-Marchand P, Dumas I, et al. Impact of treatment time and dose escalation on local control in locally advanced cervical cancer treated by chemoradiation and image-guided pulsed-dose rate adaptive brachytherapy. Radiother Oncol. 2015;114(2):257–63.
4. Klopp AH, Yeung AR, Deshmukh S, et al. Patient-reported toxicity during pelvic intensity-modulated radiation therapy: NRG Oncology-RTOG 1203. J Clin Oncol. 2018;36(24):2538–44.
5. Lawrie TA, Green JT, Beresford M, et al. Interventions to reduce acute and late adverse gastrointestinal effects of pelvic radiotherapy for primary pelvic cancers. Cochrane Database Syst Rev. 2018;1(1):CD012529.
6. Karlsson J, Dreifaldt AC, Bohr Mordhorst L, et al. Differences in outcome for cervical cancer patients treated with or without brachytherapy. Brachytherapy. 2017;16(1):133–40.
7. Banerjee R, Kamrava M. Brachytherapy in the treatment of cervical cancer: a review. Int J Women's Health. 2014;6:555–64.
8. Creutzberg CL, Nout RA, Lybeert ML, et al. Fifteen-year radiotherapy outcomes on the randomised PORTEC-1 trial for endometrial carcinoma. Int J Radiat Oncol Biol Phys. 2011;81(4):e631–8.
9. Concin N, Matias-Guiu X, Vergote I, et al. ESGO/ESTRO/ESP guidelines for the management of patients with endometrial carcinoma. Int J Gynecol Cancer. 2021;31(1):12–39.
10. Nout RA, Smit VT, Putter H, et al. Vaginal brachytherapy versus pelvic external beam radiotherapy for patients with endometrial cancer of high-intermediate risk (PORTEC-2): an open-label, non-inferiority, randomised trial. Lancet. 2010;375(9717):816–23.

11. De Boer SM, Powell ME, Mileshkin L, et al. PORTEC study group: adjuvant chemoradiotherapy versus radiotherapy alone for women with high-risk endometrial cancer (PORTEC-3): final results of an international, open-label, multicentre, randomised, phase 3 trial. Lancet Oncol. 2018;19(3):295–309.
12. Churn M, Jones B. Primary radiotherapy for carcinoma of the endometrium using external beam radiotherapy and single line source brachytherapy. Clin Oncol. 1999;11(4):255–62.
13. Gill BS, Kim H, Houser C, et al. Image-based three-dimensional conformal brachytherapy for medically inoperable endometrial carcinoma. Brachytherapy. 2014;13(6):542–7.
14. Landoni F, Maneo A, Colombo A, et al. Randomised study of radical surgery versus radiotherapy for stage Ib-IIa cervical cancer. Lancet. 1997;350(9077):535–40.
15. Perez CA, Grigsby PW, Castro-Vita H, et al. Carcinoma of the uterine cervix part 1. Impact of prolongation of overall treatment time and timing of brachytherapy on outcome of radiation therapy. Int J Radiat Oncol Biol Phys. 1999;32(5):1275–88.
16. Chemoradiotherapy for Cervical Cancer Meta-Analysis Collaboration (CCCMAC). Reducing uncertainties about the effects of chemoradiotherapy for cervical cancer: individual patient data meta-analysis. Cochrane Database Syst Rev. 2010;2010(1):CD008285.
17. Faul CM, Mirmow D, Huang Q, et al. Adjuvant radiation for vulvar carcinoma: improved local control. Int J Radiat Oncol Biol Phys. 1997;38(2):381–9.
18. Oonk MHM, Slomovitz B, Baldwin P, et al. Radiotherapy instead of inguinofemoral lymphadenectomy in vulvar cancer patients with a metastatic sentinel node: results of GROINSS-V II. Int J Gynecol Cancer. 2019;29:A14.
19. Han SC, Kim DH, Higgins SA, et al. Chemoradiation as primary or adjuvant treatment for locally advanced carcinoma of the vulva. Int J Radiat Oncol Biol Phys. 2000;47(5):235–44.
20. Thomas G, Dembo A, DePetrillo A, et al. Concurrent radiation and chemotherapy in vulvar carcinoma. Gynecol Oncol. 1989;34(3):263–7.
21. Rajagopalan MS, Xu KM, Lin JF, et al. Adoption and impact of concurrent chemoradiation therapy for vaginal cancer: a National Cancer Data Base (NCDB) Study. Gynecol Oncol. 2014;135(3):495–502.

Palliative Care in Gynaecologic Oncology

Seema Singhal, Milind Arolker, and Rakesh Garg

14.1 Introduction

World Health Organization WHO defines palliative care as an "approach that improves the quality of life (QoL) of patients with life-threatening illnesses, and their families. It prevents and relieves suffering through early identification, correct assessment, and treatment of pain and other problems, whether physical, psychosocial, or spiritual" [1]. It is an essential component of comprehensive care in oncology.

Palliative care should be incorporated in the treatment trajectory of cancer patients, from the initial treatment till the end of life, and bereavement support for the family of the deceased patient also should be provided. Published reports favor the early integration of palliative care for cancer patients. A comprehensive cancer care system should most definitely integrate palliative care, tailored to the needs of each patient. ASCO recommends that "patients with advanced cancer should be referred to palliative care services within 8 weeks of their diagnosis". A holistic early integration on the background of a multidisciplinary approach appears to be the most beneficial in improving the quality of life of cancer patients and their immediate caregivers. This should include clinical and social aspects like setting realistic expectations, understanding the course of illness, coping up with reality and smooth transition from curative care to end of life care, minimizing non-beneficial and aggressive interventions towards the end of life.

Provision of palliative care services to a patient of gynaecological cancer is not a single physician endeavor and needs to be actively embraced by all providers including gynaecological oncologists, radiation oncologists, medical oncologists, and palliative care specialists along with other supportive care and should be integrated into all areas of medical care.

This chapter will deal with the management of specific surgical and non-surgical issues in advanced gynaecological cancers from the perspective of a palliative care specialist and a gynae-oncologist.

S. Singhal
Department of Obstetrics and Gynaecology, All India Institute of Medical Sciences, New Delhi, India

M. Arolker
University of Birmingham, Birmingham, UK
e-mail: milind.arolker@heartofengland.nhs.uk

R. Garg (✉)
Department of Onco-Anaesthesiology and Palliative Medicine, Dr BRAIRCH, All India Institute of Medical Sciences, New Delhi, India

14.2 Current Status of Palliative Care Services

Approximately, 40 million people require palliative care services globally. Of these patients, 78% live in low- and middle-income countries (LMICs).

WHO reports that only 39% of countries worldwide report the availability of palliative care services in the primary health care setting and 40% in primary health centers/community settings. This figure drops to 15% in LMICs. Access to oral morphine is reported to be available in only 44% of countries, with less than 15% in countries without dedicated funding to palliation [2]. According to a study by Taylor et al. (2016) around one-third of women suffering from gynaecological cancers would die without being referred to a palliative care specialist [3]. Half of such patients had received either surgery or chemotherapy in the last 6 months of their life. Availability of specialized palliative care services has been diverse depending on the resources with maximum access at comprehensive cancer centers and limited or no access at other non-specialized hospitals. Similarly, training options are also limited and most gynaecologic oncology fellows lack exposure to the actual end-of-life care and understanding the goals of care. According to a survey conducted among the members of SGO, although the palliative care services were perceived as an essential collaboration by 97% of respondents, it was utilized appropriately only by 48% of them. Forty-two percent of responders thought that palliative care specialists should be involved when life expectancy is below 6 months, while 30% of respondents believed in collaborating at the time of recurrence. Seventy-five percent of the respondents believed the need for palliative care at all stages of disease for symptom control predominantly pain control. According to another study by Alexandre Buckley de Meritens et al. majority of gynae oncologists perceived themselves as competent to carry out the end-of-life discussions and were concerned about the false interpretation by families as the care of the patient being given up if palliative care services were being provided [4].

14.3 Provision of Palliative Care Services

Palliative care services include ambulatory palliative care clinics (integrated with comprehensive cancer care centers or independent units), inpatient consultation services, home-based palliative care services, and outpatient palliative care services. These may be accomplished by accommodating the goals under nine domains as outlined by the American Association of Hospice and Palliative Medicine –"rapport and relationship building with patients and family caregivers, symptom distress and function status management, exploration of understanding and education of prognosis, clarification of treatment goals, assessment and support of coping, assistance with medical decision making, coordination with other providers, and provision of referrals to other providers" [5].

Services for following these domains may well be offered by both the primary care team and palliative care experts, but the services offered by each of them are different.

1. **Primary Palliative care**: Basic management of symptoms including pain, anxiety, stress, depression. Communication skills concerning suffering, goals, or methods of treatment and prognosis are included.
2. **Specialty Palliative care**: Management of more complex symptoms including refractory pain, complex neuropsychiatric symptoms, conflict resolution with families, staff, and treatment teams. Setting up realistic expectations.

14.4 Timing of Palliative Care Among Gynaecological Cancer Patients

The comprehensive integration of palliative care throughout the entire spectrum of cancer care is need of the hour. Early integration for palliative care among cancer patients at the time of diagnosis remains the norm for a better quality of life. It enhances better rapport among the treating team members and also among palliative care physicians and the patient. Though the role of the palliative care team may not be much in the initial days of diagnosis for early diseases at times, patients are diagnosed late and the inclusion of a palliative care physician shall help in improving the quality of life.

It was reported that the continuation of palliative chemotherapy till late end-stage gynaecological cancers was not beneficial. Not only the duration of last chemotherapy and end of life was lesser but also the quality of life deteriorated [6]. This raised an important concern of the timely decisions with regards to best supportive therapy and appropriate goals of care with good communication with the patient and family members.

Due to the lack of integration of palliative care teaching in the existing curriculum for gynaecology teaching and training, it is essential that various triggers need to be identified by all for palliative physician involvement in patient care (Fig. 14.1).

The triggers may be labeled as primary and secondary [7]. Primary triggers include "frequent admissions, admission prompted by difficulty to control symptoms, complex care requirements, and decline in function". Secondary triggers include "metastatic or incurable cancer, chronic oxygen use, admission from a long-term care facility, and limited social support" [7]. These triggers shall help identify the definite need for palliative physician involvement. Though it remains imperative not only to have palliative care understanding by all but also early involvement of palliative care physicians remains of utmost importance.

14.5 Symptom Management

Palliative care includes all domains of management including physical, social, psychological, and spiritual. Gynaecological cancer patients may present with various symptoms at various stages of cancer. Each of these symptoms can be variedly manifested and hence needs thorough assessment with a high index of suspicion in case patient presents with the new-onset symptom(s). The basic principle of symptom management includes "reverse the reversible" while symptoms due to advanced disease require supportive care to improve the quality of life.

14.5.1 Bleeding in Advanced Gynaecological Cancers

Bleeding is one of the common problems in a gynaecological cancer patient. It can be either because of invasion of vessels by tumor or tumor neoangiogenesis or systemic pathologies like thrombocytopenia, platelet dysfunction, coagulopathy, or adverse effects related to therapy. Terminal hemorrhage leading to rapid loss of volume, blood, and subsequently death occurs in approximately 10% of cases [8]. Genitourinary tract, gastrointestinal tract, and respiratory tract

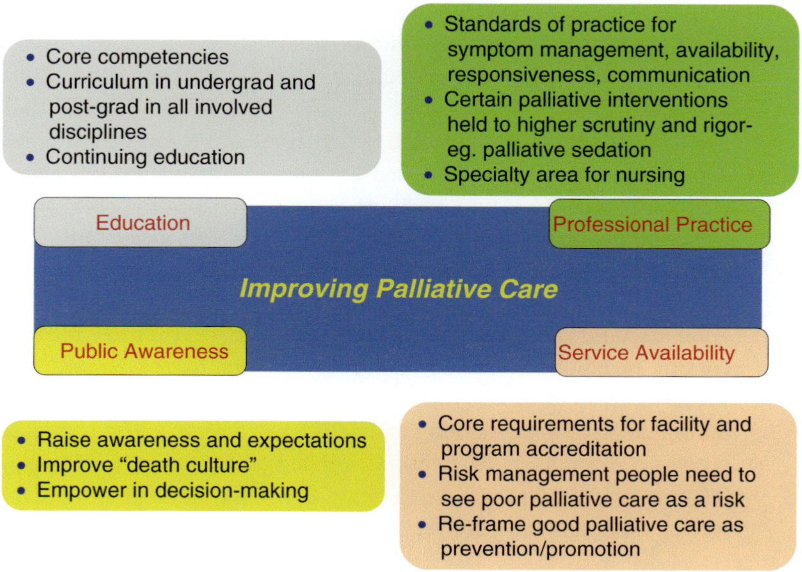

Fig. 14.1 Strategies of integration of palliative care

- Core competencies
- Curriculum in undergrad and post-grad in all involved disciplines
- Continuing education

- Standards of practice for symptom management, availability, responsiveness, communication
- Certain palliative interventions held to higher scrutiny and rigor- eg. palliative sedation
- Specialty area for nursing

Education

Professional Practice

Improving Palliative Care

Public Awareness

Service Availability

- Raise awareness and expectations
- Improve "death culture"
- Empower in decision-making

- Core requirements for facility and program accreditation
- Risk management people need to see poor palliative care as a risk
- Re-frame good palliative care as prevention/promotion

are the most frequent sites of hemorrhage in gynaecologic cancer patients.

Treatment is difficult and needs to be individualized depending on the life expectancy and quality of life. The first step is establishing the goals of care, benefits, and risks of a particular treatment option and essentially resuscitation. Bleeding should be assessed in terms of duration, onset, severity, cardiovascular collapse, and most importantly, psychosocial concerns. Reversible causes should be identified and corrected. Treatment aimed at correction of anemia may be instituted. Any systemic medication that is responsible for the bleeding tendency may be stopped. Blood transfusions should be decided based on treatment goals and patient expectations. All efforts should be done to control bleeding.

1. Local measures
   - Vaginal packing and local agents: Vaginal packing is useful for the initial control of vaginal or cervical bleeding. A roller gauze soaked in formalin or 1:1000 adrenaline solution may be used to snugly pack the vaginal canal. Monsel's paste (Ferric subsulphate) has been used for controlling bleeding from cervical and vaginal tumors. Vulvar tumors that bleed may be controlled by adherent dressing with absorbable gelatin or collagen. Infected wounds should be treated with appropriate antibiotics after taking a wound swab for culture and sensitivity.
   - Radiation therapy: Hemostatic radiotherapy has been conventionally used for controlling bleeding from tumors. Short-course palliative hypofractionated 3-D CRT in the dose of 20–25 Gy in 5 Gy daily fractions has been well-tolerated and effective with good response rates. Radiation therapy can control bleeding within 24–48 h, but it needs the patient to be lying on the table during the treatment planning and delivery process. The course of hypofractionated RT may be further extended with 2–4 weeks intervals to deliver 44.40 Gy depending on tolerance and clinical condition of the patient.
   - Transcutaneous arterial embolization: Embolization of arteries feeding the tumor with particles (e.g., polyvinyl alcohol), mechanical devices (e.g. coils), or liquids (e.g. glue, alcohol).
   - Endoscopic procedures: Endoscopic procedures like cystoscopy or proctoscopy may be considered for those with genitourinary or gastrointestinal bleed. The bleeding vessels may be managed using either cautery, Argon plasma coagulation, vascular clips, laser therapy injection of epinephrine, or sclerosing agents.
   - Surgical methods: Ligation of large vessels or excision of bleeding tissues may be considered on a case-by-case basis.
2. Systemic therapy: Antifibrinolytic drugs like tranexamic acid and aminocaproic acid injections have been successfully used for controlling heavy bleeding. After the control of the acute episode, maintenance oral doses can be continued for a span of 5–7 days. Complications include color vision abnormalities, allergic reactions, and formation of thrombosis.
3. Hematuria may be either due to invasion into vessels of the urinary tract or hemorrhagic cystitis related to alkylating agents, or infection or radiation cystitis. Initial management with bladder irrigation with cold saline, cystoscopy guided removal of clots, application of astringents, and coagulation of bleeding vessels can be done. For refractory cases infusion with 1%, alum or administration of PGE2 and silver nitrate may be considered. Formalin has been utilized as a last resort with good efficacy.

For terminal patients, it is important to discuss the risk of hemorrhage and whether the patient is a candidate for intervention or not, well in advance. The patient and family may find bleeding mentally disturbing. Hence, counseling, and psychological support to the patient and family is important. For nursing the patient, a trained health professional should be present and if possible, pressure or packing may be applied. Oxygen support and administration of sedatives or even narcotics may be considered. To avoid the visual shock of seeing a massive bleed, use of suction, dark clothing, blankets and towels should be encouraged along with the use of fast-acting sedatives like subcutaneous Midazolam.

14.5.2 Malignant Ascites

Malignant ascites is most frequently encountered in women with advanced ovarian cancer, breast cancer, and advanced endometrial cancer among gynaecological malignancies. Its presence is associated with poor prognosis and has an enormous impact on a patient's quality of life. According to the HES statistics (2007–2008) in England, around 28,000 bed-days were occupied by malignant ascites [9]. These patients frequently experience fatigue, nausea, lower limb swelling, discomfort, anorexia, breathlessness, constipation, and frequency of micturition. Pathophysiological reasons for the formation of malignant ascites include obstruction of lymphatic drainage, increased vascular permeability, and hepatic venous obstruction by tumor invasion.

The management of ascites in terminally ill cancer patients may range from simple procedures like tapping to resolve symptoms to highly morbid cytoreductive surgeries and targeted therapy. Management aims to improve the quality of life of these patients and prolong their survival without causing undue morbidity.

1. Paracentesis is the first intervention usually employed for immediate relief. It may be a one-time procedure or continuous drainage. Usually, 1–2 L of fluid is drained in every episode, with careful monitoring of the patient's vital signs. Placement of a fine tube for several hours or even days may be considered, in case of the rapid buildup of ascites. Insertion of permanent tunneled catheter drains, or peritoneal-venous shunts are preferred options for those who need frequent drainage and most of the time remain functional for a longer period as needed. Complications include electrolyte imbalance, circulatory collapse and infections leading to secondary peritonitis.

2. Pharmacological agents include diuretics, immunological agents, and are typically used as an adjunct to mechanical interventions. Spironolactone and furosemide are the most commonly used diuretics in clinical practice, though there is data that malignant ascites with a serum ascites albumin gradient (SAAG) ratio <1.1 mg/dL may not respond to diuretics [10]. Immunological agent *Catumaxomab* has been used in heavily pretreated chemotherapy-refractory cases and the intraperitoneal infusion reduced the requirement for repeated paracentesis. It is a bispecific antibody directed against epithelial cell adhesion molecule (EpCAM) and CD3 which is a T cell antigen [11]. However, it is not much utilized in clinical practice due to logistic issues. Other agents include the use of intraperitoneal bevacizumab therapy. Ascites may be a predictor for identifying the subset of ovarian cancer patients who may benefit greatly from bevacizumab therapy [12]. In a recent phase 2 trial REZOLVE (ANZGOG-1101), administration of bevacizumab intraperitoneally to chemotherapy-resistant epithelial ovarian cancer patients who had rapid re-accumulation of ascites within 28 days, were found to have longer paracentesis free days compared to the historical cohort before intervention [13].

Despite these various therapeutic and palliative options available, the management of ascitic fluid in advanced cancer patients nearing the end of life is still imperfect and warrants further research and novel therapeutic options.

14.5.3 Breathlessness

The American Thoracic Society defines it as "a subjective experience of breathing discomfort that consists of qualitatively distinct sensations that vary in intensity". Breathlessness is not an individual manifestation but seen with multitude of factors resulting from physiological, psychological, social, and environmental factors. But most importantly, the ATS emphasized that dyspnoea *per se* can only be perceived *by the person experiencing it* [14]. The causes of dyspnoea in a patient with gynaecological malignancy may be due to a variety of causes like pleural effusion, lung metastasis, lymphangitis carcinomatosis, panic attack, infection, or anemia.

It is a highly distressing symptom not only for the patients but also for the family of the patient. Management aims to identify and treat any reversible causes found and to provide symptomatic relief.

1. Non-pharmacological management
   - Included reassurance and support to the patient. A complete explanation of the situation and treatment planning may alleviate the stress and anxiety of the patient
   - Panic attacks may be relieved by teaching the patient to remain calm in a silent room, relaxing the shoulders and back, practicing pursed-lip breathing, and asking the patient to concentrate on her breath
   - Respiratory muscle strengthening exercises may help in chronically ill patients with a poor effort
   - Directing a fan towards the patient's face may provide relief
2. Pharmacological therapy
   - Oxygen: May help if the patient is hypoxic, though use is controversial. A thorough explanation of the role of invasive ventilation should be discussed with patients and caregivers who are transitioning from curative to palliative intent to avoid unnecessary procedures and allow time for rethinking decisions.
   - Benzodiazepines: These may help alleviate the feeling of breathlessness by acting on central GABA receptors and may help in panic attacks also. The side effect includes sleep disturbances. Short-acting benzodiazepines like lorazepam are preferred.
   - Opioids: Though the mechanism of action of opioids in relieving breathlessness is not completely understood, they are the first choice of drugs in the management of refractory dyspnoea. Their mechanism of action is proposed to be due to inhibition of the respiratory center, decreasing respiratory drive, and reducing anxiety.
3. Surgical management
   - Pleural effusion requires therapeutic pleural tapping of around 1–1.5 L of fluid.
   - Pleurodesis is the procedure in which the pleural cavity is partially obliterated by the addition of chemical agents within the pleural space between the visceral and parietal pleura. Various agents like talc, tetracycline, chemotherapeutic agents like cisplatin, doxorubicin, mitomycin, mitoxantrone, 5-fluorouracil can be used
   - Indwelling tunneled pleural catheter-like PleurX may be used for repeated tapping by patients or caregivers

14.5.4 Malignant Bowel Obstruction

Malignant bowel obstruction (MBO) may be seen in advanced cancer patients and usually a terminal phase of disease progression. It is more commonly associated with gastrointestinal cancer and ovarian cancer.

14.5.4.1 Pathophysiology

The various pathophysiological factors are responsible for bowel obstruction in cancer patients. The common etiological and pathological factors include:

- Extrinsic compression of bowel lumen: This is related to external compression of the bowel resulting from primary or metastatic tumour to the abdomen. This may also occur due to adhesions and fibrosis (due to prior surgery/

radiation therapy) without or without recurrence or metastasis in the abdomen.
- Intra-luminal occlusion of the lumen: This type of bowel obstruction results from primary tumor of the bowel with its intraluminal growth leading to occlusion of the bowel. At times, intratumoral bleeding or tumor lesion edema may precipitate bowel obstruction.
- Intramural lesion leading to luminal occlusion: Conditions like intestinal linitis plastica which is due to tumor in the bowel wall results in obstruction and also decreased bowel activity
- Retroperitoneal LN pushing on the pyloric antrum/duodenum
- Adynamic ileus or functional obstruction may be due to intestinal motility disorders due to tumor infiltration of the mesentery or bowel wall muscle and nerves, malignant involvement of the coeliac plexus, paraneoplastic neuropathy, chronic intestinal pseudo-obstruction (CIP), and paraneoplastic pseudo-obstruction.

The symptoms may include the inability to eat, intractable nausea and vomiting, pain, cramping, tachypnoea, dyspnoea, low-grade fever, dehydration, and obstipation. Partial obstruction may present as changing bowel habits or loose stools.

Blood investigations may show thrombocytosis, haemoconcentration, low albumin, and dys-electrolytemia like hypokalemia, hypochloremia, and metabolic alkalosis. A radiograph of the abdomen may show multiple air-fluid levels, distended bowel loops, gas under the diaphragm. Contrast-enhanced computed tomogram of the abdomen and pelvis may show the extent of disease, presence of ascites, carcinomatosis, and give information about the obstruction such as level, partial/complete, and the number of sites.

14.5.4.2 Management
A multidisciplinary team approach is essential.

1. Conservative management: The first line of treatment is conservative which includes bowel rest, hydration, intravenous fluids to correct dehydration and electrolyte imbalance. A nasogastric tube may be inserted to relieve symptoms. Institution of parenteral nutrition can be used in patients who are awaiting a more definitive treatment option but is controversial in patients nearing the end of life.
2. Medical management: Pain relief is crucial with the help of antispasmodics like hyoscine and opioids. Antiemetics may relieve vomiting and provide comfort. Steroids are usually included to decrease bowel wall edema and relieve pressure symptoms. Prokinetic drugs like metoclopramide may be used if there is no suspicion of complete obstruction. Octreotide is a somatostatin analog, which decreases secretions, hyperemia, and intraluminal pressure and thereby proving symptomatic benefit. If symptoms resolve with conservative or medical management, the patient may be discharged on the same treatment. The natural history of ovarian cancer is characterized by progressive increasing degrees of bowel obstruction in the late course of the disease that becomes increasingly difficult to manage non-surgically.
3. In patients who fail to respond to medical management, minimally invasive options like percutaneous decompression gastrostomy tube (PDGT) or percutaneous endoscopic gastrostomy (PGT). Stents can also be considered before opting for surgical management.
4. Surgical management: Surgery for MBO should be carefully decided after considering the patient status, disease sites, intent of therapy, patient expectations, and expected survival outcomes. Most patients may be poor surgical candidates due to malnutrition and underlying disease. Thorough preoperative counselling should be done in terms of high morbidity, mortality, and failure of therapy in terms of successful palliation which is measured by oral intake for at least 60 days after surgery. One-third of the patients may have re-obstruction due to disease progression. Surgical management has risks of low rates of hospital discharge and high inpatient mortality rate. Contraindications to palliative surgery include carcinomatosis causing adynamic

ileus, extensive ascites, diffusely metastatic cancer with bowel obstruction on multiple levels, obstruction at the level of proximal ileum, jejunum and duodenum involvement, long-standing obstruction, tumor cachexia, low serum albumin, multiple previous abdominal surgeries, and a rapidly progressing chemo-resistant disease. The outcomes of surgery are variable, with surgical correction possible in 84% of patients and successful palliation in 74% of patients planned for the procedure [15]. Complications occur in 22% of cases and may include enterocutaneous fistula, abscess, bacterial peritonitis, and thromboembolism. Surgery-related mortality ranges from 15 to 25%. Survival outcome for such patients who can receive chemotherapy after surgical correction is 9–10 months but is about 2–3 months for patients who were not suitable for postoperative palliative chemotherapy [16].

14.5.5 Pain

Pain remains one of the important and major symptoms in advanced gynaecologic cancer patients. Pain is not just physical but the concept of "total pain" needs to be followed (Fig. 14.2, Table 14.1).

Lack of knowledge both among physicians and patients remains one of the factors for inappropriate management of pain. It leads to poor quality of life if not managed timely and optimally. The type and nature of pain depend on the extent of the disease. A thorough clinical assessment is paramount. If available, the imaging should also be part of the assessment of pain. Various assessment tools have been described for pain assessment (Fig. 14.3).

Patients with gynaecologic cancers, pain is due to disease per se, the extent of disease (local invasion, metastasis) and side effects of therapy like chemotherapy/radiotherapy (neuropathies) [17].

The basic principles of pain assessment include:

- Believe the patient presentation
- Thorough assessment of pain
- Identify various pain domains and components
- Look for overview of disease status
- Identify various precipitating and reliving factors
- Assess and reassess.

Pain management is effectively done using the WHO analgesic ladder (Fig. 14.4). Also, various nerve and plexus blocks like hypogastric plexus blocks are administered for the pain in patients with cancers.

14.5.6 Management of Other Symptoms

Apart from the above mentioned symptoms, advanced gynaecologic cancer patients may also have other symptoms including malnutrition, brain involvement, deep vein thrombosis, edema, neurological manifestations, gastrointestinal symptoms like constipation, delirium, nausea, and vomiting, metabolic and electrolyte disturbances, etc. [18].

Advanced gynaecological malignancies can develop fistulas like vesicovaginal, recto-vaginal, or enterovaginal fistulas. The fistula formation may result from advanced disease invasion or the side effect of therapy like surgery, radiotherapy, and chemotherapy. These pathologic communications not only cause

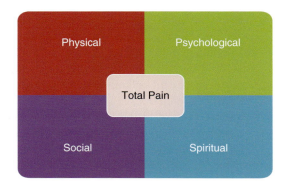

Fig. 14.2 Total pain

Table 14.1 Concept and components of total pain

Emotional pain (Affective)	Social pain (Behavioural)	Physical pain (Physiological)	Spiritual pain
• Anxiety • Depression • Anger • Sadness • Social Isolation • Fear of suffering • Experience of illness	• Financial Worries • Loss of job • Worries about future of family • Inability to Work • Loss of role and social status	• Illness (cancer) • Treatment • Unrelated to cancer	• Guilt • Regret • Fear of Dying • Anger with God • Loss/struggle with faith • Finding meaning

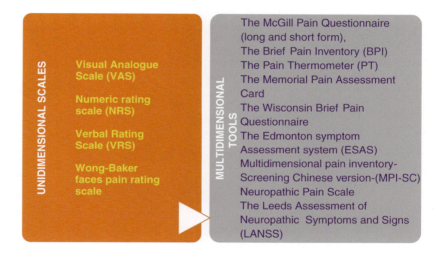

Fig. 14.3 Assessment tools for pain

systemic derangements but also disturbs the patients psychologically and socially. The patient may manifest with bleeding, vaginal discharge, urine/fecal incontinence, etc. The management requires an understanding of the underlying condition for the development of the fistula and whether curative intervention may be offered needs to be assessed. The majority of the time some palliative intervention shall be required for symptom management. Wherever the surgical intervention is not feasible, utmost care shall be provided for maintaining hygiene/skincare and thus to prevent further deterioration. The use of diapers and regular skincare is useful.

Cancers of the cervix and ovary may at times cause ureteral obstructions due to direct infiltration or compression over the ureter. In case of good, predicted survival, interventions to relieve the ureteral obstruction should be attempted using stenting or diversion procedures like nephrostomy.

Gynaecological cancers are prone to increase thrombotic episodes like deep vein thrombosis. The use of anticoagulants including low molecular weight heparin in the initial stages and oral anticoagulants remains the standard of care. Continued anticoagulation at end of life remains controversial.

14.6 End-of-Life Care

Considerations need to be provided not only to a good life but also to the 'good death'. Patients and family members need to be prepared and supported for this phase of life. The patient needs to be provided all comfort care including optimal symptom management even these days. Physical and psychosocial symptoms need to be assessed and reassessed regularly and management provided accordingly. At this stage, unnecessary investigations, imaging or medications should be avoided. This also requires honest and compas-

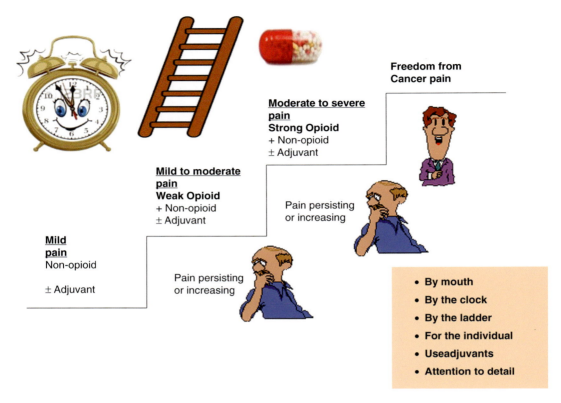

Fig. 14.4 WHO analgesic ladder for cancer pain management

sionate communication with the patient and immediate caregivers. The patient requires gentle nursing care for daily needs like positioning, urine, and bowel-related concerns. Delirium and agitation remain some of the most disturbing symptoms for the patient and caregivers and are seen in patients who are terminally ill. These require comfort care and may require sedation at this point.

14.7 Conclusion

Palliative care needs to be closely integrated with anticancer and disease-modifying therapy for gynaecological cancer patients. The team managing gynaecological cancers needs to be well coordinated for such integration and a holistic approach to provide the best goals of care is required. A thorough and proper understanding of symptom manifestations, their management options are required to counsel patients effectively in the decision-making process and treatment adherence. Understanding and respecting patient wishes, expectations, and attitudes

Key Points
- Palliative care needs to be closely integrated with anticancer and disease-modifying therapy for gynaecological cancer patients.
- Early integration for palliative care among cancer patients at the time of diagnosis remains the norm for a better quality of life.
- Palliative care shall include all domains of management including physical, social, psychological, and spiritual.

- Considerations need to be provided not only to a good life but also to the 'good death'.
- A thorough and proper understanding of symptom manifestations, their management options are required to counsel patients effectively in the decision-making process and treatment adherence.

towards end-of-life care is of utmost importance in providing a satisfactory treatment experience and increasing quality of life outcomes.

References

1. WHO definition of palliative care. World Health Organization website. www.who.int/cancer/palliative/definition/en
2. https://www.who.int/news-room/fact-sheets/detail/palliative-care
3. Taylor JS, Brown AJ, Prescott LS, Sun CC, Ramondetta LM, Bodurka DC. Dying well: how equal is end of life care among gynecologic oncology patients? Gynecol Oncol. 2016;140(2):295–300.
4. Buckley de Meritens A, Margolis B, Blinderman C, Prigerson HG, Maciejewski PK, Shen MJ, et al. Practice patterns, attitudes, and barriers to palliative care consultation by gynecologic oncologists. J Oncol Pract. 2017;13(9):e703–11.
5. Ferrell BR, Temel JS, Temin S, et al. Integration of palliative care into standard oncology care: American Society of Clinical Oncology clinical practice guideline update. J Clin Oncol. 2016;35(1):96–112.
6. Jang TK, Kim SW, Park JY, Suh DS, Kim JH, Kim YM, et al. Trends in treatment during last stages of life in end-stage gynecologic cancer patients who received active palliative chemotherapy: a comparative analysis of 10-year data I a single institution. BMC Palliat Care. 2018;17:99.
7. Mullen MM, Cripe JC, Thaker PH. Palliative care in gynecologic oncology. Obstet Gynecol Clin North Am. 2019;46:179–97.
8. Cartoni C, Niscola P, Breccia M, Brunetti G, D'Elia GM, Giovannini M, et al. Hemorrhagic complications in patients with advanced hematological malignancies followed at home: an Italian experience. Leuk Lymphoma. 2009;50(3):387–91.
9. HES statistics. HES online. Hospital episode statistics:Main procedures and interventions: 4 character. NHS. The information centre for health and social care; 2007-08. http://www.hesonline.nhs.uk/Ease/servlet/ContentServer?siteID=1937&categoryID=215
10. Pockros PJ, Esrason KT, Nguyen C, Duque J, Woods S. Mobilization of malignant ascites with diuretics is dependent on ascitic fluid characteristics. Gastroenterology. 1992;103(4):1302–6.
11. Sebastian M. Review of catumaxomab in the treatment of malignant ascites. CMAR. 2010;2:283–6.
12. Ferriss JS, Java JJ, Bookman MA, Fleming GF, Monk BJ, Walker JL, et al. Ascites predicts treatment benefit of bevacizumab in front-line therapy of advanced epithelial ovarian, fallopian tube and peritoneal cancers: an NRG Oncology/GOG study. Gynecol Oncol. 2015;139(1):17–22.
13. Sjoquist KM, Espinoza D, Mileshkin L, Ananda S, Shannon C, Yip S, et al. REZOLVE (ANZGOG-1101): a phase 2 trial of intraperitoneal bevacizumab to treat symptomatic ascites in patients with chemotherapy-resistant, epithelial ovarian cancer. Gynecol Oncol. 2021;161(2):374–81.
14. Parshall MB, Schwartzstein RM, Adams L, Banzett RB, Manning HL, Bourbeau J, et al. An official American thoracic society statement: update on the mechanisms, assessment, and management of dyspnea. Am J Respir Crit Care Med. 2012;185(4):435–52.
15. Paul Olson TJ, Pinkerton C, Brasel KJ, Schwarze ML. Palliative surgery for malignant bowel obstruction from carcinomatosis: a systematic review. JAMA Surg. 2014;149(4):383.
16. Hoppenot C, Peters P, Cowan M, Moore ED, Hurteau J, Lee NK, et al. Malignant bowel obstruction due to uterine or ovarian cancer: are there differences in outcome? Gynecol Oncol. 2019;154(1):177–82.
17. Rezk Y, Timmins PF, Smith HS. Palliative care in gynecologic oncology. Am J Hosp Palliat Med. 2011;28:356–74.
18. Landrum LM, Blank S, Chen MLM, Duska L, Baejump V, Lee PS, et al. Comprehensive care in gynecology oncology: the importance of palliative care. Gynecol Oncol. 2015;137:193–202.

Clinical Interpretation of Immunohistochemistry in Gynaecological Cancers

15

William Boyle, Matthew Evans, and Josefa Vella

15.1 Introduction

The introduction of immunohistochemistry (IHC) into histopathology in the second half of the twentieth century has transformed the specialty, allowing it to make finer and more precise discriminations between entities which cannot reliably be distinguished on routine staining. Automated immunohistochemistry staining has now become standard in pathology laboratories.

IHC is the process by which antigens (proteins) that are present in a cell are detected by the use of antibodies that bind to the antigens. A primary antibody is firstly applied to the tissue which binds to its antigen and then a secondary antibody directed against the primary antibody is applied. The site of binding of the secondary antibody is detected by an enzyme reaction which leads to deposition of an insoluble dark brown reaction end product enabling the site of binding of the primary antibody to be visualised under a microscope. The interpretation of whether an immunohistochemical stain is positive or negative involves knowledge of the subcellular localization or distribution of the targeted antigen (i.e. membranous, cytoplasmic or nuclear) so that only true staining is accepted.

Controls which are aimed to test for the specificity of the antibodies involved are essential in order for the results obtained to be valid. The specificity controls include a positive and a negative control. Positive controls are sections of tissue known to be positive for the particular antibodies being used in the test and are included in each batch of slides undergoing staining to ensure that absence of positive staining is not due to technical failure in the staining process. Negative controls consist of sections of the test sample on which no primary antibody is applied and therefore no positive reaction should be seen. If positivity is seen in negative controls, this indicates that the immunoreactivity is non-specific and the test is not valid for interpretation.

15.2 Purposes of Immunohistochemistry

IHC serves three broad purposes in tumour pathology, namely:

15.2.1 To Help Make a Diagnosis

- IHC can help to classify a tumour type. For example, it may be impossible morphologi-

W. Boyle (✉) · J. Vella
Birmingham Women's and Children's NHS Trust, Birmingham, UK
e-mail: williamboyle@nhs.net; josefavella@nhs.net

M. Evans
Black Country Pathology Services, Wolverhampton, UK
e-mail: matthew.evans7@nhs.net

cally to accurately diagnose a poorly differentiated endometrial carcinoma. However, by examining its expression of various proteins using immunohistochemistry it is usually possible to classify it as, for example, an endometrioid or serous carcinoma.
- It can help to determine the origin of a malignancy. For example, a deposit of adenocarcinoma in the omentum may have metastasised from anywhere in the body. By determining its pattern of protein expression it is usually possible to determine from which tissue is has most likely arisen.
- In select situations, it can help to identify the presence of an underlying germline cancer predisposition syndrome. The only common example of this at the moment is MMR immunohistochemistry, which can be used to screen for Lynch syndrome in patients with endometrial carcinomas.

15.2.2 To Provide Prognostic Information

- It can help to establish how intrinsically aggressive a tumour is likely to be. For example, in some tumours, the extent of Ki67 expression may roughly predict how likely the tumour is to recur and/or metastasise.
- It can help to identify adverse prognostic features in a tumour sample. For example, it can be very difficult to confidently diagnose lymphovascular invasion on routine staining. However, the use of an endothelial immunohistochemical marker (e.g. CD31) can confirm that a nodule of tumour is within a blood vessel and, by extension that the tumour may need to be treated more aggressively.

15.2.3 To Provide Predictive Information

- It can also provide predictive information, to determine how well a patient is likely to respond to a given treatment. For example, IHC testing for the presence of hormone receptors in endometrial cancers may direct towards hormone manipulation as a primary treatment tool in patients who are unfit for surgery. Another example is MMR immunohistochemistry which, in addition to screening for Lynch syndrome, can be used to determine whether patients with metastatic endometrial carcinoma are likely to respond to immune checkpoint inhibitors.

In this chapter we will discuss the use of IHC in gynaecological pathology by site in the Female genital tract.

15.3 Ovary

Ovarian neoplasms are most commonly classified into carcinomas, sex-cord stromal tumours, germ cell tumours, neuroendocrine neoplasms and metastases to ovary.

15.3.1 Carcinomas

The five most common types of ovarian carcinoma are high grade serous carcinoma, low grade serous carcinoma, endometrioid carcinoma, clear cell carcinoma and mucinous carcinoma. The immunoprofile of primary ovarian tumours depends on their specific epithelial subtype. The immunoprofiles of the main ovarian carcinoma histiotypes are outlined in Table 15.1.

15.3.1.1 p53

p53 is a tumour suppressor which is encoded by the *TP53* gene. *TP53* is the single most commonly mutated gene in human cancers. A variety of mutations can occur in *TP53*, resulting in a variety of patterns of expression of the p53 protein [2]. 'Aberrant' staining is the term used to describe any of the abnormal staining patterns (Fig. 15.1).

- Wild type expression is the normal pattern of p53 expression and is characterised by variable proportions of nuclei staining and with variable intensity.

Table 15.1 Immunoprofiles of primary tubo-ovarian carcinomas [1]

	p53	WT1	ER	Napsin A	AMACR
High-grade serous carcinoma	Aberrant	+	±	−	−
Low-grade serous carcinoma	Wild type	+	+	−	−
Endometrioid carcinoma	Wild type	−	+	−	−
Clear cell carcinoma	Wild type	−	−	+	+
Mucinous carcinoma	Wild type	−	−	−	−

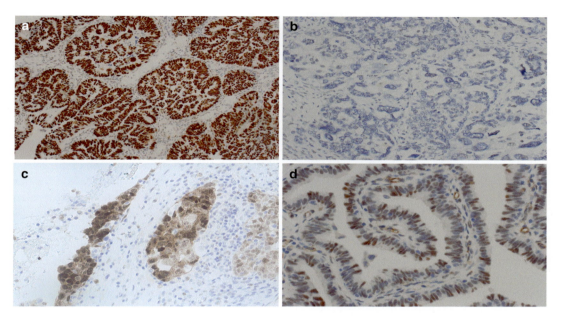

Fig. 15.1 The most common patterns of p53 staining. (**a**) p53 overexpression. (**b**) p53 null. (**c**) p53 cytoplasmic. (**d**) p53 wild type

- p53 overexpression is the commonest pattern of abnormal p53 expression and is defined as strong nuclear staining in at least 80% of tumour cell nuclei.
- p53 null expression is the next commonest pattern of abnormal p53 expression and is defined as no staining in tumour cell nuclei.
- p53 cytoplasmic staining is an uncommon pattern of abnormal p53 expression and is defined as predominant cytoplasmic staining in the absence of strong nuclear staining, in more than 80% of tumour cells.

15.3.1.2 WT1

WT1 nuclear expression has been reported in more than 90% of extra-uterine high-grade serous carcinomas [3]. In contrast, serous carcinomas originating from the endometrium are usually WT1 negative. This can help in distinguishing the origin of a serous carcinoma as either uterine or extra-uterine, however, this rule is not absolute since it is reported that up to 20% of serous carcinomas of genuine endometrial origin express WT1 [3].

15.3.2 Sex-Cord Stromal Tumours

Sex cord-stromal tumours constitute a diverse range of neoplasms and the differential diagnosis may be wide. Inhibin and calretinin are the most useful immunohistochemcial markers in demonstrating sex cord stromal differentiation. Cytokeratins are frequently expressed in sex cord-stromal tumours occasionally resulting in diagnostic confusion with carcinoma; EMA expression however is rare in sex cord-stromal tumours and therefore may help in making this distinction [4]. A summary of the immunoprofiles of the commonest entities is provided in Table 15.2.

15.3.3 Germ Cell Tumours

Most types of germ cell tumour are rare. A summary of the immunoprofiles of the more common tumour types is provided in Table 15.3.

15.3.4 Neuroendocrine Neoplasms

Neuroendocrine neoplasms in the ovary are classified as neuroendocrine tumours and neuroendocrine carcinomas. Neuroendocrine tumours are low and intermediate grade tumours, known as carcinoid and atypical carcinoid respectively. Neuroendocrine carcinomas are high grade tumours and consist of small cell neuroendocrine carcinoma (SCNEC) and large cell neuroendocrine carcinoma (LCNEC). Synaptophysin, chromogranin and CD56 are the most commonly used immunostains to demonstrate neuroendocrine differentiation. Immunohistochemical demonstration of neuroendocrine differentiation may not be seen in SCNEC. It should be noted that whilst the immunostain Ki67 is used as a prognostic marker in gastrointestinal and pancreatic neuroendocrine tumours, a similar use in neuroendocrine neoplasms of the female genital tract has not been validated.

15.3.5 Metastases

The most common sites of origin of metastatic tumours to the ovary are the gastrointestinal tract, breast, endometrium and cervix [6]. Immunohistochemistry plays a valuable role in helping to distinguish between primary ovarian carcinomas and metastatic carcinomas, which may morphologically resemble primary ovarian carcinomas. This distinction has important implications with regards to prognosis and treatment. Immunohistochemistry can give an extremely good idea of the origin of metastatic adenocarcinoma but it is not completely infallible; clinical and radiological correlation is always required. The pattern of expression of cytokeratin 7 and cytokeratin 20 is extremely helpful in broadly establishing likely tissues of origin (Table 15.4).

More specific markers may be used either alongside or (especially if tissue is limited) after cytokeratin 7 and cytokeratin 20, in order to narrow down the tissue of origin (Table 15.5).

Unlike adenocarcinomas, squamous cell carcinomas do not express markers which can be used to determine their site of origin. Determination of the site of origin of metastatic squamous cell carcinoma therefore depends essentially entirely on clinical and radiological correlation. However, it may be possible to use HPV status to distinguish between a typically hrHPV-positive site (e.g. lower female genital tract, oropharynx) and a typically hrHPV-negative site (e.g. skin, lung, oesophagus, other head and neck sites). p16 is not useful in this con-

Table 15.2 Immunoprofiles of ovarian sex-cord stromal tumours [4]

	Calretinin	Inhibin	WT1	EMA	Cytokeratin
Adult granulosa cell tumour	+	+	±	−	±
Juvenile granulosa cell tumour	+	+	±	±	+
Sertoli-Leydig cell tumour	+	+	+	−	+

Table 15.3 Immunoprofiles of ovarian germ cell tumours [5]

	SALL-4	OCT3/4	SOX2	CD117	CD30	Glypican 3	AFP	hCG
Dysgerminoma	+	+	−	+	−	−	−	−
Yolk sac tumour	+	−	−	±	−	+	+	−
Embryonal carcinoma	+	+	+	−	+	−	−	−
Choriocarcinoma	±	−	−	−	−	−	−	+

15 Clinical Interpretation of Immunohistochemistry in Gynaecological Cancers

Table 15.4 The reported proportions of malignancies which express the various combinations of cytokeratin 7 and cytokeratin 20

	n	CK7+/CK20+ (%)	CK7+/CK20− (%)	CK7−/CK20+ (%)	CK7−/CK20− (%)
Adrenal cortical neoplasm	10	0	0	0	100
Bladder, urothelial carcinoma	24	25	63	4	8
Breast, ductal carcinoma	20	0	95	0	5
Breast, lobular carcinoma	6	0	100	0	0
Cervix, squamous cell carcinoma	15	0	87	0	13
Colon, adenocarcinoma	20	5	0	95	0
Endometrium, adenocarcinoma	10	0	100	0	0
Gastrointestinal tract, carcinoid tumour	15	0	13	7	80
Head and neck, squamous cell carcinoma	30	0	27	6	67
Kidney, renal cell carcinoma	19	0	11	0	89
Liver, cholangiocarcinoma	14	43	50	0	7
Liver, hepatocellular carcinoma	11	0	9	9	82
Lung, adenocarcinoma	10	10	90	0	0
Lung, carcinoid tumour	9	0	22	0	78
Lung, small cell carcinoma	7	0	43	0	57
Lung, squamous cell carcinoma	15	0	47	0	53
Mesothelioma	17	0	65	0	35
Neuroendocrine carcinoma (all sites)	9	56	0	44	0
Oesophagus, squamous cell carcinoma	14	0	21	0	79
Ovary, adenocarcinoma	24	4	96	0	0
Pancreas, adenocarcinoma	13	62	30	0	8
Prostate, adenocarcinoma	18	0	0	0	100
Salivary gland tumour	9	0	100	0	0
Skin, Merkel cell carcinoma	9	0	0	78	12
Stomach, adenocarcinoma	8	13	25	37	25
Thymus, thymoma	8	0	0	0	100
Thyroid, carcinoma	55	0	98	0	2

The patterns of expression of cytokeratin 7 and cytokeratin 20 is a useful initial tool in establishing the likely site of origin of a carcinoma. Here, ovarian adenocarcinoma refers to an aggregation of all subtypes of ovarian carcinomas [7]

Table 15.5 The reported proportions of malignancies which express more specific localising markers

	CDX2	ER	GATA3	PAX8	TTF1
Colon	+	±	−	−	−
Lung	−	−	−	−	±
Upper gastrointestinal tract	±	−	−	−	−
Pancreatobiliary tract	±	−	±	−	−
Gynaecological tract	±	±	−	+	−
Breast	−	+	+	−	−
Renal cell carcinoma	−	−	±	+	−
Thyroid	−	−	−	+	+
Urothelial carcinomas	−	−	±	−	−

In general, gynaecological carcinomas (excluding squamous cell carcinomas) are positive or ER and PAX8, but this is certainly not absolute [8]

text, since non-hrHPV-driven cancers frequently overexpress p16. HPV ISH is more helpful, but with the caveat that lower female genital tract cancers may be hrHPV negative, and cancers thought not to be associated with hrHPV can be positive on HPV ISH.

15.3.6 Pseudomxyoma Peritoneii

Most cases of pseudomyxoma peritonei originate from the large intestine (usually the appendix) [9]. In most cases the epithelium shows positive staining with cytokeratin 20 and is negative with cytokeratin 7.

15.4 Fallopian Tube

High grade serous carcinoma is the most common malignant tumour in the fallopian tube and has an identical immunoprofile to that seen in the ovary. Tubal high grade serous carcinomas as well as the majority of so-called 'ovarian' high grade serous carcinomas are known to originate from serous intraepithelial carcinoma (STIC) in the fallopian tube.

15.5 Uterine Corpus

Typing of endometrial carcinoma provides prognostic information and determines clinical management strategies. Different endometrial carcinoma types are named for their histomorphological appearances. The most common types of endometrial cancer are:

1. Endometrioid carcinoma
2. Uterine serous carcinoma
3. Clear cell carcinoma

Endometrial cancers can normally be typed based on microscopic appearance; however, immunohistochemistry is used for cases with ambiguous morphology (Table 15.6), or to differentiate endometrial carcinomas from histological mimics, such as endocervical adenocarcinomas (Fig. 15.2) [10]. There is also a limited role for using immunohistochemistry to direct treatment, for example the use of hormone modulating agents in advanced carcinomas expressing hormone receptors in women unable to tolerate chemotherapy.

Undifferentiated carcinoma, dedifferentiated carcinoma and carcinosarcoma are uncommon, clinically aggressive subtypes of endometrial carcinoma with specific histological diagnostic criteria. These tumours show complete or partial loss of epithelial differentiation. In carcinosarcoma, this manifests as a cytologically malignant mesenchymal component. A shift in differentiation from a presumed epithelial component (or from a common progenitor cell) results in the absence of expression of immunomarkers expected in gynaecological tract carcinoma. Loss of expression of PAX8, ER, PR, pan-cytokeratin, cytokeratin 8/18 is common in undifferentiated

15 Clinical Interpretation of Immunohistochemistry in Gynaecological Cancers

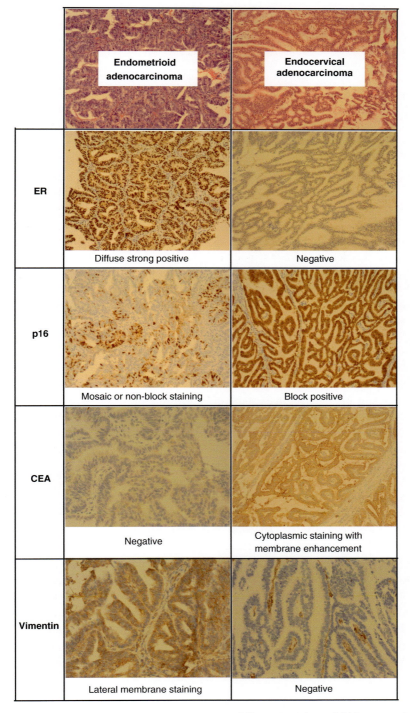

Fig. 15.2 Distinction between endometrioid endometrial adenocarcinoma and HPV-associated endocervical adenocarcinoma may require a panel of immunohistochemistry, especially on an endometrial biopsy specimen. The typical expression profiles of ER, p16, CEA and vimentin in these two adenocarcinomas is displayed

Table 15.6 Expected immunohistochemistry results in common types of endometrial carcinoma

	ER	Vimentin	PTEN	p53	Napsin A	AMACR
Endometrioid	+	+	Lost	Wild type	−	−
Serous	−	−	Retained	Aberrant	−	−
Clear cell	−	−	Retained	Wild type	+	+

The immunophenotypes are often a reflection of the biological properties of the cancer types. For example, uterine serous carcinomas arise from atrophic endometrial epithelium that has acquired loss-of-function mutation in TP53, a tumour suppressor gene. This is manifest as abnormal expression of p53, the protein encoded by TP53. Abnormal p53 expression profiles are the same as those in tubo-ovarian high grade serous carcinomas [11]

or sarcomatous elements, with PAX8 loss being reported to be more reliable [12].

As our understanding of the molecular underpinnings of endometrial carcinoma grows, endometrial cancer classification is evolving. A classification system based upon identification of genetic mutations defined in the the cancer genome atlas (TCGA) will supplement and, in the future, supplant the existing system as evidence for making treatment decisions based on subgroups emerges [13]. Immunohistochemistry is applied in this context by detecting abnormal antigen expression secondary to particular genetic mutations. Prioritising the identification of molecular characteristics of tumours resolves some of the well-known problems of tumour classification, such as inter-observer disagreement in pathological typing, and the incidence of cancers showing incongruence between prognosis and apparent tumour grade [14]. *TP53* mutation is the driver mutation in serous carcinoma but may occur as a secondary event in other cancers, including endometrioid carcinomas. Detection of a *TP53* mutation through abnormal p53 expression implies a poor prognosis regardless of the tumour's morphological appearance. Detection of abnormal mismatch repair (MMR) protein expression is associated with intermediate prognosis, with tumour behaviour akin to endometrioid carcinoma, regardless of morphology [15].

15.5.1 Mismatch Repair (MMR) Immunohistochemistry

In addition its role in tumour classification, MMR immunohistochemistry is used to screen women presenting with endometrial cancer for Lynch syndrome and predicts response to treatment with immune checkpoint inhibitors [16]. MMR comprises several protein components, chiefly MLH1, MSH2, PMS2 and MSH6, which are involved in correcting base-base mismatches and insertion/deletion mispairs generated during DNA replication. Deficient activity of MMR is seen in 25–30% of endometrial carcinomas and usually occurs as a result of either sporadic mutations in the genes encoding these proteins or somatic epigenetic silencing, mediated by MLH1 promoter hypermethylation. Lynch syndrome, caused by hereditary mutations in MMR genes, accounts for 3–5% of endometrial cancers [17].

In the presence of a mismatch repair defect, there is loss of expression of one or more of the MMR proteins. The four major MMR proteins occur as heterodimers, MLH1 pairing with PMS2 and MSH2 with MSH6. While MLH1 and MSH2 can stabilize in the cell by forming heterodimers with other proteins, PMS2 and MSH6 can only exist stably in the cell in the presence of MLH1 and MSH2 respectively. There are therefore four typical abnormal MMR IHC patterns (Fig. 15.3) [18]. In endometrial carcinoma, loss of MLH1 and PMS2 expression usually results from MLH1 promoter hypermethylation, however may less commonly occur because of a germline mutation in MLH1. For this reason, tumours showing MLH1 and PMS2 loss are tested for MLH1 promoter hypermethylation [19].

15.6 Uterine Mesenchymal Neoplasms

A panel of immunohistochemistry is often required to distinguish between mesenchymal neoplasms presenting in the uterus. A brief sum-

15 Clinical Interpretation of Immunohistochemistry in Gynaecological Cancers

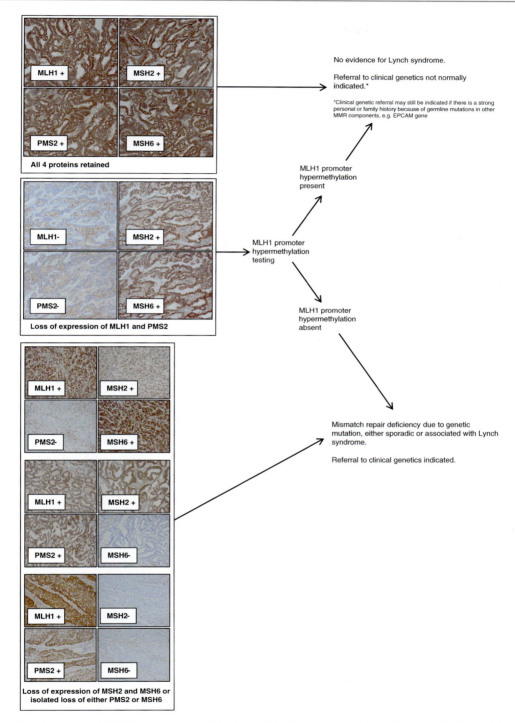

Fig. 15.3 Examples of MMR expression profiles that may be encountered in endometrial carcinomas and their respective implications for patient management. Staining is assessed in malignant epithelium with any staining in background stroma acting as an internal positive control

mary of the immunophenotypes of the more common tumour types is provided:

- Smooth muscle neoplasms are generally positive for SMA, desmin and h-caldesmon, unlike endometrial stromal neoplasms (although the latter may show areas of smooth muscle differentiation) [20].
- Endometrial stromal nodules and low-grade endometrial stromal sarcomas are usually strongly and diffusely positive for CD10 [21]. High-grade endometrial stromal sarcomas are usually positive for CD10, albeit only focally, and are often positive for cyclin D1 [22].
- Immunohistochemistry is generally unhelpful in the diagnosis of adenosarcomas, which generally show stromal staining with CD10 and ER, as per normal endometrial stroma and endometrial polyps [23].
- Uterine tumours resembling ovarian sex cord tumour (UTROSCT) usually express some combination of inhibin, calretinin, WT1 and MelanA [24]. There is frequent expression of smooth muscle markers, CD10, CD117 and cytokeratin.
- Gastrointestinal stromal tumours are typically positive for DOG1, CD34 and CD117.
- PEComas are generally positive for HMB45, MelanA, MiTF, SMA, desmin and h-caldesmon [25].

15.7 Vulva

15.7.1 Extramammary Paget's Disease (EMPD)

Although a diagnosis of EMPD can be strongly suspected on H&E staining, it can be difficult to distinguish from melanocytic lesions (including melanoma) and vulval intraepithelial neoplasia (VIN). Immunohistochemistry is therefore required before making a definitive diagnosis (Table 15.7; Fig. 15.4).

Furthermore, EMPD is divided into primary and secondary disease. Primary EMPD arises in the vulval skin itself, whereas secondary EMPD represents spread from an underlying visceral malignancy.

Table 15.7 A useful panel of markers for distinguishing EMPD from melanocytic proliferations and VIN [26]

	CAM5.2	p63	S100
EMPD	+	−	−
VIN	−	+	−
Melanocytic lesion	−	−	+

Immunohistochemistry is vital in drawing this distinction (Table 15.8); the finding of secondary EMPD should prompt careful search for an underlying malignancy, especially in the colorectum or urinary tract.

15.7.2 Vulval Squamous Neoplasia

Vulval intraepithelial neoplasia (VIN) is the in-situ precursor lesion of vulval squamous cell carcinoma. Both VIN and squamous cell carcinoma are divided into HPV-associated and HPV-independent subtypes.

HPV-independent VIN (also known as differentiated VIN) is the less common subtype of VIN. It tends to be subtle on H&E staining and can be difficult to distinguish from reactive changes in non-neoplastic squamous epithelium (e.g. from chronic trauma or inflammatory disease). Immunohistochemistry is therefore usually needed to confirm the diagnosis. p53 and Ki67 are the most useful markers [28]:

- Normally, p53 shows nuclear staining of variable intensity in the basal layers of the epithelium; in HPV-independent VIN there is either uniformly strong nuclear staining or loss of nuclear staining in the basal and parabasal layers.
- Normally, Ki67 shows staining only in the basal layers in normal resting epithelium; in HPV-independent VIN, this staining extends beyond the basal layer. This is poorly specific, however, and is also seen in reactive non-neoplastic conditions.

HPV-associated VIN is the more common form of VIN. It is divided into VIN1, VIN2 and VIN3, which are associated with an increasing risk of progression to squamous cell carcinoma. The

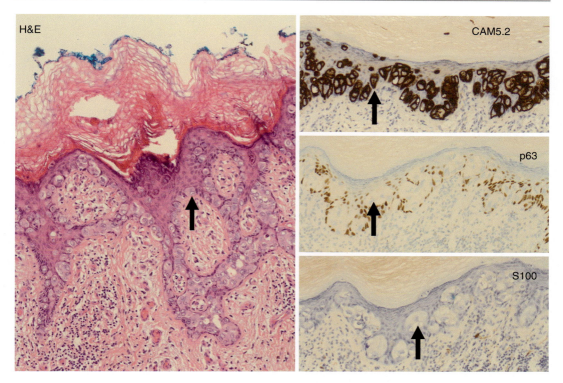

Fig. 15.4 H&E staining of a vulvectomy specimen shows Paget cells scattered throughout the epidermis (arrow); they are large cells with abundant pale cytoplasm. The Paget cells (arrows) are positive for CAM5.2 and negative for p63 and S100; this supports the diagnosis of EMPD. p63 stains the background squamous epithelial cells in the epidermis but not the Paget cells

Table 15.8 A useful panel of markers for distinguishing between primary and secondary EMPD, and for determining the site of origin of secondary EMPD [27]

	Cytokeratin 7	GCDFP-15	HER2	Cytokeratin 20	CDX2	Uroplakin
Primary EMPD	+	+	±	–	–	–
Primary EMPD, colorectal	–	–	–	+	+	–
Primary EMPD, urothelial	+	–		+		–

use of immunohistochemistry in this setting is the same as for cervical squamous neoplasia, below.

15.8 Cervix

15.8.1 Cervical Squamous Neoplasia

Cervical squamous neoplasia comprises the in-situ precursor cervical intraepithelial neoplasia (CIN) and invasive squamous cell carcinoma. CIN is graded as CIN1, CIN2 or CIN3, with CIN1 being considered low-grade and CIN2 and CIN3 high-grade.

p16 is the most useful immunohistochemical marker in this setting. p16 inhibits cell cycle progression and its expression can be upregulated through two main mechanisms:

- Indirectly, by productive high-risk HPV (hrHPV) infection which is the underlying aetiology of most cases of CIN and cervical squamous cell carcinoma;

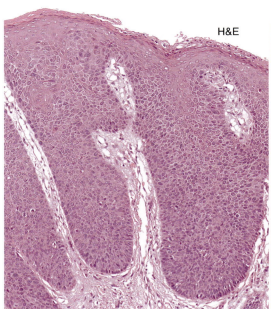 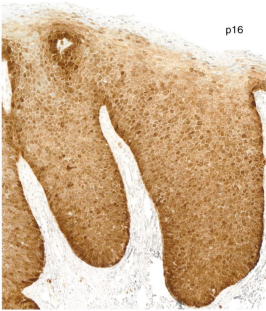

Fig. 15.5 H&E staining shows squamous epithelium in which there is loss of maturation. Immature cells with large, atypical nuclei and mitotic activity extend through much of the thickness of the epithelium, consistent with high-grade CIN. p16 immunohistochemistry shows strong nuclear and cytoplasmic staining which extends for far more than six cells in the horizontal plane and for at least two thirds of the epithelium in the vertical plane. This is block positivity and supports the morphological diagnosis of high-grade CIN

- Directly, by any form of cellular stress (e.g. rapid cell cycle progression, DNA damage).

p16 overexpression can therefore be used as a surrogate marker for productive hrHPV infection; because cervical high-grade squamous neoplasia is usually driven by productive hrHPV, p16 overexpression can be used to support a diagnosis of high-grade squamous neoplasia. However, it is not entirely specific for productive hrHPV infection because it is upregulated in any state of cellular stress. Unrestrained use of p16 immunohistochemistry will therefore result in misdiagnoses: it is essential that it is used (1) only in very specific situations where its specificity is maximised, and that (2) very strict criteria for defining 'overexpression' are used.

Many tissues will show some staining with p16 but this of course does not necessarily indicate hrHPV infection. Only a very specific pattern of staining called 'block positivity' is consistent with p16 overexpression secondary to productive hrHPV infection (Fig. 15.5). This requires all of [29]:

- Strong, continuous nuclear (± cytoplasmic) staining in epithelial cells in the basal and parabasal layers;
- Upward extension of staining involving at least the lower third of the epithelium;
- Involvement of at least six contiguous cells in the horizontal plane.

Anything less than this is considered 'non-block' staining and does not provide evidence of productive hrHPV infection (Fig. 15.6).

It is stressed that most cases of CIN can be diagnosed and graded accurately on morphological grounds alone; p16 immunohistochemistry has only a supportive role in the minority of challenging cases. There are three settings in which p16 immunohistochemistry is useful [29]:

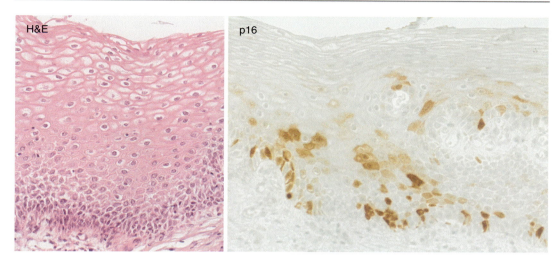

Fig. 15.6 H&E staining shows squamous epithelium containing koilocytes. The epithelium matures appropriately, however, and so there is no evidence of CIN. p16 shows nuclear and cytoplasmic staining in scattered cells throughout the epithelium ('mosaic pattern'). This falls well short of the definition of block positivity and suggests that there is no underlying productive hrHPV infection

1. Where the morphological differential diagnosis is between a benign condition (e.g. immature squamous metaplasia, atrophy) and high-grade CIN. p16 block positivity in the epithelium supports a diagnosis of high-grade CIN, although morphological assessment is still needed to grade this as CIN2 or CIN3. This is the most common setting in which p16 immunohistochemistry is useful.
2. Where morphologically there is CIN, but it is not possible to classify it as low- or high-grade because of a confounding factor (e.g. atrophy or because the epithelium has become detached). It is stressed that grading of CIN must be undertaken on morphological grounds if at all possible. p16 immunohistochemistry can be used to favour low- or high-grade CIN only as a last resort. p16 block positivity in this setting favours high-grade CIN, but this is not absolute.
3. Where the morphology suggests that there is either no neoplasia or only low-grade CIN, but there is a high risk of missing high-grade CIN (e.g. because of high-grade dyskaryosis on cytology). It is stressed that p16 here is being used purely to avoid overlooking an area of high-grade disease and that if there is absolutely no morphological evidence of high-grade CIN, p16 block positivity should not lead to a diagnosis of high-grade CIN.

Invasive squamous cell carcinoma is divided into HPV-associated and HPV-independent subtypes. It is therefore common to perform p16 immunohistochemistry routinely in cervical squamous cell carcinoma for classification purposes.

15.8.2 Cervical Glandular Neoplasia

Cervical glandular neoplasia encompasses high-grade cervical glandular intraepithelial neoplasia (HGCGIN, also known as adenocarcinoma in situ, AIN) and invasive adenocarcinoma. Most cases are HPV-associated but, unlike for cervical squamous neoplasia, a sizeable minority are HPV-independent. HPV-independent adenocarcinomas fall into a variety of subtypes which frequently require rather extensive panels of immunohistochemistry for classification.

HCGIN can sometimes be difficult to distinguish from reactive changes in endocervical glandular epithelium, and so p16 immunohistochemistry is very often performed for confirmation. Strong, continuous, diffuse nuclear (± cytoplasmic) staining in the cells suggests underlying productive hrHPV infection and, by extension, supports a diagnosis of HGCGIN. This pattern of staining is referred to as 'abnormal diffuse positivity' [29] (Fig. 15.7).

15.8.3 HPV In Situ Hybridisation (ISH)

p16 is a good, but not fully sensitive or specific, surrogate marker for productive hrHPV infection. Where more definitive determination of hrHPV status is required, HPV ISH is useful. This is similar to immunohistochemistry but, rather than using antibodies which bind to proteins of interest, ISH uses antibodies which bind to specific nucleic acid sequences. HPV ISH is therefore used to highlight the presence of hrHPV nucleic acids in neoplastic cells. While it shows superior concordance with hrHPV status by PCR, it is still not completely sensitive [30].

It is most often used where a lesion is expected to be hrHPV positive but fails to show p16 overexpression. An example is a uterine squamous cell carcinoma which shows non-block p16 staining; because only a small minority of cervical squamous cell carcinomas are genuinely hrHPV-negative, negativity with HPV ISH should prompt very careful consideration of the tumour actually being a (rare) primary endometrial squamous cell carcinoma.

15.9 Undifferentiated Malignancies

In some cases, a tumour may be so poorly differentiated that it cannot be classified as any particular tumour type on H&E staining alone. Here, immunohistochemistry is essential for accurate classification.

In theory, one could use a huge bank of immunohistochemical stains on such tumour samples from the outset in order to arrive at a diagnosis quickly. However, this is not generally good practice because it is costly and is likely to deplete tumour samples, especially in the case of biopsies. It is therefore preferable to use a series of smaller, sequential immunohistochemical panels to subclassify such tumours in a stepwise fashion. An initial panel for an undifferentiated malignancy should try to place it into a broad tumour family (Table 15.9).

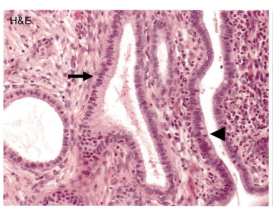
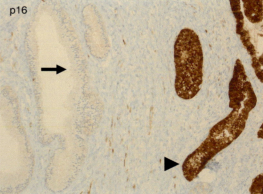

Fig. 15.7 H&E staining shows clearly benign endocervical glands whose epithelial cells have normochromatic basal nuclei and abundant mucinous cytoplasm (arrow); this contrasts with glands in which the epithelial cells have more hyperchromatic nuclei with mitotic figures and loss of cytoplasmic mucin (arrowhead). While the morphology is suggestive of HGCGIN, inflammation could also mimic this. p16 immunohistochemistry shows complete negativity in the benign epithelium (arrow); the atypical glands show strong, continuous, diffuse nuclear and cytoplasmic staining (arrowhead). This supports the diagnosis of HGCGIN

Table 15.9 A useful initial immunohistochemical panel for categorising an undifferentiated malignancy into a broad family of tumours

	Pan-cytokeratin (e.g. AE1/3, CAM5.2)	EMA	S100 (or MelanA, HMB45)	CD45 (LCA)	OCT3/4
Carcinoma	+	+	−	−	−
Melanoma	−	−	+	−	−
Lymphoma	−	−	−	+	−
Germ cell tumour	−	−	−	−	+
Sex cord stromal tumour	−	+	−	−	−
Sarcoma	±	±	±	−	−

There is no single marker which is useful for diagnosing sarcoma; a diagnosis of sarcoma is made by excluding other possibilities, by using markers specific for particular sarcomas, and by using molecular tests

Once a tumour has been placed into a broad tumour category, more specific markers can be used to arrive at a diagnosis, as discussed in the preceding sections of this chapter.

15.10 Serous Fluid Cytology

Pleural or peritoneal fluid is frequently sampled in order to identify the nature and site of origin of metastatic malignancy. Peritoneal fluid is also frequently sampled in order to establish the stage of gynaecological malignancies, particularly tubo-ovarian and primary peritoneal malignancies.

Assessment of serous fluid cytology can be challenging. Normally present mesothelial cells may frequently be difficult to distinguish from metastatic adenocarcinoma on morphological grounds. If the cytology is worrying for malignancy, it is typical to produce from the fluid a solid pellet called a cell block; this can then be used for an initial immunohistochemical panel to distinguish between mesothelial cells and metastatic adenocarcinoma (Table 15.10; Fig. 15.8).

Once an initial panel has established that a sample contains metastatic adenocarcinoma, further markers can be used to determine its site of origin and subtype.

15.11 Summary

Immunohistochemistry is a method for identifying specific antigens in tissue samples from tumours in order to help make a diagnosis, provide prognostic information and, occasionally, to predict response to particular medical therapies. IHC does not act as a replacement for histology; however, can be used as an adjunctive investigation is selected circumstances. No immunomarker is completely sensitive and specific and therefore a panel of several markers is normally required in diagnostically challenging cases. In these circumstances, the markers are chosen at the discretion of the pathologist in order to resolve a specific dilemma, for example typing a tumour with ambiguous or poorly differentiated morphology or identifying the site of origin of a metastatic deposit. Immunohistochemistry has an expanding role in the diagnosis of endometrial carcinoma: reflex testing will become standard practice in order to identify antigen expression profiles associated with emerging molecular classifications and to screen patients for Lynch syndrome.

Interpretation of immunohistochemistry is normally straightforward; however, in some situations, requires awareness of specific staining patterns. For example, aberrant over-expression, null expression or purely cytoplasmic staining with p53 implies an underlying TP53 mutation and so can be used to support a diagnosis of tubo-ovarian high grade serous carcinoma or uterine serous carcinoma, whereas variable intensity staining (wild type) is seen in normal tissues and non-serous tumours. Different patterns of p16 staining can be used in carcinomas and precursor lesions of cervix and vulva to determine the likelihood of an association with high-risk HPV.

Pathologists present immunohistochemistry results in their reports and at tumour board meetings with interpretive advice. Knowledge of the principles of immunohistochemistry and its application in female genital tract tumours will help the clinician to optimise decision-making and patient care.

Table 15.10 Many markers can be used to discriminate between mesothelial cells and metastatic adenocarcinoma, but generally a panel of two mesothelial and two adenocarcinoma markers should be used

	MOC31	BerEP4	Calretinin	WT1
Mesothelial cells	−	−	+	+
Metastatic adenocarcinoma	+	+	−	±

WT1 is frequently used as a mesothelial marker, but it is cautioned that WT1 is also positive in low-grade ovarian serous carcinomas and high-grade extrauterine serous carcinomas

15 Clinical Interpretation of Immunohistochemistry in Gynaecological Cancers

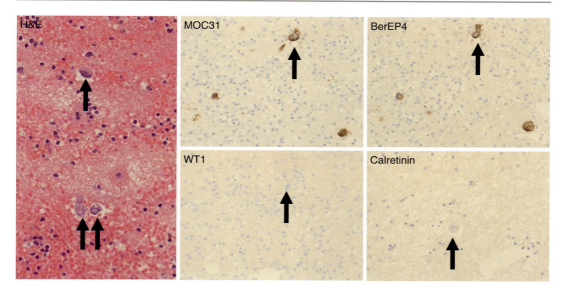

Fig. 15.8 This is a cell block produced from a pleural fluid sample. It comprises large amounts of blood and inflammatory cells with a few large atypical cells (arrows). Immunohistochemistry needs to be used to determine whether these represent metastatic adenocarcinoma or mesothelial cells. The atypical cells (arrows) are positive for MOC31 and BerEP4; they are negative for WT1 and calretinin. This confirms that they represent metastatic adenocarcinoma. Further immunohistochemistry was consistent with metastatic endometrial serous carcinoma

Key Points
1. Immunohistochemistry is an important adjunct to histology and helps to ascertain the diagnosis, site of tumour origin and provide prognostic and predictive information.
2. Aberrant over-expression, null expression or purely cytoplasmic staining with p53 implies an underlying TP53 mutation and so can be used to support a diagnosis of tubo-ovarian high grade serous carcinoma or uterine serous carcinoma, whereas variable intensity staining (wild type) is seen in normal tissues, low grade and non-serous tumours.
3. For metastatic ovarian cancer, pattern of cytokeratin 7 and cytokeratin 20 expression helps to broadly identify the tissue of origin; CDX2 is positive for colon while GATA 3 indicates metastasis from breast
4. WT-1 can help in distinguishing the origin of a serous carcinoma as either uterine or extra-uterine, as the former are usually WT-1 negative.
5. MMR immunohistochemistry (MLH1, MSH2, PMS2 and MSH6) is used to screen for Lynch syndrome and predicts response to treatment with immune checkpoint inhibitors.
6. Smooth muscle neoplasms are generally positive for SMA, desmin and h-caldesmon, unlike endometrial stromal neoplasms. Low-grade endometrial stromal sarcomas are positive for CD10 while high grade ESS show focal positivity for CD10 and are often positive for cyclin D1.
7. Different patterns of p16 staining can be used in carcinomas and precursor lesions of cervix and vulva to determine the likelihood of an association with high-risk HPV.

References

1. Köbel M, Rahimi K, Rambau PF, Naugler C, Le Page C, Meunier L, et al. An immunohistochemical algorithm for ovarian carcinoma typing. Int J Gynecol Pathol. 2016;35(5):430–41.
2. Köbel MM, McCluggage WG, Gilks CB, Singh N. Interpretation of p53 immunohistochemistry in tubo-ovarian carcinoma: guidelines for reporting. Br Assoc Gynaecol Pathol. 2016; https://www.thebagp.org/download/bagp-ukneqas-project-p53-interpretation-guide-2016/ (accessed 27.01.22)
3. Al-Hussaini M, Stockman A, Foster H, McCluggage WG. WT-1 assists in distinguishing ovarian from uterine serous carcinoma and in distinguishing between serous and endometrioid ovarian carcinoma. Histopathology. 2004;44(2):109–15.
4. Deavers MT, Malpica A, Liu J, Broaddus R, Silva EG. Ovarian sex cord-stromal tumors: an immunohistochemical study including a comparison of calretinin and inhibin. Mod Pathol. 2003;16(6):584–90.
5. Rabban JT, Zaloudek CJ. A practical approach to immunohistochemical diagnosis of ovarian germ cell tumours and sex cord-stromal tumours. Histopathology. 2013;62(1):71–88.
6. Al-Nafussi A. Ovarian epithelial tumours: common problems in diagnosis. Curr Diagn Pathol. 2004;10(6):473–99.
7. Chu P, Wu E, Weiss LM. Cytokeratin 7 and cytokeratin 20 expression in epithelial neoplasms: a survey of 435 cases. Mod Pathol. 2000;13(9):962–72.
8. Conner JR, Hornick JL. Metastatic carcinoma of unknown primary: diagnostic approach using immunohistochemistry. Adv Anat Pathol. 2015;22(3):149–67.
9. Ronnett BM, Shmookler BM, Diener-West M, Sugarbaker PH, Kurman RJ. Immunohistochemical evidence supporting the appendiceal origin of pseudomyxoma peritonei in women. Int J Gynecol Pathol. 1997;16(1):1–9.
10. McCluggage WG, Sumathi VP, McBride HA, Patterson A. A panel of immunohistochemical stains, including carcinoembryonic antigen, vimentin, and estrogen receptor, aids the distinction between primary endometrial and endocervical adenocarcinomas. Int J Gynecol Pathol. 2002;21(1):11–5.
11. Kounelis S, Kapranos N, Kouri E, Coppola D, Papadaki H, Jones MW. Immunohistochemical profile of endometrial adenocarcinoma: a study of 61 cases and review of the literature. Mod Pathol. 2000;13(4):379–88.
12. Ramalingam P, Masand RP, Euscher ED, Malpica A. Undifferentiated carcinoma of the endometrium: an expanded immunohistochemical analysis including PAX-8 and basal-like carcinoma surrogate markers. Int J Gynecol Pathol. 2016;35(5):410–8.
13. Cancer Genome Atlas Research Network, Kandoth C, Schultz N, Cherniack AD, Akbani R, Liu Y, et al. Integrated genomic characterization of endometrial carcinoma. Nature. 2013;497(7447):67–73.
14. Gilks CB, Oliva E, Soslow RA. Poor interobserver reproducibility in the diagnosis of high-grade endometrial carcinoma. Am J Surg Pathol. 2013;37(6):874–81.
15. Levine DA, Getz G, Gabriel SB, Cibulskis K, Lander E, Sivachenko A, et al. Integrated genomic characterization of endometrial carcinoma. Nature. 2013;497(7447):67–73.
16. Baretti M, Le DT. DNA mismatch repair in cancer. Pharmacol Ther. 2018;189:45–62.
17. Cerretelli G, Ager A, Arends MJ, Frayling IM. Molecular pathology of Lynch syndrome. J Pathol. 2020;250(5):518–31.
18. Stelloo E, Jansen AML, Osse EM, Nout RA, Creutzberg CL, Ruano D, et al. Practical guidance for mismatch repair-deficiency testing in endometrial cancer. Ann Oncol. 2017;28(1):96–102.
19. Bruegl AS, Djordjevic B, Urbauer DL, Westin SN, Soliman PT, Lu KH, et al. Utility of MLH1 methylation analysis in the clinical evaluation of Lynch Syndrome in women with endometrial cancer. Curr Pharm Des. 2014;20(11):1655–63.
20. Oliva E, Young RH, Amin MB, Clement PB. An immunohistochemical analysis of endometrial stromal and smooth muscle tumors of the uterus: a study of 54 cases emphasizing the importance of using a panel because of overlap in immunoreactivity for individual antibodies. Am J Surg Pathol. 2002;26(4):403–12.
21. McCluggage WG, Sumathi VP, Maxwell P. CD10 is a sensitive and diagnostically useful immunohistochemical marker of normal endometrial stroma and of endometrial stromal neoplasms. Histopathology. 2001;39(3):273–8.
22. Iwasaki S-i, Sudo T, Miwa M, Ukita M, Morimoto A, Tamada M, et al. Endometrial stromal sarcoma: clinicopathological and immunophenotypic study of 16 cases. Arch Gynecol Obstet. 2013;288(2):385–91.
23. Gallardo A, Prat J. Mullerian adenosarcoma: a clinicopathologic and immunohistochemical study of 55 cases challenging the existence of adenofibroma. Am J Surg Pathol. 2009;33(2):278–88.
24. de Leval L, Lim GSD, Waltregny D, Oliva E. Diverse phenotypic profile of uterine tumors resembling ovarian sex cord tumors: an immunohistochemical study of 12 cases. Am J Surg Pathol. 2010;34(12):1749–61.
25. Bennett JA, Braga AC, Pinto A, Van de Vijver K, Cornejo K, Pesci A, et al. Uterine PEComas: a morphologic, immunohistochemical, and molecular analysis of 32 tumors. Am J Surg Pathol. 2018;42(10):1370–83.
26. Wang EC, Kwah YC, Tan WP, Lee JS, Tan SH. Extramammary Paget disease: immunohistochemistry is critical to distinguish potential mimickers. Dermatol Online J. 2012;18(9):4.

27. Perrotto J, Abbott JJ, Ceilley RI, Ahmed I. The role of immunohistochemistry in discriminating primary from secondary extramammary paget disease. Am J Dermatopathol. 2010;32(2):137–43.
28. Mulvany NJ, Allen DG. Differentiated intraepithelial neoplasia of the vulva. Int J Gynecol Pathol. 2008;27(1):125–35.
29. Singh NG, Gilks CB, Wong RWC, McCluggage WG, Herrington CS. Interpretation of p16 immunohistochemistry in lower anogenital tract neoplasia. Br Assoc Gynaecol Pathol. 2019; https://www.thebagp.org/download/bagp-ukneqas-c1qc-projectinterpretation-guide-2018/ (accessed 27.01.22)
30. Guo M, Gong Y, Deavers M, Silva EG, Jan YJ, Cogdell DE, et al. Evaluation of a commercialized in situ hybridization assay for detecting human papillomavirus DNA in tissue specimens from patients with cervical intraepithelial neoplasia and cervical carcinoma. J Clin Microbiol. 2008;46(1):274–80.

16

Genomics in Gynaecological Cancer: What the Clinician Needs to Know

Anca Oniscu, Ayoma Attygalle, and Anthony Williams

16.1 Introduction

Molecular information is increasingly used in diagnostic practice and planning clinical management. The availability and decreased cost of molecular techniques such as next generation sequencing have enabled the development of molecular subgroup classification of tumours beyond features which can be identified by histology or immunochemistry. This information may be used in a number of ways. Specific mutations or genomic rearrangements may support or confirm the diagnosis of a particular tumour type. Efficacy of potential therapeutic strategies may be predicted, and molecular lesions identified which may be targeted by specific therapy. Although it is often impractical to obtain extensive sequencing information on diagnostic specimens, a range of specific investigations may be used to evaluate treatment options and identify molecular subgroups of tumours. These techniques are available in many pathology laboratories and used routinely in diagnostic practice.

16.2 Ovarian Tumours

16.2.1 Ovarian Carcinomas

The study of underlying molecular abnormalities has helped refine the classification of tubo-ovarian carcinomas (TOC) [1]. Due to the reliability of diagnoses based on morphology and immunohistochemistry, genomics is of limited value in the current diagnostic setting but plays an important role in influencing therapeutic options with possible wider genetic implications.

16.2.1.1 High Grade Serous Carcinoma (HGS)

HGS accounts for approximately 70% of all TOC [1]. Most originate in the fimbrial end of the fallopian tube arising from a precursor lesion, serous tubal intra-epithelial carcinoma (STIC) [2].

TP53 Mutations
Almost all HGS and STIC harbour deleterious *TP53* mutations (*TP53*muts), the driver event in pathogenesis. Gain of function (GOF)/non-synonymous *TP53*muts are more common than loss of function (LOF) (stop-gain, frameshift,

A. Oniscu
Royal Infirmary of Edinburgh, Edinburgh, UK
e-mail: anca.oniscu@doctors.org.uk

A. Attygalle
The Royal Marsden NHS Foundation Trust, London, UK
e-mail: ayoma.attygalle@rmh.nhs.uk

A. Williams (✉)
Birmingham Women's and Children's NHS Foundation Trust, Birmingham, UK
e-mail: Anthony.williams15@nhs.net

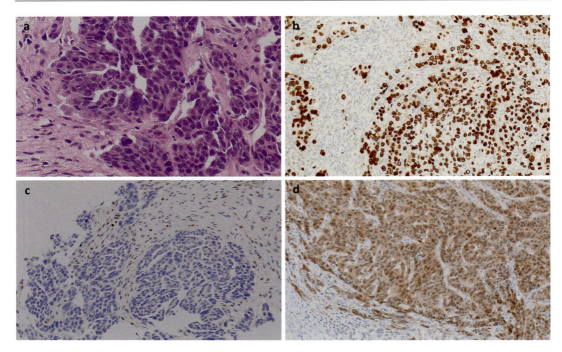

Fig. 16.1 High grade serous carcinoma stained with haematoxylin and eosin (**a**) and with antibodies to p53 demonstrating the three abnormal staining patterns associated with *TP53* mutation: Strong staining in virtually all nuclei (mutant over-expressed pattern) (**b**), Complete absence of nuclear staining (null mutant pattern) (**c**) and abnormal cytoplasmic staining (**d**)

splicing) mutations. Immunohistochemistry is a reliable method of detecting *TP53*muts (Fig. 16.1) in approximately 96% of cases, while in 4%, wild-type staining is observed despite an underlying LOF *TP53*mut [3]. Although there may be some clinical differences depending on whether tumours harbour a GOF or LOF mutation [4] there is no current clinical indication for routine *TP53* mutational analysis.

Although morphology and immunohistochemistry enable diagnosis in virtually all cases, there may be an occasional scenario where equivocal morphology and wild-type p53 staining requires mutational profiling to distinguish between HGS and low grade serous carcinoma (LGSC). This diagnostic distinction may not only influence the choice of whether to opt for primary cytoreductive surgery, but also determines the eligibility and efficacy of maintenance poly ADP ribose polymerase (PARP) inhibitor therapy.

Homologous Recombinant Deficiency (HRD)

Mutations in homologous recombinant (HR) genes result in an inability to repair double strand DNA breaks. HRD not only predisposes to the development of tubo-ovarian HGS but such tumours show increased sensitivity to platinum therapy and PARP inhibitor therapy. Although *BRCA* 1/2 genes are more commonly affected, mutations in other HR genes (germline/somatic) such as *BRIP1*, *RAD51C*, and *RAD51D*, albeit infrequently, are also associated with an increased risk of TOC with possible therapeutic implications [5].

Pathogenic *BRCA1* and *BRCA2* variant genes confer a lifetime risk of developing tubo-ovarian HGS, of up to 50% and 20% respectively. Although mostly germline, some may be somatic and confined to tumour tissue. The role of germline BRCA testing in risk stratification and genetics counselling is well recognised. More recently

PARP inhibitor therapy has been shown to significantly improve progression free survival in patients with advanced HGS harbouring *BRCA1/2* mutations and has been approved for use in this clinical setting [6]. Germline testing performed on peripheral blood (PB) does not detect the minority of cases that are somatic, where the mutation is confined to tumour tissue. Conversely, targeted next generation sequencing (NGS) employed to detect *BRCA* variants in the tumour (t*BRCA*) does not identify large genomic rearrangements. Detection of the latter, which accounts for a minority of germline BRCA variants, requires Multiplex Ligation-dependent Probe Amplification (MLPA), a technique performed on peripheral blood. Therefore, both germline and t*BRCA* testing are needed to capture all pathogenic variants [6].

16.2.1.2 Low Grade Serous Carcinoma (LGSC)

LGSC are unrelated to HGS, have an indolent clinical course and lack *TP3* mutations. A significant number arise in association with serous borderline tumours. LGSC have a high frequency of *MAPK* pathway mutations, with *KRAS, BRAF* and *NRAS* mutations being the most common (Fig. 16.2). While *BRAF* mutations are less frequently seen in high stage tumours, *KRAS* mutations are associated with tumour recurrence [1]. Less frequently, LGSC may be associated with mutations involving *USP9X* and *EIF1AX*, genes linked with mTOR regulation [7]. These molecular alterations have paved the way for targeted therapy e.g. MEK inhibitors, in the trial setting. However, mutational profile is not currently performed routinely, but may be of value in the rare setting mentioned above when distinction between HGS and LGCS is problematic.

16.2.1.3 Ovarian Endometrioid Carcinoma (OEC)

Most OECs arise from endometriosis and display a mutational profile that reflects this. Molecular profiling has played an important role in re-classifying seromucinous carcinoma as OECs with mucinous differentiation [1]. OECs and EECs have similar molecular alterations, at differing frequencies. McConechy at al detected *CTNNB1* (WNT/beta catenin pathway) mutations in 53% of OEC, *KRAS* in 33% (MAPK pathway), *ARID1A* (SWI/SNF complex) in 30%, *PIK3CA* in 40% and *PTEN* mutations in 17% (PI3K pathway) [8].

The four molecular subtypes defined by TCGA for EECs have also been proposed for OECs: ultramutated (POLE-EDM mutant) (3–10%), hypermutated (mismatch repair deficient [MMRd]) (8–19%), *TP53* mutated (17–24%) and no specific molecular profile (58–61%) [1]. If large studies validate the results of smaller series, subtyping may play a role in decisions regarding adjuvant therapy. Most OECs are stage 1 at presentation and are associated with an excellent outcome, but

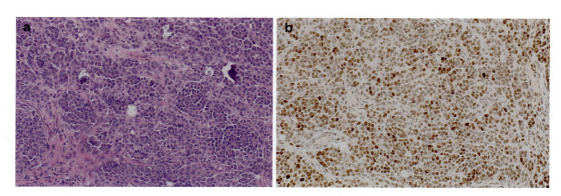

Fig. 16.2 Low grade serous carcinoma stained with haematoxylin and eosin (**a**) and with antibody to p53 (**b**) demonstrating a wild-type pattern of variable nuclear staining intensity

immunotherapy in the case of MMR deficient tumours and novel therapies for targetable alterations (e.g. ATR inhibitor for *ARID1A* mutations) are being trialled in the minority of patients with relapsed disease.

16.2.1.4 Ovarian Clear Cell Carcinoma (OCCC)

OCCCs account for 10% of ovarian carcinomas in the West. They are confined to the ovary, but prognosis is poor in advanced/relapsed disease, with a demand for novel therapies to improve outcome. *ARID1A* mutations occur in 50% of cases. *PIK3CA* mutations frequently occur in tumours also harbouring *ARID1A* mutations. MMR deficiency is uncommon (2%) [1]. Immunotherapy and targeted therapies are being trialled in relapsed/refractory OCCC. Immunohistochemistry is a reliable surrogate for *ARID1A* mutations to identify patients who may benefit from ATR inhibitor therapy [9].

16.2.1.5 Mucinous Carcinoma (MC)

Most MCs arise from borderline tumours. The commonest abnormalities, copy number loss of *CDKN2A* and *KRAS* mutations, are early events that are also present in borderline tumours. *TP53*muts occur at a higher frequency in MC suggesting that it occurs with disease progression. *ERBB2 (HER2)* amplifications may be detected of a minority of tumours harbouring *TP53*muts [10].

16.2.1.6 Undifferentiated/ De-Differentiated Carcinoma

Rare tumours, similar to those of the endometrium.

16.2.2 Sex Cord Stromal Tumours (SCST)

16.2.2.1 Adult Granulosa Cell Tumour (AGCT)

Recurrent *FOXL2* missense mutation (pCys-134Trp), detected in nearly all AGCTs is of no clinical significance, but may help distinguish AGCT from thecoma, which may express the FOXL2 antigen but usually lacks the mutation [1].

16.2.2.2 Sertoli Leydig Cell Tumour (SLCT)

There are three molecular subtypes of SLCTs (Table 16.1) [11]. The predominant *DICER1* mutant group often presents with androgenic manifestations whereas the *FOXL2* mutant group frequently presents with uterine bleeding related to oestrogenic manifestations attributed to upregulation of *CYP19A1*, encoding aromatase.

16.2.2.3 Microcystic Stromal Tumour

Nearly always benign, these tumours harbour mutually exclusive mutations in either *CTNNB1* or *APC*. The latter may rarely be associated with familial polyposis coli [1].

16.2.2.4 Juvenile Granulosa Cell Tumour and Gynandroblastoma

Germline *DICER1* mutations are detected in a minority [1].

16.2.2.5 Sex Cord Tumour with Annular Tubules (SCTAT)

Although very rare, these tumours may commonly occur in patients with Peutz-Jeghers syndrome (PJS), when they are typically small,

Table 16.1 Features of Sertoli Leydig cell tumour molecular subtypes

Molecular subtype	Genetics	Age group	Histologic features
DICER1 mutant	Hotspot mutations in RNase IIIb domain of *DICER1*	15–62 years Up to 70% germline (*DICER1* syndrome): young age	Always moderate to poorly differentiated (M-PD) All cases showing retiform differentiation (RD) and heterologous elements (HE) in this group
FOXL2 mutant	*FOXL2* c.402C>G (p. Cys134Trp)	Post-menopausal	Always M-PD RD and HE not seen
DICER1/FOXL2 wild type	*DICER1/FOXL2* wild type	17–74 years	All well differentiated tumours in this group. RD and HE not seen

bilateral and multifocal and have germline *STK11* mutations. Although non-syndromic cases, typically unilateral and larger, may be associated with extra-ovarian spread, those associated with PJS are typically benign [1].

16.2.3 Small Cell Carcinoma of Hypercalcaemic Type

These rare tumours harbour an inactivating somatic or germline mutation in *SMARCA4*, an important *SWI/SNF* chromatin remodelling gene [12]. Targeted therapy may provide hope in these and other aggressive SMARCA4 deficient tumours. Moreover, if a germline variant is detected, counselling of families with these tumours should be considered.

16.2.4 Germ Cell Tumours

Detection of chromosome 12 abnormalities in up to 80% and *KIT* mutations/amplifications in a subset have no clinical relevance [1].

Choriocarcinoma
Short tandem repeat (STR) DNA genotyping is useful to differentiate non-gestational choriocarcinoma or ovarian metastasis from uterine or tubal gestational choriocarcinoma [13].

Yolk Sac Tumour, Embryonal Carcinoma, Immature Teratoma, Mixed Germ Cell Tumours
No clinically relevant molecular alterations.

16.3 Uterine Tumours

The molecular stratification of uterine tumours, both carcinomas and mesenchymal tumours of the uterus has been a focus of research and clinical trials for a number of years from different perspectives. One focused on identifying Lynch syndrome in patients diagnosed with endometrial carcinomas and the second was driven by the strong clinical need to provide a molecular classification of endometrial carcinomas with subsequent risk and therapeutic stratification.

The access to ancillary techniques such as immunohistochemistry (IHC) and fluorescence in-situ hybridisation (FISH) in addition to genomic mutation profiling is providing the pathologist with additional information which integrated with the morphology helps stratify uterine tumours in recognised molecular subtypes.

16.3.1 Endometrial Carcinomas

Endometrial carcinomas are stratified based on their morphological features with their molecular subtypes incorporated in the WHO classification of tumours [1]. These molecular signatures provide an insight into some of the variants previously unexplained. The use of immunohistochemistry (such as p53, ER, PR and mismatch repair proteins) and, if required, DNA mutation (p53, POLE, MMR) and MLH1 hypermethylation testing help in the assessment of tumours with equivocal morphology or high grade solid morphology of dedifferentiated/undifferentiated type (Fig. 16.3).

The new WHO classification groups endometrial carcinomas into several distinct morphological and molecular subtypes [1]. A comprehensive genomic analysis by The Cancer Genome Atlas provides a molecular classification of the endometrial carcinomas into four main subtypes, all of clinical importance as they provide prognostic and therapeutic value:

(a) *POLE* mutant group also known as ultramutated
(b) Mismatch repair deficient (MMRd) group also known as hypermutated
(c) Copy number low
(d) Copy number high (p53 mutant and serous or serous-like tumours which define a type II group of endometrial tumours)

16.3.1.1 Endometrioid Carcinomas of the Endometrium

This is the most common subtype of endometrial carcinoma and accounts for up to 85% of endometrial tumours. Several differentiation patterns are described such as mucinous, squamous morular, villoglandular or branching papillary but these have no diagnostic or

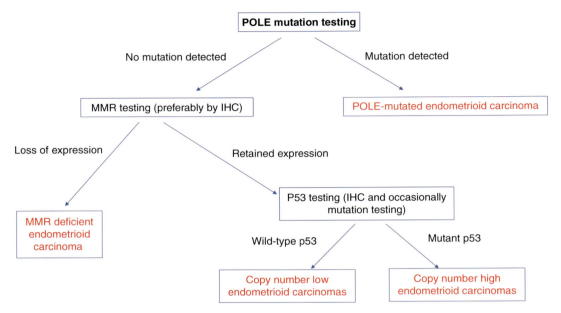

Fig. 16.3 Diagnostic algorithm for integrating the molecular classification of endometrial tumours into routine reporting using a combination of IHC and DNA mutation testing. This algorithmic approach is followed since p53 mutations (typically subclonal) may occur as secondary events in both *POLE* mutated and MMRd tumours. Mutations due to the ultramutated (POLE) and hypermutated (MMRd) genotypes do not have the prognostic implications of a primary driver p53 mutation as occurs in the copy number high tumours

therapeutic implications. Maintained glandular architecture and bland nuclear features are in the majority of cases pointing the pathologist towards a low grade tumour. Any case with nuclear pleomorphism and significant atypia should prompt additional investigations as this may suggest a non-endometrioid subtype and potentially a more aggressive molecular subtype: *TP53* mutant—copy number high (Fig. 16.1).

Endometroid carcinoma and its precursor lesion, endometrial atypical hyperplasia/endometrial intraepithelial neoplasia, have been recognised for a long time to occur on a background of unopposed oestrogenic stimulation of the endometrium either endogenous or exogenous. Most low grade tumours, classified as grade 1 and grade 2 based on the amount of gland formation, are tumours with a similar molecular phenotype: POLE, MMRd or copy number low changes and have a generally good prognosis. In contrast, high grade/grade 3 tumours may demonstrate *TP53* mutations, and in almost 20% of cases are classed as copy number high or serous-like tumours.

Most frequent abnormalities described in endometrioid carcinomas are alterations in the PI3K–PTEN–AKT–mTOR, RAS–MEK–ERK and WNT–β-catenin pathways (Fig. 16.4), microsatellite instability (MSI) indicative of MMRd and a relatively high rate of *POLE* mutations. *ARID1A* mutations have been described but with a lower prevalence. The frequent activation of the PI3K–PTEN–AKT–mTOR pathway has generated interest in the targeted therapies field and clinical trials are underway evaluating the efficacy of mTOR inhibitors, PI3K inhibitors or AKT inhibitors.

Of particular clinical value is the *POLE* or *TP53* mutation status in endometrial carcinomas as these patients may benefit from tailored chemotherapy regimens. The PORTEC-3 trial has demonstrated a clear need for molecular stratification of endometrial tumours as it provides a

16 Genomics in Gynaecological Cancer: What the Clinician Needs to Know

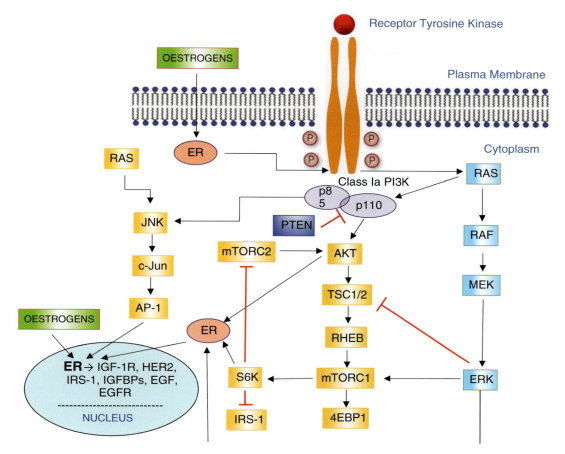

Fig. 16.4 Molecular interactions of the PI3K/AKT/mTOR pathway in endometrial cancer: Class Ia PI3Ks is composed of a catalytic (p110) and a regulatory subunit (p85) which can interact with the receptor tyrosine kinase (RTK). AKT is recruited to the membrane, phosphorylated and activated by mTORC2. AKT phosphorylates and inactivates the TSC complex, and allows for further mTORC1 activation. RTK signalling also activates the RAS pathway; ERK phosphorylates and suppresses TSC. Arrows represent activation signals and red lines highlight where inhibition occurs. Abbreviations: *4EBP1* eukaryotic initiation factor 4E-binding protein 1, *AP-1* activator protein 1, *EGFR* EGF receptor, *IGF-1R* insulin-like growth factor 1 receptor, *IGFBP* insulin-like growth factor binding protein, *IRS-1* insulin receptor substrate 1, *JNK* c-Jun N-terminal kinase, *mTORC1/2* mTOR complex 1/2, *Rheb* RAS homolog enriched in the brain, *S6K* S6 kinase, *TSC* tuberous sclerosis protein)

strong prognostic value in high-risk p53 mutant tumours which show improved recurrence free survival (RFS) while POLE mutations are associated with excellent RFS [14].

MMRd is present in approximately 20–30% of endometrioid carcinomas and, in sporadic tumours, the MMRd status is a consequence of epigenetic silencing through hypermethylation of the MLH1 promoter. While there is no significant association between the MMR status and clinical outcome, the MMR status is predictive of response to neoadjuvant chemotherapy and immune check point inhibitors in advanced-stage patients. MMR testing is also an effective screening method to identify patients with Lynch syndrome as 2–3% of endometrial cancers are familial due to inherited genetic susceptibility. Confirmation of Lynch syndrome also leads to screening of family members and helps implement effective prophylactic measures to prevent cancer developing in affected family members.

Mismatch repair deficiency could be tested by polymerase chain reaction (PCR) using tumour and normal tissue DNA and this detects microsatellite instability (MSI) by comparing the length of nucleotide repeats in tumour cells versus normal cells. A tumour is microsatellite unstable when more than 30% of the tested microsatellite regions exhibit microsatellite instability. Tumours with no instability or instability in less than 30% of regions tested are categorized as stable or microsatellite-low. Immunohistochemistry (IHC) is an alternative testing method and it is currently the testing methodology recommended by the European Society of Medical Oncology and the National Institute for Clinical Excellence (NICE) for MMRd in endometrial carcinomas. A panel of four antibodies is widely used in pathology laboratories to detect the presence or absence of nuclear protein expression for MLH1, PMS2, MSH2 and MSH6. Since these proteins are present in complexes, the loss of one of the markers causes destabilisation of its heterodimer partner. As such, loss of MLH1 expression caused by methylation silencing or by a germline mutation also leads to loss of PMS2 by immunohistochemistry (Fig. 16.5). A tumour with loss of expression for MLH1 and PMS2 but retained expression for MSH2 and MSH6 (Fig. 16.6) requires further molecular testing to investigate the presence of MLH1 promoter hypermethylation and confirmation of a sporadic nature of the tumour prior to referring the patient to Clinical Genetics services to investigate potential germline mutations in MLH1 or PMS2.

Alternatively, tumours with loss of MSH2 tend to also show loss of MSH6. Unlike MSI, MMR IHC can also help identify the gene which may carry the germline mutations. For example, a tumour showing loss of MSH2 and MSH6 nuclear expression but retained MLH1 and PMS2 expression is more likely to carry a germline MSH2 mutation (Fig. 16.7).

Testing for mismatch repair deficiency is currently recommended to be performed by IHC due to potential false negative results related to the design of commercial kits in use for testing microsatellite instability. These kits have been developed to detect microsatellite instability in colorectal tumours and their utility in endometrial tumours has only been explored in recent years due the expansion of Lynch syndrome testing to endometrial tumours. A particular pheno-

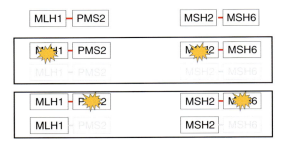

Fig. 16.5 Immunohistochemical patterns of mismatch repair (MMR) protein loss. As these proteins are present as heterodimer complexes, the lack of the upstream partner causes destabilization and inactivation of the downstream heterodimer partner. Therefore loss of MLH1 leads to loss of expression of both MLH1 and PMS2 while loss of MSH2 leads to loss of expression of both MSH2 and MSH6. However, abnormalities in one of the downstream partners of the heterodimers (PMS2 or MSH6) do not affect the expression of the upstream heterodimer partner (which may form complexes with other proteins), and demonstrate a pattern of isolated loss of PMS2 or MSH6

type in endometrioid tumours characterised by loss of MSH6 only on IHC and microsatellite-low or microsatellite stable on DNA testing would be missed if only MSI testing would be performed (Fig. 16.8).

On occasions, POLE mutation testing may be considered when there is a mismatch between the MSI and the MMR IHC status, p53 staining is ambiguous or germline testing has not identified a pathogenic mutation in any of the MMR genes [15]. The lack of a germline mutation in patients referred to clinical genetics for germline testing may also be due to double somatic hits in the MMR genes [16].

16.3.1.2 Serous Carcinomas of the Endometrium

These are aggressive tumours with a poor prognosis which are characterised by high rates of copy number alterations. More than 85% of these tumours harbour mutations in the *TP53* gene. In daily practice this is confirmed by IHC. A mutation phenotype is observed when the tumour shows strong nuclear staining or lack of nuclear staining also reported as a null-aberrant phenotype. Occasionally the pattern of expression may

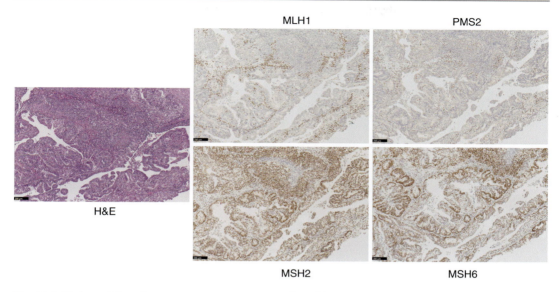

Fig. 16.6 Endometrial carcinoma stained with antibodies to MLH1, PMS2, MSH2 and MHS6. There is nuclear staining loss of MLH1 and PMS2 which may be the result of methylation of *MLH1* leading to subsequent inactivation of the gene or mutation of the *MLH1* gene. This leads to lack of expression of both MLH1 protein and its downstream heterodimer partner PMS2

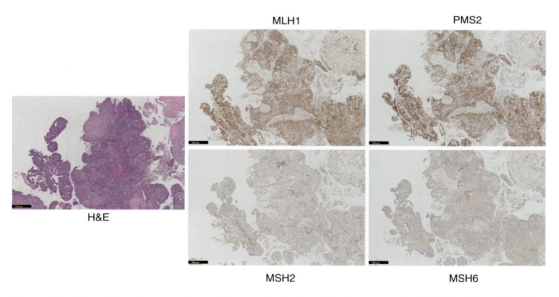

Fig. 16.7 Endometrial carcinoma stained with antibodies to MLH1, PMS2, MSH2 and MHS6. There is nuclear staining loss of MSH2 and MSH6. This pattern is likely to be Lynch Syndrome associated and therefore such patients should be referred to Clinical Genetics services for consideration of germline testing

show both nuclear and cytoplasmic staining and this has recently been recognised as another mutated phenotype (Fig. 16.1). However, due to the variation in staining intensity and distribution of staining mutation testing is recommended in such cases to guide the management of these patients.

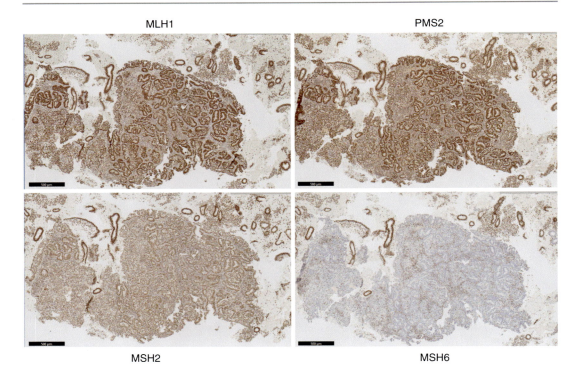

Fig. 16.8 Tumour with loss of MSH6 only and weak expression for MSH2 in a 35 year old patient. Loss of nuclear expression for MSH6 and/or MSH2 should prompt a referral to Clinical Genetics services to investigate the possibility of a pathogenic germline mutation in these genes

In addition to *TP53* mutation other molecular events implicated in the pathogenesis of serous carcinoma include somatic mutations in *PPP2R1A*, *FBXW7*, *SPOP*, *CHD4*, and *TAF1*; amplification and/or overexpression of *ERBB2*, *MYC*, and *CCNE1* (cyclin-E); and overexpression of p16. Alterations in the PI3K pathway are described with mutations in *PIK3CA* in particular (in 17–43% of tumours) and at lower frequencies mutations in *PTEN* and *PIK3R1*.

16.3.1.3 Clear Cell Carcinomas of the Endometrium

Clear cell carcinomas are rare and account for approximately 5% of endometrial tumours. Despite p53 IHC having diagnostic utility in conjunction with the hormone ER status and Napsin A, a significant number of studies report that *TP53* is the most frequently mutated gene in clear cell carcinomas, undergoing somatic mutations in 31–50% of cases and exhibiting a p53 aberrant protein expression in up to 34% of cases. Other cancer genes mutated in clear cell carcinoma are *PPP2R1A*, *PIK3CA*, *FBXW7*, *PTEN*, *KRAS*, *ARID1A*, *SPOP* and *POLE* (up to 6%). MSI or abnormal MMR protein expression have been reported in up to 19% and loss of BAF250A (*ARID1A*) expression has been observed in 26% of cases.

16.3.1.4 Carcinosarcomas

These are tumours with biphasic morphology and an immunophenotype with both epithelial and mesenchymal differentiation. However, despite showing immunophenotypic differences, both components are very similar in their molecular alterations, leading to the accepted concept that these morphological changes are due to epithelial mesenchymal interactions and transdifferentiation. Genomic studies revealed that based on their molecular phenotype approximately 70% of carcinosarcomas resemble uterine serous carcinomas and 30% are more similar to endometrioid carcinomas explaining the IHC differences sometimes encountered. Some of the endometrioid types may display MMRd or POLE mutations and follow the TCGA classification of the endometrioid carcinomas.

16.3.2 Uterine Sarcomas with Focus on Common Tumours such as Leiomyosarcomas and Uterine Stromal Sarcomas

16.3.2.1 Leiomyosarcomas

These are malignant tumours arising from the myometrial smooth muscle. They are the most common uterine sarcoma and their morphology varies from a spindle cell type with a smooth muscle fascicular arrangement to a high grade tumour pleomorphic with no morphological recognition of the low grade or smooth muscle component. In such cases ancillary tests such as IHC may help identify a phenotype suggestive of smooth muscle differentiation with smooth muscle actin, desmin or caldesmon positivity. Molecular abnormalities commonly described in these tumours are mutations and deletions in *TP53*, *RB1*, *α-thalassemia/mental retardation syndrome X-linked* (*ATRX*) and *mediator complex subunit 12* (*MED12*) but they are not specific and in high grade tumours where IHC is not discriminatory, testing does not provide diagnostic value.

16.3.2.2 Uterine Stromal Sarcomas

Endometrial stromal sarcomas could be classified based on their morphology and molecular phenotype into low-grade and high-grade stromal sarcomas. The low-grade ESS are associated in a significant proportion of cases with gene rearrangement leading to a *JAZF 1-SUZ12* fusion. Other fusions have been described and these involve the *PHF1* gene with various partners [1].

High-grade endometrial stromal sarcomas are also described to harbour several gene rearrangements and such as *YWHAE-NUTM*2A/B fusions or *ZC3H7B-BCOR* fusions. Depending on the fusion present the morphology and immunophenotype may show variation, a proportion of the *YWHAE-NUTM*2A/B sarcomas show IHC positivity for Cyclin D1 KIT, CD56 or CD99 while the *ZC3H7B-BCOR* fusion sarcomas may show Cyclin D1, CD10 and possible ER and PR positivity. Demonstrating a fusion may be helpful for diagnostic purposes. Moreover, high-grade ESS with metastasis with *YWHAE* rearrangement shows a relatively favourable prognosis and may be responsive to anthracycline-based therapy [1].

16.4 Cervical Tumours

16.4.1 Cervical Epithelial Neoplasia

The majority of cervical epithelial neoplasms are associated with high risk HPV (HR HPV) infection and the WHO 2020 classification system distinguishes between HPV associated (HPVA) and HPV independent (HPVI) tumours. Although most cervical cancers are squamous cell carcinomas, amongst which HPV independent tumours are rare, adenocarcinomas are increasing in both relative and absolute incidence accounting for up to 25% of tumours in populations where cervical screening is well established. Approximately 15% of endocervical adenocarcinomas are HPV independent. These include gastric, clear cell mesonephric and endometrioid type tumours which harbor distinct molecular alterations. Regard to these specific abnormalities may enable the identification of predictive biomarkers and specific therapeutic intervention, with areas of interest including *ERBB2* (*HER2*) mutations and PDL1 expression.

16.5 Vulval and Vaginal Tumours

16.5.1 Vulval Squamous Neoplasia

The majority (90–95%) of malignant vulval tumours are squamous cell carcinomas (SCC). Two distinct pathways of pathogenesis are described, HPV associated (HPVA) and HPV independent (HPVI), which differ in epidemiology, clinical features, precursor lesions, histological and molecular characteristics [1]. Distinction between the two categories of tumours may be achieved by a combination of morphology, supplementary immunochemistry and testing for HPV. There are a variety of testing strategies and targets for HPV detection in tissue including HPV DNA, HPV E6/E7 mRNA following integration, or altered expression of cellular proteins, particularly overexpression of the p16 protein. Complementary overexpression of p16 accompanies Rb protein degradation following binding of the HPV E7 oncoprotein and may be detected as confluent nuclear and cytoplasmic staining on immunohistochemistry.

Around 65% of vulval SCC arise via an HPV independent pathway and show more aggressive behaviour. Many of these tumours are characterised by *TP53* mutation which may be recognized by abnormal patterns of immunohistochemical nuclear staining. A subset of HPVI tumours have wild type *TP53* and some show *NOTCH1* and *HRAS* mutations.

16.5.2 Malignant Melanoma

Melanoma is the second most common malignancy arising in the vulva, accounting for up to 10% of primary vulval malignancies. Primary vulval melanoma is uncommon compared with those at ultraviolet exposed sites and is diagnosed at older age. Up to 40% of women present with regional or distant metastasis and compared with cutaneous and non-gynaecological mucosal melanoma, prognosis is relatively poor. Information concerning molecular alterations within melanoma has led to expansion of treatment options and increased survival. Vulvovaginal melanoma differs from both cutaneous melanoma and that from other mucosal origins, with *KIT* mutations in 20–44%. Detection of *KIT* alterations may allow patients with advanced disease to undergo treatment with tyrosine kinase. *BRAF* mutation is commonly detected in melanoma on the trunk and extremities; rates of such mutation are generally lower in vulval melanoma, although identified more frequently in recent series perhaps due to more sensitive detection methods. Activating mutations such as the most common V600E mutation are seen less frequently in vulval melanoma but results in eligibility for treatment with BRAF inhibitor therapy [17, 18].

16.5.3 Mesenchymal Tumours

A broad range of soft tissue neoplasms may arise in the vulva and vagina and the majority are uncommon. Diagnosis is achieved by morphologic assessment, supplemented with immunochemistry, but a range of neoplasms have characteristic genetic abnormalities, identification of which may aid diagnosis and direct targeted therapy.

Benign mesenchymal tumours commonly have diploid karyotypes or a single characteristic chromosomal rearrangement whilst in malignancy two broad categories are seen: Sarcomas with simple karyotypes, associated with recurrent mutation or translocation and sarcomas with complex karyotypes with multiple chromosomal abnormalities, lacking recurrent mutations, except for loss of function mutations in genes such as *TP53* or *RB1* [1].

16.6 Summary

Gynaecological cancers include a large and diverse range of neoplasms. Further subgroups have been identified on the basis of molecular information and this may be of value in determining management. As the volume of molecular and clinical trial data accumulates, the challenge is to incorporate investigation into diagnostic practice to enable increasingly personalised treatment which is timely and cost efficient.

Key Points
- Molecular information supports recognition of specific cancer types, identifies subgroups of tumours and informs management strategies
- *TP53* mutations may be detected by immunochemistry and are typical in STIC, High Grade Serous Carcinoma

and some endometrial and vulval carcinomas
- Homologous recombinant deficiency including *BRCA1* and *BRCA2* mutations is common in high grade serous carcinoma and guides therapeutic management
- Ovarian endometrioid carcinomas share similar molecular alterations to endometrial carcinomas although at different frequencies
- Sertoli Leydig cell tumours may be divided into three molecular subgroups on the basis of *DICER1* and *FOXL2* mutations
- Endometrial carcinomas are divided into four molecular subgroups which may be recognised in diagnostic practice using pragmatic molecular classifiers
- Mismatch repair deficiency can be detected by immunochemistry for the proteins MLH1, PMS2, MSH2 and MSH6
- Low grade and high grade uterine stromal sarcomas may be distinguished by characteristic gene rearrangements
- Cervical and vulval carcinomas include HPV associated and diverse HPV independent tumours

References

1. WHO Classification of Tumours Editorial Board. Female genital tract, WHO classification of tumours. 5 ed. IARC. 2020.
2. Singh N, McCluggage WG, Gilks CB. High-grade serous carcinoma of tubo-ovarian origin: recent developments. Histopathology. 2017;71(3):339–56.
3. Köbel M, Piskorz AM, Lee S, Lui S, LePage C, Marass F, Rosenfeld N, Mes Masson AM, Brenton JD. Optimized p53 immunohistochemistry is an accurate predictor of TP53 mutation in ovarian carcinoma. J Pathol Clin Res. 2016;2(4):247–58.
4. Kang HJ, Chun SM, Kim KR, Sohn I, Sung CO. Clinical relevance of gain-of-function mutations of p53 in high-grade serous ovarian carcinoma. PLoS One. 2013;13:8.
5. Pennington KP, Walsh T, Harrell MI, Lee MK, Pennil CC, Rendi MH, Thornton A, Norquist BM, Casadei S, Nord AS, Agnew KJ, Pritchard CC, Scroggins S, Garcia RL, King MC, Swisher EM. Germline and somatic mutations in homologous recombination genes predict platinum response and survival in ovarian, fallopian tube, and peritoneal carcinomas. Clin Cancer Res. 2014;20(3):764–75.
6. Sundar S, Manchanda R, Gourley C, George A, Wallace A, Balega J, Williams S, Wallis Y, Edmondson R, Nicum S, Frost J, Attygalle A, Fotopoulou C, Bowen R, Bell D, Gajjar K, Ramsay B, Wood NJ, Ghaem-Maghami S, Miles T, Ganesan R. British Gynaecological Cancer Society/British Association of Gynaecological Pathology consensus for germline and tumor testing for BRCA1/2 variants in ovarian cancer in the United Kingdom. Int J Gynecol Cancer. 2021;31(2):272–8.
7. Hunter SM, Anglesio MS, Ryland GL, Sharma R, Chiew YE, Rowley SM, Doyle MA, Li J, Gilks CB, Moss P, Allan PE, Stephens AN, Huntsman DG, de Fazio A, Bowtell DD, Australian Ovarian Cancer Study Group, Gorringe KL, Campbell IG. Molecular profiling of low grade serous ovarian tumours identifies novel candidate driver genes. Oncotarget. 2015;6(35):37663–77.
8. McConechy MK, Ding J, Senz J, Yang W, Melnyk N, Tone AA, Prentice LM, Wiegand KC, McAlpine JN, Shah SP, Lee CH, Goodfellow PJ, Gilks CB, Huntsman DG. Ovarian and endometrial endometrioid carcinomas have distinct CTNNB1 and PTEN mutation profiles. Mod Pathol. 2014;27(1):128–34.
9. Khalique S, Naidoo K, Attygalle AD, Kriplani D, Daley F, Lowe A, Campbell J, Jones T, Hubank M, Fenwick K, Matthews N, Rust AG, Lord CJ, Banerjee S, Natrajan R. Optimised ARID1A immunohistochemistry is an accurate predictor of ARID1A mutational status in gynaecological cancers. J Pathol Clin Res. 2018;4(3):154–66.
10. Cheasley D, Wakefield MJ, Ryland GL, Allan PE, Alsop K, Amarasinghe KC, Ananda S, Anglesio MS, Au-Yeung G, Böhm M, Bowtell DDL, Brand A, Chenevix-Trench G, Christie M, Chiew YE, Churchman M, DeFazio A, Demeo R, Dudley R, Fairweather N, Fedele CG, Fereday S, Fox SB, Gilks CB, Gourley C, Hacker NF, Hadley AM, Hendley J, Ho GY, Hughes S, Hunstman DG, Hunter SM, Jobling TW, Kalli KR, Kaufmann SH, Kennedy CJ, Köbel M, Le Page C, Li J, Lupat R, McNally OM, McAlpine JN, Mes-Masson AM, Mileshkin L, Provencher DM, Pyman J, Rahimi K, Rowley SM, Salazar C, Samimi G, Saunders H, Semple T, Sharma R, Sharpe AJ, Stephens AN, Thio N, Torres MC, Traficante N, Xing Z, Zethoven M, Antill YC, Scott CL, Campbell IG, Gorringe KL. The molecular origin and taxonomy of mucinous ovarian carcinoma. Nat Commun. 2019;10(1):3935.
11. Karnezis AN, Wang Y, Keul J, Tessier-Cloutier B, Magrill J, Kommoss S, Senz J, Yang W, Proctor L, Schmidt D, Clement PB, Gilks CB, Huntsman DG,

Kommoss F. DICER1 and FOXL2 mutation status correlates with clinicopathologic features in ovarian Sertoli-Leydig cell tumors. Am J Surg Pathol. 2019;43(5):628–38.
12. Witkowski L, Carrot-Zhang J, Albrecht S, Fahiminiya S, Hamel N, Tomiak E, Grynspan D, Saloustros E, Nadaf J, Rivera B, Gilpin C, Castellsagué E, Silva-Smith R, Plourde F, Wu M, Saskin A, Arseneault M, Karabakhtsian RG, Reilly EA, Ueland FR, Margiolaki A, Pavlakis K, Castellino SM, Lamovec J, Mackay HJ, Roth LM, Ulbright TM, Bender TA, Georgoulias V, Longy M, Berchuck A, Tischkowitz M, Nagel I, Siebert R, Stewart CJ, Arseneau J, McCluggage WG, Clarke BA, Riazalhosseini Y, Hasselblatt M, Majewski J, Foulkes WD. Germline and somatic SMARCA4 mutations characterize small cell carcinoma of the ovary, hypercalcemic type. Nat Genet. 2014;46(5):438–43.
13. Zhang X, Yan K, Chen J, Xie X. Using short tandem repeat analysis for choriocarcinoma diagnosis: a case series. Diagn Pathol. 2019;14(1):93. https://doi.org/10.1186/s13000-019-0866-5.
14. de Boer SM, Powell ME, Mileshkin L, Katsaros D, Bessette P, Haie-Meder C, Ottevanger PB, Ledermann JA, Khaw P, Colombo A, Fyles A, Baron MH, Jürgenliemk-Schulz IM, Kitchener HC, Nijman HW, Wilson G, Brooks S, Carinelli S, Provencher D, Hanzen C, Lutgens LCHW, Smit VTHBM, Singh N, Do V, D'Amico R, Nout RA, Feeney A, Verhoeven-Adema KW, Putter H, Creutzberg CL. PORTEC study group. Adjuvant chemoradiotherapy versus radiotherapy alone for women with high-risk endometrial cancer (PORTEC-3): final results of an international, open-label, multicentre, randomised, phase 3 trial. Lancet Oncol. 2018;19(3):295–309.
15. Stelloo E, Jansen AML, Osse EM, Nout RA, Creutzberg CL, Ruano D, Church DN, Morreau H, Smit VTHBM, van Wezel T, Bosse T. Practical guidance for mismatch repair-deficiency testing in endometrial cancer. Ann Oncol. 2017;28(1):96–102.
16. Hampel H, Pearlman R, de la Chapelle A, Pritchard CC, Zhao W, Jones D, Yilmaz A, Chen W, Frankel WL, Suarez AA, Cosgrove C, Backes F, Copeland L, Fowler J, O'Malley D, Salani R, McElroy JP, Stanich PP, Goodfellow P, Cohn DE. Double somatic mismatch repair gene pathogenic variants as common as Lynch syndrome among endometrial cancer patients. Gynecol Oncol. 2021;160(1):161–8.
17. Curti BD, Faries MB. Recent advances in the treatment of melanoma. N Engl J Med. 2021;384(23):2229–40.
18. Hou JY, Baptiste C, Hombalegowda RB, Tergas AI, Feldman R, Jones NL, Chatterjee-Paer S, Bus-Kwolfski A, Wright JD, Burke WM. Vulvar and vaginal melanoma: a unique subclass of mucosal melanoma based on a comprehensive-molecular analysis of 51 cases compared with 2253 cases of nongynecologic melanoma. Cancer. 2017;123(8):1333–44.

17. Role of Genetics in Gynaecological Cancers

Ashwin Kalra, Monika Sobocan, Dan Reisel, and Ranjit Manchanda

17.1 Introduction

Advances in testing technologies, bioinformatics, falling costs, growing clinical applicability and increasing societal awareness has led to a surge in genetic testing for cancer susceptibility genes (CSGs). Over the years, genetic testing for gynaecological cancers has expanded rapidly, offering unprecedented insights into the heritability of certain cancer types, as well as new opportunities for diagnosis, treatment, and prevention. Understanding of key aspects of the genetics of gynaecological cancer and its applicability to clinical care has now become an essential part of clinical practice. In this chapter, we describe what a clinician working in women's health and oncology needs to know about genetics of gynaecological cancers, to offer optimal care to their patients.

Around 2.9 million women worldwide and ~88,000 UK women are diagnosed with ovarian cancer (OC), breast cancer (BC), endometrial cancer (EC), or colorectal cancer (CRC) every year. Around 1.05 million women worldwide and 25,000 women in the UK will die from these cancers each year [1–3]. These cancers account for ~50% cancers in women [3]. GLOBOCAN predicts these cancer cases will rise by 20–36% and deaths by 36–47% in UK women; while cases will increase by 27–53% and deaths by 49–69% in women worldwide over the next 20 years [2], leading to a huge increase in disease burden.

Studies from twins suggest that inheritable factors account for ~22% of ovarian cancer (OC), ~27% of breast cancer (BC) and ~35% of CRC risk [4]. Inheritable 'pathogenic and likely pathogenic variants' or 'mutations', here forth called 'Pathogenic variants' or 'PVs' in moderate to high penetrance CSGs account for around 15–20% OC [5, 6], 4% BC [7, 8], 3% EC [9] and 4% CRC [10, 11] with a majority being potentially preventable. See Table 17.1 for a list of relevant genes, associated cancer risks and corresponding risk management options.

Ashwin Kalra, Monika Sobocan and Dan Reisel contributed equally with all other contributors.

A. Kalra · M. Sobocan
Wolfson Institute of Population Health, Queen Mary, University of London, London, UK
e-mail: a.kalra@qmul.ac.uk; m.sobocan@qmul.ac.uk

D. Reisel
Department of Women's Cancer, Institute for Women's Health, University College London, London, UK

R. Manchanda (✉)
Wolfson Institute of Population Health, Queen Mary, University of London, London, UK

Department of Gynaecological Oncology, Barts Health NHS Trust, London, UK

Department of Health Services Research, Faculty of Public Health & Policy, London School of Hygiene & Tropical Medicine, London, UK
e-mail: r.manchanda@qmul.ac.uk

Table 17.1 Genes, relevant cancer risks and management options

GENE	Cancer risks % BC	OC	CRC	EC	Risk management options BC	OC	CRC	EC	Other
[a]*BRCA1*/ [12]	~72	~44			RRM [13], CP (SERM), [14] [b]Screening (MRI, Mammogram) [15]	RRSO [16] RRESDO [17, 18]			Lifestyle Reproduction Contraception, PND, PGD
BRCA2	69	17							
[a]*PALB2* [19]	53	5							
[a]*RAD51C* [20]	21–	11–			[b]Screening (Mammogram) [15]				
RAD51D	20	13							
[c]*BRIP1* [21]		6							
[d]*MLH1* [22–24]		11	48	37		Hysterectomy and BSO [25]	Screening (Colonoscopy) [26]Surgical Prevention, CP (Aspirin) [27]	Hysterectomy [25] Annual USS, hysteroscopy and endometrial biopsy
[d]*MSH2*		17	47	49					
[d]*MSH6*		11	20	41					
[d]*PMS2*[e]		3	10	13					

RRM Risk Reducing Mastectomy, *RRSO* Risk reducing Salpingo-oophorectomy, *RRESDO* Risk reducing early salpingectomy and delayed oophorectomy, *BSO* Bilateral Salpingo-oophorectomy, *Hyst* hysterectomy, *SERM* Selective Estrogen Receptor Modulators, *PGD* Pre-implantation Genetic Diagnosis, *PND* Prenatal Diagnosis, *CP* chemoprevention

[a]Breast and Ovarian cancer genes
[b]NHS High risk Breast Cancer Screening Programme
[c]Ovarian cancer gene
[d]MMR or Lynch Syndrome genes
[e]BSO is not recommended for *PMS2* as ovarian cancer risk is similar to population level risk

17.2 Cancer Syndromes

The common cancer syndromes encountered in gynaecological practice are associated with autosomal dominant gene mutations. These include Hereditary Breast and Ovarian Cancer (HBOC), Hereditary ovarian cancer (HOC) and Lynch Syndrome (LS). Other rarer conditions which contribute only a small proportion to the spectrum include Cowden's, Peutz-Jeghers and Li-Fraumeni syndromes. See Table 17.2 for a list of syndromes and associated cancers.

Hereditary Breast and Ovarian Cancer (HBOC) Includes families with multiple cases of breast and ovarian cancer. Important genes implicated include high penetrance *BRCA1*, *BRCA2*, *PALB2*, and moderate penetrance *RAD51C*, *RAD51D* genes.

Hereditary Ovarian Cancer (HOC) Includes families with multiple cases of ovarian cancer only. Important genes implicated include high penetrance *BRCA1*, *BRCA2*, *PALB2*; and moderate penetrance *RAD51C*, *RAD51D*, *BRIP1* genes.

Lynch Syndrome (LS) The tumour spectrum comprises a number of cancers of which colorectal cancer (CRC), EC, and OC are the commonest. Additionally, it includes gastric, small bowel, hepatobiliary, brain, ureteric and renal pelvic (upper urologic tract) cancers. LS is caused by a mutation in one of the MMR genes [23, 25]. MMR genes include *MLH1*, *MSH2*, *MSH6* and *PMS2*. Historically the Amsterdam criteria-2 (AC-2) were used to identify LS [28]. This follows a 3:2:1 rule and includes, (a) ≥3 relatives related by a first degree relationship with an LS cancer (described above), (b) These LS cancers should span ≥2 generations and (c) one (or more) of these cancers is <50 years [28]. Given the poor sensitivity of AC-2, Bethesda criteria were introduced and used at cancer diagnosis to determine which tumour samples should undergo molecular analysis via microsatellite instability (MSI) or immunohistochemistry (IHC) to identify MMR deficiency and enable subsequent triage for MMR gene testing. However, both AC-2 and Bethesda criteria miss a number of MMR PV carriers.

Cowden's Syndrome
Cowden's Syndrome is caused by PVs in the *PTEN* gene. These PVs are associated with a 10–28% risk of EC [29, 30]. However, the risk of OC is not increased. It is also associated with a 50% risk of BC and 3–10% risk of thyroid cancer.

Peutz-Jeghers Syndrome (PJS)
PJS is caused by PVs in the *STK11/LKB1* genes. PJS is characterised by polyps throughout the gastrointestinal tract and muco-cutaneous pigmentation. PJS is associated with an increased risk of adenoma malignum which is a rare cervical cancer. Additionally, benign sex cord stromal ovarian

Table 17.2 Relevant cancer syndromes

	HBOC	HOC	Lynch syndrome	Cowden's syndrome	Peutz-Jeghers syndrome
Genes	*BRCA1, BRCA2, RAD51C, RAD51D, PALB2*	*BRCA1, BRCA2, RAD51C, RAD51D, BRIP1*	MMR (*MLH1/MSH2/MSH6/PMS2*)	*PTEN*	*STK11/LKB1*
Cancers gynaecological	Ovary Breast	Ovary	Ovary Endometrium	Breast Endometrium	Breast Cervix
Cancers other			Colon, gastric, ureteral, small bowel, ureteric, renal pelvic, biliary, pancreatic, glioblastoma	Colon, thyroid, benign hamartomas	Bowel hamartomas, gastric, pancreatic

tumours have been reported in PJS. Although EC and OC cases have been reported in some series these are uncommon [31, 32]. It is also associated with an increased risk of breast and gastrointestinal cancers. PJS-associated cervical cancer is difficult to screen for and preventive hysterectomy is not warranted.

Li-Fraumeni Syndrome (LFS) LFS is caused by germline *TP53* mutations, and is highly penetrant with up to 90% of carriers developing cancer by age 60 [33]. It is associated with young-onset sarcomas, breast cancer, colon cancer, adrenocortical carcinoma, leukaemia, lymphoma and childhood tumours. It does not increase the risk of ovarian, endometrial or cervical cancers.

17.3 Classes of Variants

Variants can be of 5 classes (see Table 17.3) [34]. Pathogenic and Likely pathogenic variants are clinically actionable (together called PVs). A small proportion of Variants of Uncertain Significance (VUS) may get reclassified as PVs in the future. However, currently no clinical intervention should be based on VUS alone.

17.4 Advantages of Genetic Testing

Effective preventive therapy options including risk reducing surgery, chemoprevention and screening are available to reduce PV carriers' cancer risks are available (see Table 17.1).

Women can also make lifestyle, contraceptive and reproductive choices impacting cancer risk including pre-natal or preimplantation genetic diagnosis (PGD) to prevent transmission to their children [35].

Women at increased risk of ovarian cancer can opt for risk-reducing salpingo-oophorectomy (RRSO) which is the most effective option to reduce their OC risk once their family is complete [16, 36]. Traditionally it has been offered to *BRCA1/BRCA2* carriers and been shown to reduce OC incidence and mortality. There is a very small residual risk of primary peritoneal cancer. Additionally, 5% women may have STIC (serous tubular intraepithelial carcinoma) or early invasive cancer detected at histology, necessitating further investigations and surgical staging. RRSO has been found to be cost-effective above a 4–5% lifetime ovarian cancer risk threshold [37, 38]. At this level of OC risk it can add another 10 years to a woman's life who would have otherwise developed OC. This provides clinical utility for RRSO to be undertaken for the moderate penetrance genes too [39]. RRSO is now offered to women with moderate penetrance OC genes who are at intermediate (5–10%) risk of OC. Women undergoing premenopausal oophorectomy if not contraindicated, should be offered HRT until the average age of natural menopause (51 years) to minimize the detrimental consequences of early menopause. Women should be provided with evidence-based information, HRT advice, specialist counselling and long-term support to deal with

Table 17.3 Class of variants

Variant description	Variant class	Probability of being pathogenic	Clinical recommendations
Pathogenic	5	>0.99	Eligible for risk management options
Likely pathogenic	4	0.95–0.99	Eligible for risk management options
Variant of uncertain significance (VUS)	3	0.05–0.949	No clinical implication (on its own). Needs follow up. A small proportion may get reclassified as Class 4 or 5 in the future
Likely benign or likely not pathogenic	2	0.001–0.049	No clinical implication
Benign or not pathogenic	1	<0.001	No clinical implication

the health consequences of early menopause. Broad acceptance of the tubal hypothesis has led to risk-reducing early salpingectomy and delayed oophorectomy (RRESDO) as a new OC prevention strategy for premenopausal women. This has high acceptability in premenopausal women concerned about the side effects of early surgical menopause [17, 40]. However, given the lack of long-term outcome data it is currently advocated in the context of a clinical trial [18]. Annual screening for ovarian cancer in a low-risk population has not shown a mortality benefit [41]. In high-risk women 4-monthly CA125 based screening using a longitudinal mathematical algorithm has been investigated and showed a significant stage shift [42], but these studies were not designed to assess survival or mortality. There is no national OC screening programme for high-risk women. Testing women with OC offers the opportunity for tailored chemotherapy treatment at first line (and relapse) settings, which can improve progression-free survival (see below) [43].

Women at increased risk of BC can opt for MRI/mammography screening and chemoprevention with selective estrogen receptor modulators (SERM) to reduce their BC risk [14]. Surgical prevention in the form of risk-reducing mastectomy (RRM) is the most effective option for reducing BC risk [13].

Options for LS/MMR carriers include prophylactic hysterectomy and bilateral salpingo-oophorectomy as the most effective intervention to prevent EC and OC. This is usually offered after the age of 40 years once a carrier's family is complete. Oophorectomy is not recommended in women with PMS2 PVs or Cowden's syndrome. Additionally 1–2 yearly colonoscopy for colorectal cancer screening and daily aspirin [27, 44] is advised to reduce CRC risk [26]. Although the evidence base for EC screening in high-risk women is limited, case series [45–48] show it can detect both precancer (complex atypical hyperplasia) and early cancer, although interval cancers may occur. EC screening may have a role to play in LS/Cowden's for women who wish to delay surgical prevention, and is usually undertaken from 35 years of age. EC screening options involve annual transvaginal ultrasound scanning (TVS) and endometrial sampling alone or outpatient hysteroscopy plus endometrial sampling (OHES). TVS alone without endometrial sampling is not effective.

17.5 Disadvantages of Genetic Testing

Some of the disadvantages described include some women feeling anxious or distressed after receiving a positive test result; feeling guilty about transmission to children and their risk; implications for family dynamics; marriageability (in some communities) and stigmatization (reported in a minority). Additionally, some women may receive an uncertain result called a variant of uncertain significance (VUS). Other issues to consider include potential implications for insurance/employment. In the US the GINA (Genetic Information Non-discrimination Act) and in the UK a code on genetic testing and insurance provides a moratorium between Department of Health and Association of British Insurers to protect against use of test results for setting insurance premiums (https://www.abi.org.uk/data-and-resources/tools-and-resources/genetics/code-on-genetic-testing-and-insurance/).

17.6 The Traditional Family History (FH) Based Approach to Genetic Testing

Traditionally, women carrying moderate to high penetrance PVs in CSGs have been identified by the FH based approach to genetic testing. This involves obtaining a detailed three generation FH, including both maternal and paternal sides of the family, ethnicity, types of cancer, ages of onset, ages of death, histology and any genetic testing undertaken. Results of any molecular testing undertaken on tumour tissue and prophylactic surgical history should also be documented. Various FH models and clinical criteria have been used to predict probability of carrying a PV and to identify those who are at increased risk and should be offered genetic testing. This is dependent on knowledge and accuracy of FH. Commonly used models include the Manchester Scoring System (MSS), BOADICEA or CANRISK, Tyrer-Cuzick and BRCAPRO. In the UK *BRCA1/BRCA2* testing is offered to those who have an *apriori* ≥10% combined *BRCA1+BRCA2* probability. MSS is an easy-to-use table providing a score based on FH of BC, OC, prostate and pancreatic cancers on the same side of the family [49]. A combined score of 15 corresponds to the 10% testing threshold and a score of 20 to the 20% threshold. However, MSS cannot be used for Ashkenazi Jewish (AJ) families. Laxer clinical criteria are used for AJ families given the higher *BRCA* prevalence in this population [50].

Genetic testing may be diagnostic or predictive. A diagnostic genetic test is when the test is used to identify a PV in the family for the first time. This is often undertaken in an individual with cancer. Predictive genetic test is when the genetic test is used to identify a known PV in the family in another untested and usually unaffected family member.

17.7 Limitations to the Traditional FH Approach

FH or clinical criteria-based testing is moderately effective at identifying individuals with PVs but poor at ruling out the presence of one. This approach has involved testing affected individuals from high-risk families via high-risk cancer genetic clinics after face-to-face pre-test genetic counselling by geneticists/genetic counsellors. For this to be effective, it is important for individuals and their doctors to recognise the significance of their FH and act on it. However, a number of PV carriers are unaware of their FH or its significance, are not proactive in seeking advice, may lack a strong enough FH, or may not get referred and get excluded. This pathway has often been complex, varies regionally and internationally, and is associated with restricted uptake and under-utilisation of genetic testing [51–53]. An analysis across Greater London shows that over 97% of *BRCA* carriers remain undetected despite 25 years of NHS testing [52].

Around 50% of BC/OC CSG carriers do not fulfil current clinical or FH-based criteria for genetic testing and are missed [5, 50, 54, 55]. Far greater numbers are missed through unselected population ascertainment. Bethesda and Amsterdam-II clinical criteria miss, 12–30% and 55–70% of MMR (Lynch Syndrome) carriers respectively [9, 56, 57]. Advances in testing technology and bioinformatics has now enabled large-scale delivery of high-throughput genetic testing. The limitations of the FH approach can be addressed by (a) unselected genetic testing at cancer diagnosis and (b) population testing. Unselected testing at cancer diagnosis improves genetic testing access and PV carrier identification in affected women. It has been implemented for OC [58] and CRC [59]; is now being implemented for EC [60]; and there have been calls for considering this for BC [54].

17.8 Unselected Genetic Testing at Ovarian Cancer Diagnosis

Around 11–18% of OC patients have germline *BRCA1/BRCA2* PV and another 6–9% have a somatic *BRCA1/BRCA2* PV in the tumour tissue alone which is not inherited [5, 61]. Thus two-thirds of PVs in tumour tissue originate from the germline, but one-third are somatic. *BRCA1/BRCA2* genes code proteins which are required in the homologous recombination repair (HRR) pathway of double stranded DNA breaks. PARP (poly ADP ribose polymerase) is an essential component of single-strand DNA repair. Inhibition of PARP leads to more double strand breaks and prevents HRR deficient (HRD) tumour cells from surviving chemotherapy induced DNA damage [62]. HRD may occur due to a large number of genes mutations in the HRR pathway, including *RAD51C*, *RAD51D*, *BRIP1* and *PALB2*. Tumours that are HRD deficient, regardless of the HRD deficiency is inherited or sporadic, are more susceptible to systemic therapy with 'PARP inhibitors' (PARPi) and platinum agents. This trait is referred to as "BRCAness". Approximately 50% of high grade serous OC are characterised by HRD and HRD assays are now being used in clinical practice [63]. Germline as well as somatic *BRCA* mutated OC have been shown to benefit from PARP-i therapy with improved progression free survival in both first line and recurrent settings [43, 62, 64–66]. This need to identify women who can benefit from first line PARPi therapy has given an impetus to genetic testing in all women with high grade epithelial non-mucinous OC. Testing on the basis of FH would miss around 50% of the germline PVs. A non-genetic cancer clinician driven 'mainstreaming approach' where counselling and genetic testing for all OC patients is undertaken by the medical oncologist/surgical oncologist/clinical nurse specialist is now part of standard NHS clinical practice [5, 67]. PV carrier identification enables cascade testing and primary cancer screening and prevention in unaffected relatives (see Table 17.1) along with secondary cancer prevention and access to novel drugs (e.g. PARP-inhibitors) or clinical trials to improve survival in affected carriers [43]. Parallel germline and somatic testing is recommended as ~10% of PVs are large genomic rearrangement (LGR) germline PVs and are missed by somatic testing. Germline testing for a panel of relevant OC genes can identify another 2–3% non-*BRCA* PVs whose family members can benefit from cascade testing and subsequent screening and prevention. It is important that only genes with well-established 'clinical utility' are tested for. We are against indiscriminate panel testing as in large commercial panels. A valid OC panel today could include *BRCA1*, *BRCA2*, *RAD51C*, *RAD51D*, *BRIP1*, *PALB2* and MMR genes. The lack of an effective OC screening strategy in low-risk women [41] further amplifies the need for identifying high risk women for precision prevention.

17.9 Unselected Genetic Testing at Endometrial Cancer Diagnosis

Given the number of LS cases missed by clinical criteria-based restricted access, the current recommendation is to test all EC tumours for MMR gene deficiency. This guideline was recently introduced into NHS practice by NICE in 2020 [60]. Tumours can be found to be MMR deficient by IHC or MSI. Both IHC and MSI show comparable sensitivity and high concordance. However, as IHC has been found to be more cost-effective and is easily accessible to pathologists, IHC is now used as first line to test endometrial cancer tissue for MLH1, MSH2, MSH6, and PMS2 gene expression. While 25–30% of ECs are found to be MMR deficient, only around 3% have LS [9]. If the EC tumour IHC shows somatic MSH2 or MSH6 deficiency (negative stain for MSH2/MSH6), germline testing for LS genes is indicated. If IHC shows MLH1 (often combined with PMS2) deficiency, MLH1 promotor hypermethylation testing needs to be performed first as the majority of these are due to sporadic silencing of the MLH1 gene by hypermethylation of the MLH1 promotor region within tumour cells and do not reflect the presence of LS [68]. A result of low hypermethylation (negative test) indicates requirement for germline testing, while a result of high hypermethylation (positive test) suggests a false positive result and excludes the need for germline MMR gene testing. Figure 17.1 depicts a recommended flow chart for IHC-based triage for MMR gene testing for LS. Figure 17.2 illustrates the numbers of LS patients that would be identified along with number of false positives if 1000 EC cases were tested [9, 69, 70]. All gynaecologists and gynaecological oncologists involved in the diagnosis and treatment of women with EC will need to be able to interpret these results as

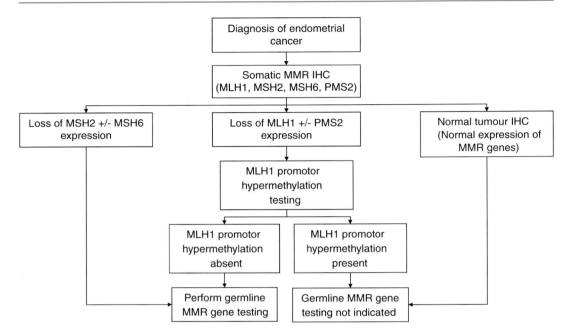

Fig. 17.1 Flow chart for IHC based triage for MMR gene testing for LS at diagnosis of endometrial cancer

well as counsel women and undertake genetic testing for LS. A similar mainstreaming approach has previously been implemented for OC cases across treatment pathways. Identified PV carriers need to be referred to clinical genetics and family members should be offered predictive testing. LS women with EC should be offered bowel screening (annual colonoscopy) and aspirin for chemoprevention. Unaffected family members can avail of screening or prevention options highlighted in Table 17.1.

17.10 Population Testing

The inadequacies and limitations of our current clinical approach to genetic testing, given the effective risk management/preventive options available for high-risk women, highlights the massive scale of missed opportunities for cancer prevention. Unselected unaffected population testing can overcome these limitations. The strongest evidence base for population testing comes from the Jewish population. Population-based *BRCA* testing in Ashkenazi Jews compared to FH/clinical criteria based *BRCA* testing is feasible, acceptable, safe, doesn't harm quality-of-life or psychological well-being, reduces long-term anxiety, identifies 150% additional *BRCA*-carriers [50, 71], can be delivered in a community setting [72, 73] and is extremely cost-effective [74, 75]. This supports changing paradigm to population-based *BRCA*-testing in the Jewish population [76, 77] and this approach has now very recently been implemented in Israel. It is important that other countries follow suit. Unselected germline testing in a non-Jewish general population has also been shown to be cost-effective, but this remains a matter of ongoing research [78–81].

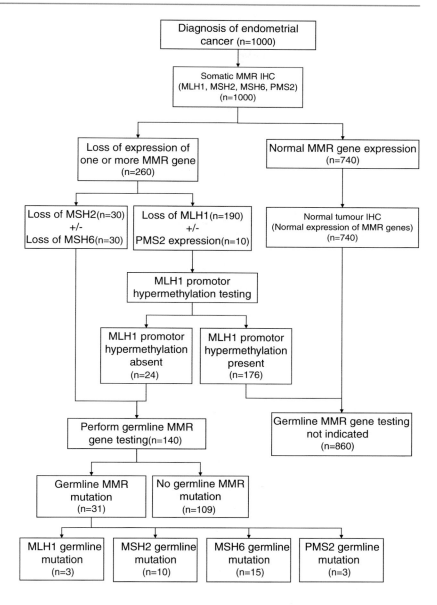

Fig. 17.2 Flow chart for number of LS patients identified if 1000 endometrial cancer cases were tested[9, 69]

17.11 Summary

Ovarian, breast, endometrial, and colorectal cancer cases are projected to rise over the next 20 years. 20% of ovarian cancers, 4% of breast cancers, 3% of endometrial cancers, and 4% of colorectal cancers are due to pathogenic variants in cancer susceptibility genes. CSG identification offers many opportunities to PV carriers including enhanced screening for early detection, prevention options including chemoprevention or risk-reducing surgery, along with pre-implantation genetic diagnosis to prevent variant transmission. Traditional genetic testing eligibility was based on family history and/or clinical criteria but is underutilised and misses 50% of PV carriers even with ideal usage. Unselected genetic testing is now recommended for all women with endometrial cancer following IHC triage. Unselected parallel panel germline and somatic genetic testing is now recommended for all women with high grade epithelial ovarian cancer. Germline PVs and HRR deficient ovarian cancers are eligible for PARPi therapy. PV identification can enable secondary cancer prevention in cancer patients and cascade testing in family members to identify unaffected PV carriers who can benefit from precision prevention. Population-based *BRCA* genetic testing is now recommended for the Ashkenazi Jewish population.

Key Points

- Pathogenic variants in moderate to high penetrance cancer susceptibility genes of clinical utility account for around 15–20% OC, 4% BC, 3% EC and 4% CRC with a majority being potentially preventable.
- Family history-based clinical criteria for genetic testing miss >50% pathogenic variants in cancer susceptibility genes.
- Unselected genetic testing at cancer diagnosis is now recommended for all women with high grade epithelial ovarian cancer. Both germline and somatic testing should be undertaken in parallel to maximise variant identification. Germline PVs and HRR deficient tumours are eligible for PARPi therapy. Family members of germline PVs can undergo cascade testing for precision prevention.
- Unselected IHC testing at diagnosis and subsequent triage for MMR gene testing is now recommended for all women with endometrial cancer.
- Early recognition of cancer susceptibility gene carriers for *BRCA1/BRCA2*, *PALB2*, *RAD51C*, *RAD51D*, *BRIP1*, *MLH1*, *MSH2*, *MSH6* and *PMS2*, can offer women important opportunities for screening/early diagnosis and cancer prevention.
- RRSO is the most effective method of preventing ovarian cancer in women at increased risk of ovarian cancer. Hysterectomy and bilateral salpingo-oophorectomy is recommended in women with Lynch Syndrome. Early salpingectomy and delayed oophorectomy should currently only be offered in the context of a clinical trial.
- Population testing is now recommended for the Ashkenazi Jewish population and has recently been implemented in Israel.

References

1. CRUK. Ovarian cancer statistics. Ovarian cancer incidence. 2017. Available from: http://www.cancer-researchuk.org/health-professional/cancer-statistics/statistics-by-cancer-type/ovarian-cancer. Accessed 30 Aug 2017.
2. International Agency for Research on Cancer. Cancer Tomorrow. A tool that predicts the future cancer incidence and mortality burden worldwide from the current estimates in 2018 up until 2040. 2018. Available from: http://gco.iarc.fr/tomorrow/home. Accessed 20 Jan 2019.
3. CRUK. Cancer incidence statistics. Cancer cases and rates by country in the UK. 2018. Available from: https://www.cancerresearchuk.org/health-professional/cancer-statistics/incidence#heading-Five. Accessed 10 Feb 2019.
4. Lichtenstein P, Holm NV, Verkasalo PK, Iliadou A, Kaprio J, Koskenvuo M, et al. Environmental and heritable factors in the causation of cancer—analyses of cohorts of twins from Sweden, Denmark, and Finland. N Engl J Med. 2000;343(2):78–85.
5. George A, Riddell D, Seal S, Talukdar S, Mahamdallie S, Ruark E, et al. Implementing rapid, robust, cost-effective, patient-centred, routine genetic testing in ovarian cancer patients. Sci Rep. 2016;6:29506.
6. Norquist BM, Harrell MI, Brady MF, Walsh T, Lee MK, Gulsuner S, et al. Inherited mutations in women with ovarian carcinoma. JAMA Oncol. 2016;2(4):482–90.
7. Buys SS, Sandbach JF, Gammon A, Patel G, Kidd J, Brown KL, et al. A study of over 35,000 women with breast cancer tested with a 25-gene panel of hereditary cancer genes. Cancer. 2017;123(10):1721–30.
8. Breast Cancer Association Consortium, Dorling L, Carvalho S, Allen J, Gonzalez-Neira A, Luccarini C, et al. Breast cancer risk genes—association analysis in more than 113,000 women. N Engl J Med. 2021;384(5):428–39.
9. Ryan NAJ, Glaire MA, Blake D, Cabrera-Dandy M, Evans DG, Crosbie EJ. The proportion of endometrial

cancers associated with Lynch syndrome: a systematic review of the literature and meta-analysis. Genet Med. 2019;21(10):2167–80.
10. Salovaara R, Loukola A, Kristo P, Kaariainen H, Ahtola H, Eskelinen M, et al. Population-based molecular detection of hereditary nonpolyposis colorectal cancer. J Clin Oncol. 2000;18(11):2193–200.
11. Hampel H, Frankel WL, Martin E, Arnold M, Khanduja K, Kuebler P, et al. Feasibility of screening for Lynch syndrome among patients with colorectal cancer. J Clin Oncol. 2008;26(35):5783–8.
12. Kuchenbaecker KB, Hopper JL, Barnes DR, Phillips KA, Mooij TM, Roos-Blom MJ, et al. Risks of breast, ovarian, and contralateral breast cancer for BRCA1 and BRCA2 mutation carriers. JAMA. 2017;317(23):2402–16.
13. Rebbeck TR, Friebel T, Lynch HT, Neuhausen SL, van't Veer L, Garber JE, et al. Bilateral prophylactic mastectomy reduces breast cancer risk in BRCA1 and BRCA2 mutation carriers: the PROSE Study Group. J Clin Oncol. 2004;22(6):1055–62.
14. Cuzick J, Sestak I, Bonanni B, Costantino JP, Cummings S, DeCensi A, et al. Selective oestrogen receptor modulators in prevention of breast cancer: an updated meta-analysis of individual participant data. Lancet. 2013;381(9880):1827–34.
15. NICE. Familial breast cancer: classification, care and managing breast cancer and related risks in people with a family history of breast cancer. 2017. https://www.nice.org.uk/guidance/cg164. Available from: https://www.nice.org.uk/guidance/cg164. Accessed 16 Mar 2019.
16. Rebbeck TR, Kauff ND, Domchek SM. Meta-analysis of risk reduction estimates associated with risk-reducing salpingo-oophorectomy in BRCA1 or BRCA2 mutation carriers. J Natl Cancer Inst. 2009;101(2):80–7.
17. Gaba F, Blyuss O, Chandrasekaran D, Osman M, Goyal S, Gan C, et al. Attitudes towards risk-reducing early salpingectomy with delayed oophorectomy for ovarian cancer prevention: a cohort study. BJOG. 2020;128(4):714–26.
18. Gaba F, Robbani S, Singh N, McCluggage WG, Wilkinson N, Ganesan R, et al. Preventing ovarian cancer through early Excision of Tubes and late Ovarian Removal (PROTECTOR): protocol for a prospective non-randomised multi-center trial. Int J Gynecol Cancer. 2020;31(2):286–91.
19. Yang X, Leslie G, Doroszuk A, Schneider S, Allen J, Decker B, et al. Cancer risks associated with germline PALB2 pathogenic variants: an international study of 524 families. J Clin Oncol. 2019;38(7):674–85.
20. Yang X, Song H, Leslie G, Engel C, Hahnen E, Auber B, et al. Ovarian and breast cancer risks associated with pathogenic variants in RAD51C and RAD51D. J Natl Cancer Inst. 2020;112(12):1242–50.
21. Ramus SJ, Song H, Dicks E, Tyrer JP, Rosenthal AN, Intermaggio MP, et al. Germline mutations in the BRIP1, BARD1, PALB2, and NBN genes in women with ovarian cancer. J Natl Cancer Inst. 2015;107(11):djv214.
22. Moller P. Prospective Lynch Syndrome Database (PLSD)—cumulative risk for cancer by age, genetic variant, and gender. 2019. Available from: http://www.lscarisk.org/
23. Barrow E, Hill J, Evans DG. Cancer risk in lynch syndrome. Fam Cancer. 2013;12(2):229–40.
24. Dominguez-Valentin M, Sampson JR, Seppala TT, Ten Broeke SW, Plazzer JP, Nakken S, et al. Cancer risks by gene, age, and gender in 6350 carriers of pathogenic mismatch repair variants: findings from the Prospective Lynch Syndrome Database. Genet Med. 2019;22(1):15–25.
25. Crosbie EJ, Ryan NAJ, Arends MJ, Bosse T, Burn J, Cornes JM, et al. The Manchester International Consensus Group recommendations for the management of gynecological cancers in Lynch syndrome. Genet Med. 2019;21(10):2390–400.
26. Vasen HF, Blanco I, Aktan-Collan K, Gopie JP, Alonso A, Aretz S, et al. Revised guidelines for the clinical management of Lynch syndrome (HNPCC): recommendations by a group of European experts. Gut. 2013;62(6):812–23.
27. Burn J, Gerdes AM, Macrae F, Mecklin JP, Moeslein G, Olschwang S, et al. Long-term effect of aspirin on cancer risk in carriers of hereditary colorectal cancer: an analysis from the CAPP2 randomised controlled trial. Lancet. 2011;378(9809):2081–7.
28. Vasen HF, Moslein G, Alonso A, Bernstein I, Bertario L, Blanco I, et al. Guidelines for the clinical management of Lynch syndrome (hereditary non-polyposis cancer). J Med Genet. 2007;44(6):353–62.
29. Bubien V, Bonnet F, Brouste V, Hoppe S, Barouk-Simonet E, David A, et al. High cumulative risks of cancer in patients with PTEN hamartoma tumour syndrome. J Med Genet. 2013;50(4):255–63.
30. Tan MH, Mester JL, Ngeow J, Rybicki LA, Orloff MS, Eng C. Lifetime cancer risks in individuals with germline PTEN mutations. Clin Cancer Res. 2012;18(2):400–7.
31. Hearle N, Schumacher V, Menko FH, Olschwang S, Boardman LA, Gille JJ, et al. Frequency and spectrum of cancers in the Peutz-Jeghers syndrome. Clin Cancer Res. 2006;12(10):3209–15.
32. Beggs AD, Latchford AR, Vasen HF, Moslein G, Alonso A, Aretz S, et al. Peutz-Jeghers syndrome: a systematic review and recommendations for management. Gut. 2010;59(7):975–86.
33. Malkin D. Li-fraumeni syndrome. Genes Cancer. 2011;2(4):475–84.
34. Eccles DM, Mitchell G, Monteiro AN, Schmutzler R, Couch FJ, Spurdle AB, et al. BRCA1 and BRCA2 genetic testing-pitfalls and recommendations for managing variants of uncertain clinical significance. Ann Oncol. 2015;26(10):2057–65.
35. Menon U, Harper J, Sharma A, Fraser L, Burnell M, Elmasry K, et al. Views of BRCA gene mutation carriers on preimplantation genetic diagnosis as a

reproductive option for hereditary breast and ovarian cancer. Hum Reprod. 2007;22(6):1573–7.
36. Finch A, Beiner M, Lubinski J, Lynch HT, Moller P, Rosen B, et al. Salpingo-oophorectomy and the risk of ovarian, fallopian tube, and peritoneal cancers in women with a BRCA1 or BRCA2 Mutation. JAMA. 2006;296(2):185–92.
37. Manchanda R, Legood R, Antoniou AC, Gordeev VS, Menon U. Specifying the ovarian cancer risk threshold of 'premenopausal risk-reducing salpingo-oophorectomy' for ovarian cancer prevention: a cost-effectiveness analysis. J Med Genet. 2016;53(9):591–9.
38. Manchanda R, Legood R, Pearce L, Menon U. Defining the risk threshold for risk reducing salpingo-oophorectomy for ovarian cancer prevention in low risk postmenopausal women. Gynecol Oncol. 2015;139(3):487–94.
39. Manchanda R, Legood R, Antoniou AC, Pearce L, Menon U. Commentary on changing the risk threshold for surgical prevention of ovarian cancer. BJOG. 2017;125(5):541–4.
40. Gaba F, Goyal S, Marks D, Chandrasekaran D, Evans O, Robbani S, et al. Surgical decision making in premenopausal BRCA carriers considering risk-reducing early salpingectomy or salpingo-oophorectomy: a qualitative study. J Med Genet. 2021; https://doi.org/10.1136/jmedgenet-2020-107501.
41. Menon U, Gentry-Maharaj A, Burnell M, Singh N, Ryan A, Karpinskyj C, et al. Ovarian cancer population screening and mortality after long-term follow-up in the UK Collaborative Trial of Ovarian Cancer Screening (UKCTOCS): a randomised controlled trial. Lancet. 2021;397(10290):2182–93.
42. Rosenthal AN, Fraser LSM, Philpott S, Manchanda R, Burnell M, Badman P, et al. Evidence of stage shift in women diagnosed with ovarian cancer during phase II of the United Kingdom familial ovarian cancer screening study. J Clin Oncol. 2017;35(13):1411–20.
43. Moore K, Colombo N, Scambia G, Kim BG, Oaknin A, Friedlander M, et al. Maintenance olaparib in patients with newly diagnosed advanced ovarian cancer. N Engl J Med. 2018;379(26):2495–505.
44. Burn J, Sheth H, Elliott F, Reed L, Macrae F, Mecklin JP, et al. Cancer prevention with aspirin in hereditary colorectal cancer (Lynch syndrome), 10-year follow-up and registry-based 20-year data in the CAPP2 study: a double-blind, randomised, placebo-controlled trial. Lancet. 2020;395(10240):1855–63.
45. Dove-Edwin I, Boks D, Goff S, Kenter GG, Carpenter R, Vasen HF, et al. The outcome of endometrial carcinoma surveillance by ultrasound scan in women at risk of hereditary nonpolyposis colorectal carcinoma and familial colorectal carcinoma. Cancer. 2002;94(6):1708–12.
46. Gerritzen LH, Hoogerbrugge N, Oei AL, Nagengast FM, van Ham MA, Massuger LF, et al. Improvement of endometrial biopsy over transvaginal ultrasound alone for endometrial surveillance in women with Lynch syndrome. Familial Cancer. 2009;8(4):391–7.
47. Manchanda R, Saridogan E, Abdelraheim A, Johnson M, Rosenthal AN, Benjamin E, et al. Annual outpatient hysteroscopy and endometrial sampling (OHES) in HNPCC/Lynch syndrome (LS). Arch Gynecol Obstet. 2012;286(6):1555–62.
48. Renkonen-Sinisalo L, Butzow R, Leminen A, Lehtovirta P, Mecklin JP, Jarvinen HJ. Surveillance for endometrial cancer in hereditary nonpolyposis colorectal cancer syndrome. Int J Cancer. 2007;120(4):821–4.
49. Evans DG, Harkness EF, Plaskocinska I, Wallace AJ, Clancy T, Woodward ER, et al. Pathology update to the Manchester Scoring System based on testing in over 4000 families. J Med Genet. 2017;54(10):674–81.
50. Manchanda R, Burnell M, Gaba F, Desai R, Wardle J, Gessler S, et al. Randomised trial of population-based BRCA testing in Ashkenazi Jews: long-term outcomes. BJOG. 2020;127(3):364–75.
51. Childers CP, Childers KK, Maggard-Gibbons M, Macinko J. National estimates of genetic testing in women with a history of breast or ovarian cancer. J Clin Oncol. 2017;35(34):3800–6.
52. Manchanda R, Blyuss O, Gaba F, Gordeev VS, Jacobs C, Burnell M, et al. Current detection rates and time-to-detection of all identifiable BRCA carriers in the Greater London population. J Med Genet. 2018;55(8):538–45.
53. Kurian AW, Ward KC, Howlader N, Deapen D, Hamilton AS, Mariotto A, et al. Genetic testing and results in a population-based cohort of breast cancer patients and ovarian cancer patients. J Clin Oncol. 2019;37(15):1305–15.
54. Sun L, Brentnall A, Patel S, Buist DSM, Bowles EJA, Evans DGR, et al. A cost-effectiveness analysis of multigene testing for all patients with breast cancer JAMA. Oncol. 2019;5(12):1718–30.
55. Beitsch PD, Whitworth PW, Hughes K, Patel R, Rosen B, Compagnoni G, et al. Underdiagnosis of hereditary breast cancer: are genetic testing guidelines a tool or an obstacle? J Clin Oncol. 2018;37(6):453–60.
56. Hampel H, Frankel WL, Martin E, Arnold M, Khanduja K, Kuebler P, et al. Screening for the Lynch syndrome (hereditary nonpolyposis colorectal cancer). N Engl J Med. 2005;352(18):1851–60.
57. Pinol V, Castells A, Andreu M, Castellvi-Bel S, Alenda C, Llor X, et al. Accuracy of revised Bethesda guidelines, microsatellite instability, and immunohistochemistry for the identification of patients with hereditary nonpolyposis colorectal cancer. JAMA. 2005;293(16):1986–94.
58. Sundar S, Manchanda R, Gourley C, George A, Wallace A, Balega J, et al. British Gynaecological Cancer Society/British Association of Gynaecological Pathology consensus for germline and tumor testing for BRCA1/2 variants in ovarian cancer in the United Kingdom. Int J Gynecol Cancer. 2021;31(2):272–8.
59. NICE. Molecular testing strategies for Lynch syndrome in people with colorectal cancer. Diagnostic Guidance 27. 2017. https://www.nice.org.uk/guidance/dg27. Available from: https://www.nice.org.

uk/guidance/dg27/resources/molecular-testing-strategies-for-lynch-syndrome-in-people-with-colorectal-cancer-pdf-1053695294917
60. NICE. Testing strategies for Lynch syndrome in people with endometrial cancer (DG42) 2020. Available from: https://www.nice.org.uk/guidance/dg42
61. Sundar S, Manchanda R, Gourley C, George A, Wallace A, Balega J, et al. British Gynaecological Cancer Society/British Association of Gynaecological Pathology consensus for germline and tumour testing for BRCA1/2 variants in ovarian cancer in the United Kingdom 2020. Available from: https://www.bgcs.org.uk/wp-content/uploads/2020/09/BGCS-BAGP-070920-final-v1.pdf. Accessed 13 Sept 2020.
62. Schettini F, Giudici F, Bernocchi O, Sirico M, Corona SP, Giuliano M, et al. Poly (ADP-ribose) polymerase inhibitors in solid tumours: systematic review and meta-analysis. Eur J Cancer. 2021;149:134–52.
63. Miller RE, Leary A, Scott CL, Serra V, Lord CJ, Bowtell D, et al. ESMO recommendations on predictive biomarker testing for homologous recombination deficiency and PARP inhibitor benefit in ovarian cancer. Ann Oncol. 2020;31(12):1606–22.
64. Ledermann J, Harter P, Gourley C, Friedlander M, Vergote I, Rustin G, et al. Olaparib maintenance therapy in patients with platinum-sensitive relapsed serous ovarian cancer: a preplanned retrospective analysis of outcomes by BRCA status in a randomised phase 2 trial. Lancet Oncol. 2014;15(8):852–61.
65. Coleman RL, Oza AM, Lorusso D, Aghajanian C, Oaknin A, Dean A, et al. Rucaparib maintenance treatment for recurrent ovarian carcinoma after response to platinum therapy (ARIEL3): a randomised, double-blind, placebo-controlled, phase 3 trial. Lancet. 2017;390(10106):1949–61.
66. Pujade-Lauraine E, Ledermann JA, Selle F, Gebski V, Penson RT, Oza AM, et al. Olaparib tablets as maintenance therapy in patients with platinum-sensitive, relapsed ovarian cancer and a BRCA1/2 mutation (SOLO2/ENGOT-Ov21): a double-blind, randomised, placebo-controlled, phase 3 trial. Lancet Oncol. 2017;18(9):1274–84.
67. Systematic genetic testing for personalised ovarian cancer therapy (SIGNPOsT). 2017. Available from: https://www.isrctn.com/ISRCTN16988857?q=&filters=conditionCategory:Cancer&sort=&offset=4&totalResults=1950&page=1&pageSize=10&searchType=basic-search. Accessed 8 Oct 2017.
68. Singh NWR, Tchrakian N, Allen S, Clarke B, Gilks CB. Interpretation and reporting terminology for mismatch repair protein immunohistochemistry in endometrial cancer. Br Assoc Gynaecol Pathol. 2020;39(3):233–7.
69. Goodfellow PJ, Billingsley CC, Lankes HA, Ali S, Cohn DE, Broaddus RJ, et al. Combined microsatellite instability, MLH1 methylation analysis, and immunohistochemistry for lynch syndrome screening in endometrial cancers from GOG210: an NRG oncology and gynecologic oncology group study. J Clin Oncol. 2015;33(36):4301–8.
70. Ryan NAJ, McMahon R, Tobi S, Snowsill T, Esquibel S, Wallace AJ, et al. The proportion of endometrial tumours associated with Lynch syndrome (PETALS): a prospective cross-sectional study. PLoS Med. 2020;17(9):e1003263.
71. Manchanda R, Loggenberg K, Sanderson S, Burnell M, Wardle J, Gessler S, et al. Population testing for cancer predisposing BRCA1/BRCA2 mutations in the Ashkenazi-Jewish community: a randomized controlled trial. J Natl Cancer Inst. 2015;107(1):379.
72. Manchanda R, Burnell M, Gaba F, Sanderson S, Loggenberg K, Gessler S, et al. Attitude towards and factors affecting uptake of population-based BRCA testing in the Ashkenazi Jewish population: a cohort study. BJOG. 2019;126(6):784–94.
73. Manchanda R, Burnell M, Loggenberg K, Desai R, Wardle J, Sanderson SC, et al. Cluster-randomised non-inferiority trial comparing DVD-assisted and traditional genetic counselling in systematic population testing for BRCA1/2 mutations. J Med Genet. 2016;53(7):472–80.
74. Manchanda R, Legood R, Burnell M, McGuire A, Raikou M, Loggenberg K, et al. Cost-effectiveness of population screening for BRCA mutations in Ashkenazi jewish women compared with family history-based testing. J Natl Cancer Inst. 2015;107(1):380.
75. Gabai-Kapara E, Lahad A, Kaufman B, Friedman E, Segev S, Renbaum P, et al. Population-based screening for breast and ovarian cancer risk due to BRCA1 and BRCA2. Proc Natl Acad Sci U S A. 2014;111(39):14205–10.
76. Manchanda R, Gaba F. Population based testing for primary prevention. A systematic review. Cancers (Basel). 2018;10(11):424.
77. Manchanda R, Lieberman S, Gaba F, Lahad A, Levy-Lahad E. Population screening for inherited predisposition to breast and ovarian cancer. Annu Rev Genomics Hum Genet. 2020;21:373–412.
78. Manchanda R, Patel S, Gordeev VS, Antoniou AC, Smith S, Lee A, et al. Cost-effectiveness of population-based BRCA1, BRCA2, RAD51C, RAD51D, BRIP1, PALB2 mutation testing in unselected general population women. J Natl Cancer Inst. 2018;110(7):714–25.
79. Manchanda R, Sun L, Patel S, Evans O, Wilschut J, De Freitas Lopes AC, et al. Economic evaluation of population-based BRCA1/BRCA2 mutation testing across multiple countries and health systems. Cancers (Basel). 2020;12(7):1929.
80. Gaba F, Blyuss O, Liu X, Goyal S, Lahoti N, Chandrasekaran D, et al. Population study of ovarian cancer risk prediction for targeted screening and prevention. Cancers (Basel). 2020;12(5):1241.
81. Evans O, Manchanda R. Population-based genetic testing for precision prevention. Cancer Prev Res (Phila). 2020;13(8):643–8.

Radiology Investigations and Interventions in Gynaeoncology

18

Lohith Ambadipudi

18.1 Introduction

Radiological investigations in gynaecological malignancies have a role in screening, tumour detection, staging, treatment planning, and post-treatment surveillance. Imaging is also useful in performing interventions and evaluating complications. Ultrasound (US), magnetic resonance imaging (MRI), computed tomography (CT) and fluorine 18 fluoro 2 deoxy D glucose positron emission tomography computed tomography FDG PET CT are the main imaging modalities employed in gynaeoncology.

Although FIGO (The International Federation of Gynaecology and Obstetrics) staging of gynaecological malignancies is either clinical (cervical) or surgical/pathological (ovarian and endometrial), imaging provides useful information in prognostication and treatment planning. Recent 2018 FIGO revision of cervical cancer staging incorporates radiological input with a prefix of '*r*'.

This chapter provides an overview of the basic techniques and protocols of these modalities, their relevance and use in mainly cervical, endometrial and ovarian malignancies, recommended imaging management pathways, and the role of image guided interventions. Less common gynaecological malignancies and recent advances in imaging will also be discussed briefly.

18.2 Ultrasound

Ultrasound is widely available, quick, and low-cost investigation which does not use radiation or contrast. However, it is operator dependent and could be difficult to image the pelvis optimally in patients with large body habitus or due to excess bowel gas. Transabdominal ultrasound, performed with a full bladder, provides an overview of the pelvic anatomy and transvaginal ultrasound, performed with an empty bladder, is a must in pelvic assessment. US mentioned in this chapter refers to transvaginal sonography (TVS) unless specified otherwise. Colour Doppler study can be performed at the same time to assess vascularity of the tumour. Perineal and transrectal ultrasound examinations can also be used to evaluate pelvis but are not common in routine practice.

Ovarian Ultrasound is most often the first investigation used in assessment of adnexal masses and various scoring/classification systems and risk prediction models like RMI [1] (Risk of Malignancy Index), IOTA (International ovarian tumour analysis) models [2–6] and O-RADS [7, 8] (Ovarian-Adnexal Reporting and Data System) are used. They are briefly discussed in Table 18.1. All IOTA models and RMI are

L. Ambadipudi (✉)
Department of Radiology, University Hospital of North Durham, County Durham and Darlington NHS Foundation Trust, Durham, UK
e-mail: lohith.ambadipudi@nhs.net

© The Author(s), under exclusive license to Springer Nature Switzerland AG 2022
K. Singh, B. Gupta (eds.), *Gynecological Oncology*, https://doi.org/10.1007/978-3-030-94110-9_18

Table 18.1 US based diagnostic models for adnexal masses

RMI	IOTA[a]			O-RADS[b]
	Simple rules	LR2	ADNEX	
Calculated using the product of CA-125 level, menopausal status (M) and ultrasound score(U) RMI = CA-125 × M × U M score 1 and 3 for premenopausal and postmenopausal status respectively U score of 0, 1 and 3 based on number of features of malignancy identified on transvaginal ultrasound. Multilocular cyst, solid components, bilateral lesions, metastases, and ascites are the features 0 = no features 1 = one feature 3 = two or more features RMI >200 is taken as a cut off to identify lesions with high risk of malignancy (sensitivity and specificity of 85% and 97% respectively) warranting a staging CT and gynaeoncology referral[c]	Simple Rules (SR) are used for classifying ovarian tumours into benign and malignant by using a set of ten US features. Five benign features (B) and five malignant features (M). Benign tumours have only B features whereas malignant tumours have only M features. Tumours are classified as inconclusive (approximately 25% of lesions) if none or both features apply and, in these cases, subjective assessment by a US specialist is required. In addition, MRI could be used as a problem-solving tool SR model does not predict the malignancy risk. To address this, a Simple Rules Risk calculator was introduced later which provides an estimated likelihood of cancer using logistic regression analysis based on SR and type of centre where US was performed (oncology centre or not)	Logistic regression models LR1 and LR2 were developed by the IOTA group for risk prediction. These models estimate the probability that an adnexal tumour is malignant. LR1 is based on 12 variables, 4 clinical and 8 US. LR2 is the simpler, more common version used which is based on six predictors, one clinical and five US based	This model not only estimates if the adnexal mass is benign or malignant, but also stratifies lesions as benign, borderline, stage I cancer, stage II–IV cancer, or secondary metastatic cancer. Nine predictors are used, three clinical and six US. ADNEX is the preferred diagnostic model and showed better performance than earlier models	Developed by an international multidisciplinary committee sponsored by the American College of Radiology US based risk stratification and management system applying the standardized reporting tool based on the lexicon published in 2018. Six groups of O-RADS (0–5) for risk stratification ranging from normal to high risk of malignancy and there are guidelines for management proposed for each of the categories. Combines pattern-based approach, which relies on the US predictive descriptors described in the lexicon with the algorithmic-style ADNEX model of IOTA group. Unlike earlier models, O-RADS is the only lexicon and classification system that encompasses all risk categories with their proposed management pathways

RMI Risk of Malignancy Index, *IOTA* International Ovarian Tumour Analysis, *LR2* Logistic Regression Model 2, *ADNEX* Assessment of Different NEoplasias in the adneXa, *O-RADS* Ovarian-Adnexal Reporting and Data System

Year of publication: RMI—1990, Simple Rules—2008 and SR Risk calculator—2016, LR1 and LR2—2005, ADNEX—2014, and O-RADS—2019

[a]The US parameters used in all the IOTA models are based on the terms, definitions and measurements published by the IOTA group in 2000 [2]. IOTA models are available on their official website and/or also available in the electronic format as Apps on Android and iPhone. Some ultrasound machines have built-in functionalities to use these models

[b]Except O-RADS all the other models were developed based on women undergoing surgery, excluding those selected for expectant management

[c]Some authors consider RMI value of 25–200 as indeterminate requiring further investigation with MRI to characterize the indeterminate adnexal mass

externally validated by numerous studies. The IOTA diagnostic models for evaluating adnexal masses are relatively easy to use and can be relied upon by inexperienced US operators when expert opinion is not available. However, subjective assessment of adnexal tumours by an expert US practitioner is shown to have the best diagnostic accuracy [9–11] compared to RMI and IOTA diagnostic models which clearly highlights the importance of US training and experience. RMI is still advocated by many national guidelines, however there is sufficient evidence in the literature demonstrating better performance by the ADNEX model [9–12]. O-RADS is a comprehensive system which is quite promising but is relatively new and awaits further external validation.

Ultrasound features suggestive of malignancy include thick irregular wall and/or septations, papillary projections, solid areas, size >4 cm, neovascularity in the lesion, bilaterality, ascites and peritoneal deposits.

Endometrial Postmenopausal bleeding should be investigated with transvaginal sonography to assess endometrial thickness measured in the sagittal plane but ultrasound has no role in staging. Different thresholds have been suggested in the literature for abnormal endometrial thickening in a postmenopausal woman with vaginal bleeding which would warrant further evaluation and the cut off values proposed range from 3 to 5 mm. However, thickness of >4 mm can be considered abnormal in routine practice and presence of malignancy can be confirmed by tissue sampling.

And in postmenopausal women without vaginal bleeding, the acceptable range of endometrial thickness is less well established, and a threshold of 8–11 mm has been suggested. Since the guidelines in this cohort are less clear, a follow up transvaginal ultrasound or gynaecology referral would be reasonable. In women on HRT or Tamoxifen a slightly larger cut off value is suggested with an upper limit of 5 mm, whether symptomatic or not [13–15].

In premenopausal women, endometrial thickness varies significantly with different stages of menstrual cycle along with a change in ultrasound appearance. Endometrium is thinnest during menstruation measuring approximately 2–4 mm, increasing to 5–7 mm during the early proliferative phase and reaching up to 7 mm in the late proliferative/preovulatory phase. It is thickest during the secretory phase measuring up to 16 mm (range 7–16 mm) [13, 16]. These values are only a guide as there can be considerable variation from individual to individual and the ultrasound findings should be flagged only in appropriate clinical context. When endometrial thickness is being evaluated on ultrasound fluid in the cavity should be excluded from measurements.

Cervical There is no real-world use of ultrasound in assessment of cervical cancer. Complications like hydrometra/haematometra and hydronephrosis, however, can be easily identified on ultrasound.

18.3 Computed Tomography

CT is inferior to MRI in local staging of gynaecological cancers. However, it is useful in identifying extent of peritoneal disease, distant metastases, and recurrence. Ionising radiation, contrast reactions, reduced image quality with a large body habitus and artefacts from metallic hip implants obscuring pelvic structures are the drawbacks associated with this modality.

Exposure to ionizing radiation is linked to the development of cancer and although the risk to an individual patient may be small, the increasing number of CT scans per patient and in the population overall could result in many cancer cases which are directly linked to radiation exposure. For instance, an adult patient would receive an approximate effective radiation dose of 7.7 mSv (millisievert) [17, 18] from a single-phase CT of abdomen and pelvis which is comparable to natural background radiation exposure for a duration of 2.6 years or approximately hundred times the dose of a chest X-ray. It is therefore imperative that CT scans are requested only when deemed essential and, in most places, to avoid unnecessary scans, imaging study requests received from the referrers are routinely vetted and protocolled by the radiology team before they can be slotted in for a scan. Information provided on the radiology request form should include clinical history and examination findings, relevant laboratory investigations, pregnancy status in reproductive age group women, menopausal status, and suspected aetiology.

Iodinated water-soluble contrast agents are used in CT for both intravenous (IV) and oral administration. Intravenous contrast is excreted by the kidneys whereas oral contrast mostly passes out unabsorbed with approximately 1–2% of absorption by the gut. A documented previous severe reaction to iodinated contrast agent is an absolute contraindication while renal dysfunction, previous mild contrast reaction and high risk of allergies are the relative contraindications. It is advisable to have local protocols for prevention of contrast induced nephropathy (CIN) and risk stratifying patients based on eGFR helps determine the appropriate management pathway. Adequate hydration before and after the CT is the most important step in prevention of CIN. Intravenous contrast is avoided when estimated glomerular filtration rate (eGFR) is less than 30 mL/min and contrast CT can be performed in such patients if the benefits outweigh the risk of CIN, only after ensuring optimal peri-procedural hydration following discussions with the radiologist. Usage of iso-osmolar contrast and reduction in the volume of contrast administered can also be considered if possible.

Oral contrast used in gynaeoncology patients can be iodinated contrast agent diluted in water ('positive' contrast appearing bright/hyperdense on the images) or plain water (neutral contrast) which distends the bowel lumen and helps separating bowel loops, making identification of serosal surface deposits easier. Oral contrast protocols differ between institutions, but it is routinely given in elective procedures with the time duration between start of oral contrast and actual CT scan depending on part of bowel in focus and is usually about 2 h. Rectal and urinary bladder contrast administration can also be performed in special cases for demonstrating fistulous communications.

CT without IV contrast does not provide adequate diagnostic information and should be replaced by another modality like MRI if there is history of severe allergy to iodinated contrast. In this chapter wherever CT is mentioned it refers to a contrast enhanced CT (CECT) study.

Staging CT involves scanning of chest, abdomen and pelvis following IV and oral contrast administration in the portal venous phase. This single-phase CT is sufficient for evaluation of gynaecological malignancies in most cases. However, when incidental lesions are identified, for example hepatic, pancreatic or adrenal masses, which cannot be adequately characterized on the single-phase CT, an additional CT study with a protocol specific to the organ/lesion will be required which could be a dual/triple phase or dual contrast bolus scan with different timings of image acquisition.

There is no need to perform a high-resolution CT (HRCT) of the chest to look for metastases which is primarily used in evaluating interstitial lung diseases. A routine contrast enhanced CT scan of the chest, abdomen and pelvis would suffice for staging gynaecological malignancies, which can be performed on all present-day CT scanners. With improvements in CT scanner technology, the spatial resolution has increased resulting in detection of smaller and smaller indeterminate lung nodules in the range of 1 mm. These very small nodules are non-specific and are presumed to have a very low risk of cancer, however, in the presence of a primary malignancy they are considered indeterminate and require follow up. New onset nodules or growing nodules are considered metastatic in the setting of a primary malignancy. It would be ideal to prepare management pathways for incidental pulmonary nodules based on local or national guidelines.

Most CT studies in gynaeoncology are performed electively and emergency CT will sometimes be required in cases of acute abdomen to look for bowel perforation, intra-abdominal infection and associated fluid collections that can be drained and to differentiate between ileus and

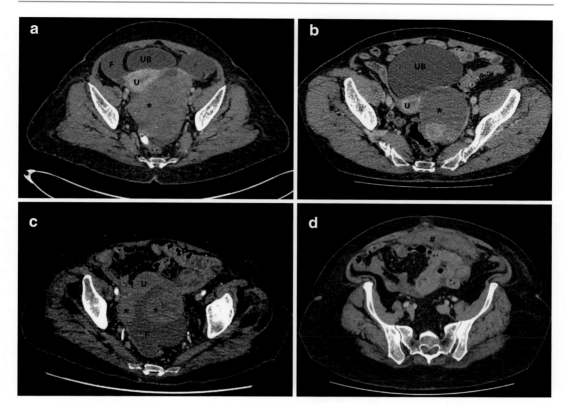

Fig. 18.1 Axial contrast enhanced CT images of ovarian cancer in different patients (**a–d**): left ovarian solid mass displacing the uterus (**a**), left ovarian cystic mass with solid component (**b**) and bilateral solid ovarian masses (**c**) are labelled as (*). Thick omental cake (#) seen immediately below anterior abdominal wall in (**d**) would be suitable for an ultrasound guided biopsy. *U* uterus, *F* ascites and *UB* urinary bladder

obstruction. Other causes of acute abdomen unrelated to the malignancy may also be picked up.

Ovarian CT is currently the investigation of choice for evaluation of ovarian cancer (Fig. 18.1). Preoperative assessment with staging based on imaging findings can be performed to determine the details of primary tumour, location and size of peritoneal implants and metastatic lymphadenopathy. This will help decide the feasibility of primary debulking surgery and in the presence of nonresectable disease (Table 18.2) patient would benefit from neoadjuvant chemotherapy. Drawback of CT is diffuse small volume peritoneal disease, which is potentially inoperable, is not seen or difficult to appreciate. CT chest is also performed along with abdomen and pelvis to look for dissemination above the diaphragm which would make it stage IV disease.

Table 18.2 Disease locations that affect the resectability in ovarian cancers[a]

- Subdiaphragmatic disease along the dome of liver
- Subcapsular liver deposits
- Fissures for ligamentum teres and venosum of the liver
- Porta hepatis and lesser omentum
- Lesser sac
- Gastrosplenic ligament
- Root of mesentery
- Serosal disease on small bowel
- Lymph nodes above the renal hilum

[a]Criteria for resectability may vary between institutions based on the surgical expertise available and treatment planning should always be made at a specialist multidisciplinary meeting

Endometrial MRI is the investigation of choice for local staging and CT is useful in detecting enlarged nodes, distant spread and in evaluation of recurrence.

Cervical While MRI is useful in evaluation of the primary tumour CT could be used in cases of advanced cervical cancer to look for disseminated disease, however, PET CT is the preferred investigation.

18.4 MRI

MRI is the imaging investigation of choice for local staging of endometrial and cervical malignancies owing to its excellent contrast resolution. It is used as a problem-solving tool for the evaluation of indeterminate adnexal masses. MRI does not use ionising radiation, but scan times are much longer; a routine MRI pelvis may take between 30 and 45 min while CT study is completed in a few minutes. MRI and CT have specific use cases and can be used in place of the other only in some scenarios and these have been described in various sections of this chapter. MRI is contraindicated in patients with claustrophobia, MRI is unsafe in patients with cardiac pacemakers and metallic implants, cochlear implants, intraocular foreign bodies, and some vascular clips.

MRI scanners currently in use are either 1.5 or 3 Tesla machines and the unit Tesla (T) refers to the magnetic field strength of the scanner. A 3 T scanner produces better image quality than 1.5 T scanner. These 1.5 and 3 T scanners are closed scanners having a donut shape with the patient placed in the central 'bore' surrounded by the magnet. Open MRI scanners are open on 2 or 3 sides, which are useful in patients with claustrophobia and those with a large body habitus who may be difficult to fit in the bore, but these magnets can only produce field strengths ranging from 0.3 to 0.7 T which significantly reduces the diagnostic quality of images obtained and are therefore not recommended for local staging. Using wide bore MRI scanners and sedation can mitigate these issues in some cases.

During an MRI scan, patient lies within the primary magnetic field while radiofrequency signal pulses are transmitted to the body and the emitted signals are detected by a radiofrequency receiver (coil). These signals are then converted into images by a computer attached to the scanner. The complex interplay between the number, frequency and direction of these radiofrequency pulses and gradient (secondary) magnetic fields results in production of different sets of images, each with a particular appearance referred to as a sequence.

T2-weighted imaging (T2 WI) is the most important sequence of pelvic MRI which is supplemented by T1-weighted imaging (T1 WI), diffusion-weighted imaging (DWI) and dynamic contrast imaging (DCE) sequences. An easy way to distinguish between T1 and T2-weighted sequences is fluid appears bright/hyperintense on T2 and dark/hypointense on T1. Contrast enhanced sequences are T1-weighted. Limited sequences of abdomen are also performed at most institutes, along with pelvic examination, to look for enlarged para-aortic lymph nodes.

Pelvic MRI can be performed on 1.5 or 3 T scanners using multichannel phased-array coils. Fasting for 3–6 h prior to the scan will reduce bowel peristalsis thereby reducing motion artefacts and a partially filled urinary bladder displaces small bowel loops from the pelvis. An antiperistaltic agent (hyoscine butyl bromide or glucagon) is routinely administered intravenously or intramuscularly before the procedure unless contraindicated.

MRI clearly displays the zonal anatomy of uterus on T2 WI with endometrium appearing hyperintense surrounded by hypointense inner myometrium/junctional zone while the outer myometrium is of intermediate signal. Similarly, endocervical mucosa, fibrous stroma and outer loose stroma appear bright, dark, and intermediate in signal respectively (Fig. 18.2). Fluid has a brighter signal than endometrial or endocervical lining. T1 WI helps in assessment of fat, haemorrhage, and bone marrow. While T1 and T2 sequences provide morphological data, functional imaging sequences like DWI and DCE have a complimentary role to the standard T2-weighted imaging as they help improve the diagnostic confidence of tumour extent and in identifying small lesions. DWI is part of the pelvic MRI protocol in most places however DCE is not routinely performed.

T2-weighted imaging helps delineate endometrial and cervical tumours from surrounding

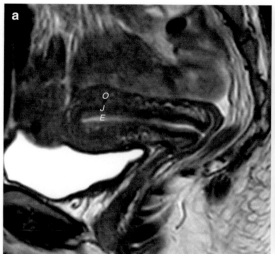

Fig. 18.2 Normal MRI anatomy of premenopausal uterus in 25-year (**a**) and 45-year (**b**) old women. T2-weighted sagittal sequences demonstrate anteverted, anteflexed uteri with well-defined zonal anatomy of endometrium (*E*), junctional zone (*J*), and outer myometrium (*O*) which continues into the cervix. Fluid/mucous in the endocervical canal in (**a**) is hyperintense, like urine in the bladder

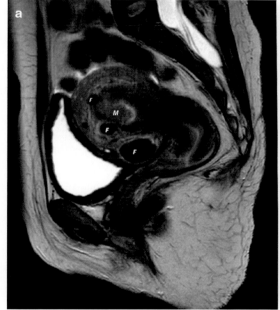
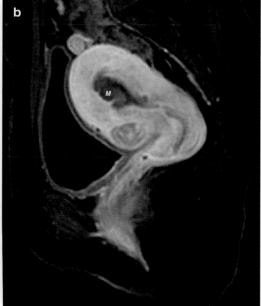

Fig. 18.3 Endometrial cancer. MRI T2-weighted sagittal sequence (**a**) shows intermediate signal endometrial mass (*M*) near the fundus invading the anterior junctional zone. The lesion enhances less than the normal myometrium making it more conspicuous on the T1-weighted post contrast sequence (**b**). Depth of myometrial invasion is less than 50% FIGO stage Ia. Intramural fibroids (*F*) are also seen

normal tissue. Endometrial cancer is of an intermediate signal compared to high signal of endometrial lining and appears hyperintense relative to the myometrium (Fig. 18.3). Cervical cancer is intermediate to high signal on T2-weighted images compared to the dark signal of stroma

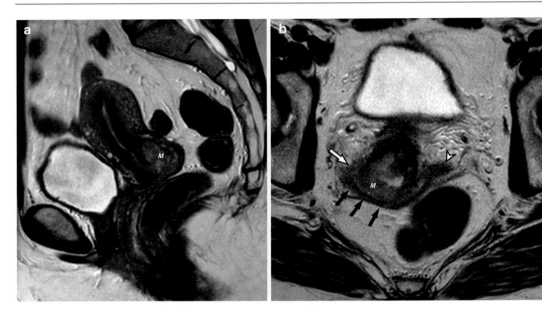

Fig. 18.4 Cervical cancer. MRI T2-weighted sagittal sequence (**a**) shows intermediate signal posterior cervical mass (*M*) replacing the normal dark signal of fibrous stroma. T2-weighted high resolution oblique axial sequence (**b**) through this lesion shows involvement of right lateral vaginal wall and early parametrial extension (white arrow). Normal posterior vaginal wall (black arrows) and left lateral fornix (white arrowhead) are seen

(Fig. 18.4). It is important to obtain high-resolution small field of view (FOV) T2 oblique axial sequence with imaging plane perpendicular to the true axis of uterus or cervix depending on the location of cancer, which will provide an accurate assessment of parametrial and pelvic sidewall extension. High resolution small FOV T2 oblique coronal sequence parallel to the long axis of uterus/cervix is also performed routinely in some protocols. A pelvic MRI protocol consists of following sequences: large FOV T1 and T2 axial, T2 sagittal, high resolution T2 oblique axial, axial and/or oblique axial DWI ± DCE.

Ovarian MRI can characterise adnexal lesions better than ultrasound and CT and its role in identifying ovarian malignancies, staging and treatment response is well established [19–24] and despite that MRI is mainly used for evaluation of indeterminate adnexal masses identified on ultrasound particularly in younger women with a normal or mildly elevated CA-125 and in some cases of staging as a problem-solving tool. MRI and CT fare equally well in identifying peritoneal implants of ovarian cancer larger than 1 cm but MRI is more accurate in identifying smaller deposits. There is ongoing research comparing multiparametric MRI against the current standard of CT for ovarian cancer staging and management, for example the MROC trial in the UK [25]. In the future MRI could potentially replace CT as the investigation of choice in ovarian cancer management. Post-treatment follow-up is with CA-125 monitoring and CECT, even though MRI is superior.

Primary features suggestive of malignancy on MRI are lesion size greater than 4 cm, solid mass with necrotic areas, cyst with enhancing solid component, thick >3 mm wall, thick septa >3 mm presence of enhancing nodules/papillae [26]. Secondary features include involvement of pelvic sidewall and/or adjacent pelvic organs, lymphadenopathy, ascites, and peritoneal deposits. Malignancy may develop within endometriotic cysts or teratomas and is commonly seen as enhancing mural nodule [27]. Digital subtraction of pre-contrast image from postcontrast image would suppress the background signal and make the enhancing nodule conspicuous. O-RADS

MRI system, like O-RADS US, and the lexicon are published recently [28, 29] and await large scale external validation studies.

Endometrial MRI is not used in detecting endometrial malignancy, which is done with transvaginal sonography and endometrial sampling. MRI is the investigation of choice for radiological staging as it accurately determines the depth of myometrial invasion, which is considered the most important prognosticator for disease spread based on its correlation with tumour grade, cervical invasion, and nodal metastasis. MRI guides treatment planning by differentiating between those requiring lymphadenectomy versus lymph node sampling and may help consider preoperative radiotherapy in very advanced disease. Myometrial invasion can be well identified on T2 weighted images as the cancer has a higher signal than myometrium. Addition of DCE sequence better demonstrates small tumours and myometrial invasion than T2 sequence alone (Fig. 18.3).

Cervical MRI, where available, is used as part of FIGO staging guidelines. It is the investigation of choice for local staging and obviates the need of invasive procedures like cystoscopy and proctoscopy if optimal quality MRI study is performed. MRI should be delayed for 7–10 days post-conization procedure to avoid over estimating tumour size because of presence of peritumoral oedema [30].

MRI helps in identifying parametrial invasion, pelvic lymph node metastasis, in treatment planning for radiotherapy and in patient selection for radical trachelectomy by providing accurate measurements. The cancer demonstrates an intermediate to high signal on T2-weighted images and DCE, although not routinely performed, helps better demonstrates small tumours. Treat response after chemoradiation is assessed with MRI. Recurrence after primary treatment can be seen in up to a third of patients which is usually central involving the vaginal vault after surgery and in the cervix post-chemoradiation.

18.5　FDG PET CT

PET is a functional imaging study performed by using radionuclides combined with tracers which target metabolic processes in the body. ^{18}F-FDG (fluorine 18 fluoro-2-deoxy-D-glucose) is the most common radiotracer used in present day imaging which is taken up by areas with increased glycolysis. This can be fused with CT, a hybrid imaging technique, providing better anatomical localisation. The study is performed after fasting for 4–6 h and intravenous injection of radiotracer. Antispasmodic can reduce normal bowel uptake. Emptying of urinary bladder before the study is better for assessment of pelvic disease.

^{18}F-FDG PET CT (will be referred to as FDG PET CT in this chapter) as compared to conventional cross-sectional imaging techniques like CT and MRI has the advantage of combining both anatomical and metabolic information. Normal FDG uptake is noted in the digestive tract, thyroid gland, myocardium, skeletal muscles, bone marrow and in the urinary tract as it is excreted by kidneys. Physiological endometrial uptake is also seen during ovulatory and menstrual phases while FDG activity in post-menopausal uterus and ovaries is considered abnormal. FDG PET CT can identify disseminated cancer and is routinely used in gynaecological malignancies.

Both PET and CT components have the disadvantage of ionising radiation. Breathing motion artefacts limit evaluation of disease along the under surface of diaphragm. Sub-centimetre peritoneal deposits and lung nodules may also miss detection. Bowel peristalsis may lead to misregistration between PET and CT images. FDG uptake in infection and inflammation can cause false positive results. Distended urinary bladder filled with excreted FDG may obscure pelvic disease. Benign lesions may sometimes show increased FDG uptake while some tumours like mucinous carcinomas and necrotic lymph nodes may show very low or no uptake [31]. Attenuation correction artefacts from metallic implants and devices may also limit interpretation.

Ovarian FDG PET CT can reliably diagnose malignant pelvic mass with a high sensitivity and specificity and could be used in identification of ovarian cancer before surgery in postmenopausal women with rising CA-125 levels and equivocal imaging. However, it is not routinely used in primary staging of ovarian cancer. Metastatic lymph nodes can be easily identified but small volume peritoneal disease is difficult to diagnose because of low spatial resolution, poor anatomical localisation, and physiological uptake in the bowel. Although FDG PET CT can evaluate treatment response, it is not used because of limited availability and high cost. It can be used to identify relapse in patients with rising CA-125 titres with equivocal cross-sectional imaging. Recurrence can be identified earlier than using CT alone however early commencement of salvage therapy in the form of localised radiotherapy or secondary debulking surgery did not improve overall survival [32].

Endometrial FDG PET CT has no role in primary staging and can be used to detect recurrence when cross-sectional imaging is inconclusive. It is also performed in patients being considered for pelvic exenteration to rule out extra pelvic disease.

Cervical FDG PET CT is routinely used in primary staging as well as restaging of cervical cancers. It is indicated in patients being considered for salvage therapy, for assessment of treatment response after chemoradiotherapy in locally advanced cervical cancer and in cases of symptomatic suspected recurrence with equivocal cross-sectional imaging.

18.6 Lymph Node Evaluation

Conventional cross-sectional imaging modalities use size criterion of ≥10 mm short axis diameter for a lymph node to be considered pathological, which has a high specificity (93–95%) but poor sensitivity (40–60%) and metastasis in normal sized lymph nodes could be missed. Additional imaging features such as necrosis, irregular margins, rounded appearance with loss of fatty hilum and signal intensity matching primary tumour can be used to identify small metastatic nodes. DWI sequence is also useful as the involved nodes show restricted diffusion, but false positives can occur, and metastatic involvement may be difficult to ascertain.

18.7 Image Guided Interventions

Interventional radiology has a role in obtaining diagnosis and treating complications. Pleural fluid aspiration for cytology can be performed under ultrasound guidance. Biopsy of omental cake or peritoneal deposits and even the primary pelvic mass can be performed using ultrasound or CT depending on feasibility and the availability of expertise and resources. Biopsy of inguinal or superficially located external iliac lymph nodes can be performed with ultrasound while deep-seated retroperitoneal para-aortic lymph nodes can be biopsied under CT guidance. Liver biopsies are rarely performed and can be undertaken with ultrasound or CT guidance depending on the location of the lesion. Lung nodules if sufficiently large can be biopsied with CT guidance. Image guided drainage of collections where necessary can be considered, mainly encountered in post-operative cases. It would be useful to discuss the feasibility of an image guided intervention beforehand with the radiologist who will be performing the procedure.

Emergency transarterial embolization of the pelvic arteries in cases of severe life-threatening haemorrhage, commonly encountered in advanced stages of cervical and uterine cancers, should be considered when conservative management fails and is a safe and effective treatment option [33, 34]. Pulmonary embolism (PE) is one of the leading causes of death in women with gynaecological malignancies as they are at a high risk of venous thromboembolism, and it can be prevented by inserting an inferior vena cava (IVC) filter when the traditional methods of PE prophylaxis with anticoagulants, intermittent pneumatic compression and graduated compression stockings have proven ineffective. Studies have shown that IVC filter is safe and effective in preventing PE, even in those who have already developed lower limb deep vein thrombosis (DVT) [35, 36]. Common indications for IVC filter placement are perioperative period, contraindication to anticoagulants due to haemorrhage and failed anticoagulation. These filters are usually planned as permanent devices but there are optional filters which can be retrieved in the future. Majority of patients receiving the IVC filter are those with ovarian cancer.

18.8 Recommended Imaging Pathways

Ovarian Transvaginal ultrasound is the first line investigation. CT chest, abdomen and pelvis is used for staging purposes to identify peritoneal deposits, lymph node metastasis and supradiaphragmatic disease. MRI is mainly used as a problem-solving tool. Image guided biopsy can be performed in patients with nonresectable disease for histological diagnosis prior to chemotherapy. CT is the cross-sectional imaging investigation of choice for follow-up after treatment and in evaluation of recurrence. MRI has proved to be better for staging and post-treatment surveillance as compared to CT in multiple small-scale studies and may become the primary investigation in the future. FDG PET CT is useful in cases of suspected recurrence with rising tumour markers and inconclusive cross-sectional imaging.

Endometrial Transvaginal ultrasound is the primary imaging modality used for diagnosis and MRI is utilised in cases where endometrial sampling cannot be done due to failed hysteroscopy or when the biopsy result is inconclusive. MRI is the investigation of choice for locoregional staging and it also provides valuable information for prognostication and planning treatment. Limited MRI sequences of the abdomen are also performed at the same time to look for enlarged retroperitoneal lymph nodes. CT of chest, abdomen and pelvis is useful in evaluation of distant spread, especially in cases with type II histology as these are more prone for metastases. MRI is the best modality for evaluation of pelvic recurrence while CT is used to determine distant metastasis. FDG PET CT is useful in patients with suspected recurrence, but cross-sectional imaging is inconclusive and in cases where salvage surgery is planned.

Cervical Ultrasound has no role in evaluating cervical malignancy. MRI is the investigation of choice for local staging, providing precise tumour measurements and helps differentiate between early disease treated with surgery and advanced disease treated with chemoradiotherapy. FDG PET CT is the investigation of choice evaluating nodal and distant spread and if PET CT is not available, CT chest abdomen and pelvis could be used. FDG PET CT is also used in evaluating treatment response following chemoradiotherapy, in cases of suspected recurrence with inconclusive CT/MRI and before salvage surgery.

18.9 Other Malignancies

Imaging principles and pathways for uncommon ovarian epithelial malignancies (clear cell adenocarcinoma, carcinosarcoma), non-epithelial germ cell and sex cord stromal tumours, and other rare tumours remain the same as those employed for commoner serous and mucinous epithelial malignancies.

Uterine sarcomas, like leiomyosarcoma, endometrial stromal sarcoma and adenosarcoma, demonstrate aggressive behaviour with a poor prognosis and are staged separately by FIGO. MRI has a role in evaluation of these tumours and CT can help identify distant spread. It is often difficult to differentiate leiomyosarcoma from an atypical or degenerating leiomyoma due to considerable overlap in the imaging features, however rapid growth, aggressive infiltrative nature of the tumour with irregular nodular borders, extensive necrosis, diffusion restriction on DWI MRI and intense postcontrast enhancement can help identify leiomyosarcoma.

Primary vulval and vaginal malignancies are rare, seen in elderly women and are mainly squamous cell carcinomas. Secondary involvement of vagina from cervical and uterine cancers is far more common than primary malignancy. Like all other gynaecological malignancies, FIGO staging is used for these sites except in cases of vulval/vaginal melanomas where AJCC (American Joint Committee on Cancer) staging of cutaneous melanomas is adopted. MRI is the investigation of choice as it clearly delineates the extent of tumour and identifies involvement of pelvic floor, urethra, anal canal, urinary bladder, and rectum which add to the findings of examination under anaesthesia and help plan surgical resection. Enlarged inguinal and pelvic lymph nodes can be detected on imaging. Fat saturated T2 sequence is a useful adjunct to the MRI protocol [37, 38]. Inguinal lymph node biopsy can be done under ultrasound guidance. MRI is also useful in local assessment post treatment. CT can be used for staging advanced cancers and FDG PET CT is an alternative.

18.10 Advances in Imaging

All present-day CT scanners can acquire volumetric scans which enable the radiologist to review images in multiple planes and produce 3D reconstructions when needed, although its usage in gynaeoncology is limited. A novel technique available in modern ultrasound machines is US-CT fusion where CT images of the patient can be transferred and fused with the US scan to localize and correlate the abnormal findings which can help in image guided interventions.

MRI lymphography is a novel technique where dextran coated ultra-small superparamagnetic iron oxide particles are used as lymph node-specific contrast agent to identify lymph node metastases, currently used mainly in research setting [39]. FDG PET MRI is a hybrid imaging technique like FDG PET CT which can potentially serve as a single step imaging assessment providing information on local tumour staging as well as nodal and distant metastases.

Radiomics is a relatively new field of study which deals with evaluating quantitative imaging features using software algorithms that cannot be identified by human vision, which could have the potential in improving diagnosis, prognostication and in predicting treatment response [40]. Radiogenomics deals with the relationship between these quantitative imaging biomarkers and various genetic or molecular features [41]. A recent study demonstrates the potential of employing radiogenomic signatures in treatment monitoring of ovarian tumours [42]. Artificial intelligence techniques are being used in Radiomics making the process automated. Extensive research is currently ongoing in these fields which undoubtably has exciting prospects.

18.11 Conclusion

Multiple imaging modalities are used in diagnosis, staging, treatment planning and post-treatment surveillance of gynaecological malignancies. Ultrasound, CT, MRI and FDG PET CT complement each other, and it is therefore essential to understand the basic techniques, indications, and limitations of these investigations to achieve an optimal standardised imaging management proto-

Key Points
- Transvaginal US and MRI are the main imaging modalities to evaluate female pelvis. T2 weighted imaging is the most important MRI sequence. CT is used for evaluation of disease spread beyond pelvis.
- US is the first investigation performed for suspected ovarian malignancy and if the risk of malignancy is high based on one of the diagnostic models a CT thorax, abdomen and pelvis is performed to assess the extent of disease. Treatment response and recurrence are also assessed by CT. MRI is mainly used for

- characterization of indeterminate adnexal masses.
- Initial evaluation of suspected endometrial cancer is by transvaginal US and local staging is by MRI. CT is done to evaluate distant spread in those with stage IB or higher and/or tumour with aggressive histology (type II). MRI is used to assess local recurrence while CT is for distant disease. FDG PET CT is used in equivocal cases of recurrence and when salvage therapy is planned.
- In cervical cancer, MRI is the investigation of choice for local staging. FDG PET CT is the preferred modality for detection of nodal and distant spread. MRI is used for monitoring treatment response.

col. Future advances in radiology will enable us to provide tailored personalised treatment options and further improve the overall care.

References

1. Jacobs I, Oram D, Fairbanks J, Turner J, Frost C, Grudzinskas J. A risk of malignancy index incorporating CA 125, ultrasound and menopausal status for the accurate preoperative diagnosis of ovarian cancer. Br J Obstet Gynaecol. 1990;97(10):922–9. https://doi.org/10.1111/J.1471-0528.1990.TB02448.X.
2. Timmerman D, Valentin L, Bourne T, Collins W, Verrelst H, Vergote I. Terms, definitions and measurements to describe the sonographic features of adnexal tumors: a consensus opinion from the International Ovarian Tumor Analysis (IOTA) Group. Ultrasound Obstet Gynecol. 2000;16(5):500–5. https://doi.org/10.1046/J.1469-0705.2000.00287.X.
3. Timmerman D, Testa A, Bourne T, et al. Simple ultrasound-based rules for the diagnosis of ovarian cancer. Ultrasound Obstet Gynecol. 2008;31(6):681–90. https://doi.org/10.1002/UOG.5365.
4. Timmerman D, Van Calster B, Testa A, et al. Predicting the risk of malignancy in adnexal masses based on the Simple Rules from the International Ovarian Tumor Analysis group. Am J Obstet Gynecol. 2016;214(4):424–37. https://doi.org/10.1016/J.AJOG.2016.01.007.
5. Timmerman D, Testa A, Bourne T, et al. Logistic regression model to distinguish between the benign and malignant adnexal mass before surgery: a multicenter study by the International Ovarian Tumor Analysis Group. J Clin Oncol. 2005;23(34):8794–801. https://doi.org/10.1200/JCO.2005.01.7632.
6. Van CB, Van HK, Valentin L, et al. Evaluating the risk of ovarian cancer before surgery using the ADNEX model to differentiate between benign, borderline, early and advanced stage invasive, and secondary metastatic tumours: prospective multicentre diagnostic study. BMJ. 2014;349:g5920. https://doi.org/10.1136/BMJ.G5920.
7. Andreotti RF, Timmerman D, Strachowski LM, et al. O-RADS US risk stratification and management system: a consensus guideline from the ACR Ovarian-Adnexal Reporting and Data System Committee. Radiology. 2019;294(1):168–85. https://doi.org/10.1148/RADIOL.2019191150.
8. Andreotti RF, Timmerman D, Benacerraf BR, et al. Ovarian-adnexal reporting lexicon for ultrasound: a white paper of the ACR Ovarian-Adnexal Reporting and Data System Committee. J Am Coll Radiol. 2018;15(10):1415–29. https://doi.org/10.1016/J.JACR.2018.07.004.
9. Meys E, Jeelof L, Achten N, et al. Estimating risk of malignancy in adnexal masses: external validation of the ADNEX model and comparison with other frequently used ultrasound methods. Ultrasound Obstet Gynecol. 2017;49(6):784–92. https://doi.org/10.1002/UOG.17225.
10. Kaijser J, Bourne T, Valentin L, et al. Improving strategies for diagnosing ovarian cancer: a summary of the International Ovarian Tumor Analysis (IOTA) studies. Ultrasound Obstet Gynecol. 2013;41(1):9–20. https://doi.org/10.1002/UOG.12323.
11. Meys EMJ, Kaijser J, Kruitwagen RFPM, et al. Subjective assessment versus ultrasound models to diagnose ovarian cancer: a systematic review and meta-analysis. Eur J Cancer. 2016;58:17–29. https://doi.org/10.1016/J.EJCA.2016.01.007.
12. Kaijser J, Sayasneh A, Van Hoorde K, et al. Presurgical diagnosis of adnexal tumours using mathematical models and scoring systems: a systematic review and meta-analysis. Hum Reprod Update. 2014;20(3):449–62. https://doi.org/10.1093/HUMUPD/DMT059.
13. Nalaboff KM, Pellerito JS, Ben-Levi E. Imaging the endometrium: disease and normal variants. Radiographics. 2001;21(6):1409–24. https://doi.org/10.1148/RADIOGRAPHICS216.g01nv211409.
14. Fong K, Kung R, Lytwyn A, et al. Endometrial evaluation with transvaginal US and hysterosonography in asymptomatic postmenopausal women with breast cancer receiving tamoxifen. Radiology. 2001;220(3):765–73. https://doi.org/10.1148/radiol2203010011.
15. Sahdev A. Imaging the endometrium in postmenopausal bleeding. BMJ. 2007;334(7594):635–6. https://doi.org/10.1136/BMJ.39126.628924.BE.
16. Williams PL, Laifer-Narin SL, Ragavendra N. US of abnormal uterine bleeding. RadioGraphics.

2003;23(3):703–18. https://doi.org/10.1148/RG233 025150.
17. Smith-Bindman R, Lipson J, Marcus R, et al. Radiation dose associated with common computed tomography examinations and the associated lifetime attributable risk of cancer. Arch Intern Med. 2009;169(22):2078. https://doi.org/10.1001/archinternmed.2009.427.
18. Patient Safety—Radiation Dose in X-Ray and CT Exams. Accessed May 5, 2021. https://www.radiologyinfo.org/en/info/safety-xray
19. DeSouza N, Rockall A, Freeman S. Functional MR imaging in gynecologic cancer. Magn Reson Imaging Clin N Am. 2016;24(1):205–22. https://doi.org/10.1016/j.mric.2015.08.008.
20. Sohaib SAA, Reznek RH. MR imaging in ovarian cancer. Cancer Imaging. 2007;7(Special issue A):S119. https://doi.org/10.1102/1470-7330.2007.9046.
21. Nougaret S, Tirumani SH, Addley H, Pandey H, Sala E, Reinhold C. Pearls and pitfalls in MRI of gynecologic malignancy with diffusion-weighted technique. AJR Am J Roentgenol. 2013;200(2):261–76. https://doi.org/10.2214/AJR.12.9713.
22. Rockall AG. Diffusion weighted MRI in ovarian cancer. Curr Opin Oncol. 2014;26(5):529–35. https://doi.org/10.1097/CCO.0000000000000112.
23. Winfield JM, Wakefield JC, Dolling D, et al. Diffusion-weighted MRI in advanced epithelial ovarian cancer: apparent diffusion coefficient as a response marker. Radiology. 2019;293(2):374–83. https://doi.org/10.1148/radiol2019190545.
24. Iyer VR, Lee SI. MRI, CT, and PET/CT for ovarian cancer detection and adnexal lesion characterization. AJR Am J Roentgenol. 2010;194(2):311–21. https://doi.org/10.2214/AJR.09.3522.
25. ISRCTN—ISRCTN51246892: MR in ovarian cancer. Accessed Oct 10, 2021. https://www.isrctn.com/ISRCTN51246892
26. Forstner R, Meissnitzer MW, Schlattau A, Spencer JA. MRI in ovarian cancer. Imaging Med. 2012;4(1):59–75. https://doi.org/10.2217/IIM.11.69.
27. McDermott S, Oei TN, Iyer VR, Lee SI. MR imaging of malignancies arising in endometriomas and extraovarian endometriosis. Radiographics. 2012;32(3):845–63. https://doi.org/10.1148/RG.323115736.
28. Reinhold C, Rockall A, Sadowski EA, et al. Ovarian-adnexal reporting lexicon for MRI: a white paper of the ACR Ovarian-Adnexal Reporting and Data Systems MRI Committee. J Am Coll Radiol. 2021;18(5):713–29. https://doi.org/10.1016/J.JACR.2020.12.022.
29. Thomassin-Naggara I, Poncelet E, Jalaguier-Coudray A, et al. Ovarian-Adnexal Reporting Data System Magnetic Resonance Imaging (O-RADS MRI) score for risk stratification of sonographically indeterminate adnexal masses. JAMA Netw Open. 2020;3(1):e1919896. https://doi.org/10.1001/JAMANETWORKOPEN.2019.19896.
30. Sheu MH, Chang CY, Wang JH, Yen MS. MR staging of clinical stage I and IIa cervical carcinoma: a reappraisal of efficacy and pitfalls. Eur J Radiol. 2001;38(3):225–31. https://doi.org/10.1016/S0720-048X(00)00278-3.
31. Lakhani A, Khan SR, Bharwani N, et al. FDG PET/CT pitfalls in gynecologic and genitourinary oncologic imaging. Radiographics. 2017;37(2):577–94. https://doi.org/10.1148/RG.2017160059.
32. Narayanan P, Sahdev A. The role of 18F-FDG PET CT in common gynaecological malignancies. Br J Radiol. 2017;90(1079):20170283. https://doi.org/10.1259/BJR.20170283.
33. Field K, Ryan MJ, Saadeh FA, et al. Selective arterial embolisation for intractable vaginal haemorrhage in genital tract malignancies. Eur J Gynaecol Oncol. 2016;37(5):736–40. https://doi.org/10.12892/EJGO3160.20L6.
34. Meyer-Wilmes P, Powerski M, Fischbach F, Omari J, Damm R, Pech M. Transarterial embolisation for the treatment of acute gynecological cancer bleeding. Arch Gynecol Obstet. 2019;300(5):1391–7. https://doi.org/10.1007/S00404-019-05316-4.
35. Dewdney S, Benn T, Rimel B, et al. Inferior vena cava filter placement in the gynecologic oncology patient: a 15-year institutional experience. Gynecol Oncol. 2011;121(2):344–6. https://doi.org/10.1016/J.YGYNO.2011.01.004.
36. Babu SB, Khan AM, Coates PJ. Three-year experience of prophylactic placement of inferior vena cava filters in women with gynecological cancer. Int J Gen Med. 2013;6:671. https://doi.org/10.2147/IJGM.S44191.
37. Parikh JH, Barton DPJ, Ind TEJ, Sohaib SA. MR imaging features of vaginal malignancies. Radiographics. 2008;28(1):49–63. https://doi.org/10.1148/RG.281075065.
38. Viswanathan C, Kirschner K, Truong M, Balachandran A, Devine C, Bhosale P. Multimodality imaging of vulvar cancer: staging, therapeutic response, and complications. AJR Am J Roentgenol. 2013;200(6):1387–400. https://doi.org/10.2214/AJR.12.9714.
39. Jahan N, Narayanan P, Rockall A. Magnetic resonance lymphography in gynaecological malignancies. Cancer Imaging. 2010;10(1):85. https://doi.org/10.1102/1470-7330.2010.0006.
40. Lambin P, Leijenaar RTH, Deist TM, et al. Radiomics: the bridge between medical imaging and personalized medicine. Nat Rev Clin Oncol. 2017;14(12):749–62. https://doi.org/10.1038/nrclinonc.2017.141.
41. Aerts H, Velazquez E, Leijenaar R, et al. Decoding tumour phenotype by noninvasive imaging using a quantitative radiomics approach. Nat Commun. 2014;5:4006. https://doi.org/10.1038/NCOMMS5006.
42. Martin-Gonzalez P, Crispin-Ortuzar M, Rundo L, et al. Integrative radiogenomics for virtual biopsy and treatment monitoring in ovarian cancer. Insights Imaging. 2020;11(1):1–10. https://doi.org/10.1186/S13244-020-00895-2.

Post-operative Care in Gynaecological Oncology

19

Christine Ang

19.1 Introduction

Ensuring the best outcome for patients relies on careful assessment, early recognition of high risk factors, pre-treatment optimisation, individualised treatment plans, and specifically in surgery, good post-operative care. This has been made increasingly difficult in recent years because of an aging, obese and more co-morbid population, increasingly complex and subspecialised surgery, greater expectations and education of patients and their relatives, an increasing number of interventions and therapies, less experienced medical and nursing staff compounded by a workforce shortage. The progressive nature of cancer is often accompanied by physiological derangement, massive fluid shifts and poor nutrition, which can make post-operative care challenging and difficult. This chapter will concentrate on the post-operative care of Gynaecological Oncology patients, in both the immediate period following surgery and while the patient remains in hospital.

19.2 Identifying the Patient at Risk

Most patients with gynaecological cancer are high risk women undergoing high risk surgery, and when they deteriorate clinically post-op, it is usually a combination of the effects of surgery on pre-existing disease, exacerbated by a complication that results in an imbalance of oxygen, fluid and nutritional requirements, delivery and utilisation.

Many centres these days use cardiopulmonary exercise testing (CPEX) as an objective assessment of cardiovascular and pulmonary reserve to assess fitness for surgery. This enables more thorough and detailed counselling regarding morbidity and mortality risk, helps dictate the level of intra-operative monitoring required and allows a decision to be made regarding the need for elective admission to high dependency after surgery. Factors determining admission to critical care depend on co-morbidities, pre-assessment outcomes (CPEX, NSQIP[1] scores), the mode of surgery (open vs. minimal access), and the extent of surgery.

C. Ang (✉)
Northern Gynaecological Oncology Centre,
Queen Elizabeth Hospital, Gateshead, UK
e-mail: christine.ang@nhs.net

[1] The National Surgical Quality Improvement Program (NSQIP) of the American College of Surgeons provides risk-adjusted surgical outcome measures for participating hospitals that can be used for performance improvement of surgical mortality and morbidity [1].

Physiological parameter	Score						
	3	2	1	0	1	2	3
Respiration rate (per minute)	≤8		9–11	12–20		21–24	≥25
SpO₂ Scale 1 (%)	≤91	92–93	94–95	≥96			
SpO₂ Scale 2 (%)	≤83	84–85	86–87	88–92 ≥93 on air	93–94 on oxygen	95–96 on oxygen	≥97 on oxygen
Air or oxygen?		Oxygen		Air			
Systolic blood pressure (mmHg)	≤90	91–100	101–110	111–219			≥220
Pulse (per minute)	≤40		41–50	51–90	91–110	111–130	≥131
Consciousness				Alert			CVPU
Temperature (°C)	≤35.0		35.1–36.0	36.1–38.0	38.1–39.0	≥39.1	

A NEW score of ≥ 5 should trigger an urgent clinical review;
A NEW score of ≥ 7 or more should trigger an emergency clinical review.

Fig. 19.1 National Early Warning Score (NEWS)

Early warning scores such as the National Early Warning Score (NEWS) help assess the need for and level of medical and nursing intervention required when patients become unwell. It incorporates a combination of clinical observations that trigger an appropriate response according to severity based on a scoring system (Fig. 19.1) [2].

19.3 Cardiovascular Complications

This section addresses the needs and types of haemodynamic support that may be required post-op and is not uncommon after extensive and prolonged oncological surgery. Cardiovascular dysfunction is seen in patients with underlying cardiovascular disease when there is an exacerbation of pre-existing disease secondary to the stress of surgery or a new insult. Cardiac disturbances are not uncommon post-op, can be broadly categorised into three groups:

1. Pre-cardiac—most commonly due to hypovolaemia secondary to haemorrhage or unreplaced fluid losses.
2. Cardiac—intrinsic problems with the heart such as ischaemia, infarction and arrhythmias.
3. Post-cardiac—due to increased or decreased afterload in conditions such as sepsis.

The initial signs and symptoms of cardiovascular compromise may be subtle, so acute awareness in combination with early recognition and timely and appropriate intervention is key. It is also important to remember that younger and fitter patients will compensate more readily, and that by the time clinical signs and symptoms are noticed, a large insult may already have occurred.

19.3.1 Arterial and Central Venous Pressure Measurements

Non-invasive intermittent measurements of arterial blood pressure can be performed using an automated sphygmomanometer and are useful in demonstrating trends in blood pressure. They are reliable in most stable patients as well as easy to use in a ward setting, but can be erroneous if the cuff size or cuff positioning is incorrect. Better accuracy with continuous monitoring can be achieved by inserting an arterial line, and is used in unstable patients or patients deemed high risk due to pre-existing co-morbidities and/or those undergoing extensive surgical procedures. Arterial lines also allow for frequent blood sampling and close monitoring of pH, PaO_2, haemoglobin and lactate.

Central venous pressure (CVP) is the pressure within the superior vena cava as it enters the right atrium, and reflects the ability of the right heart to accept and deliver circulating volume. CVP measurements are used in situations that require accurate measurement of fluid balance (co-morbid patients, extensive surgery) and patients in whom fluid balance is difficult to assess (acute kidney injury, massive fluid shifts). It is influenced by various factors, including venous return, right heart compliance, intrathoracic pressure and patient positioning. The normal range of CVP measurements are between 0–8 mmHg and 0–10 cmH_2O, and although absolute measurements of CVP are useful, it is the trend and response to fluid challenges or therapeutic manoeuvres that is important.

19.3.2 Factors Influencing Need for Haemodynamic Support

Hypovolaemia secondary to haemorrhage is the commonest cause of patients requiring haemodynamic support post-operatively. The effects of haemorrhage will depend on the duration and severity of the blood loss, the patient's age and any underlying cardiac dysfunction. Blood loss is often underestimated, and significant blood loss may only be apparent following surgery when the patient's clinical parameters fail to normalise despite apparent adequate fluid replacement. It is also important to remember that immediate post-op bleeding is almost always due poor surgical haemostasis such as the failure to secure an arterial or venous bleed within a pedicle or tissue, and in most cases will require a return to theatre within the first 12 h. A more gradual but sustained fall in haemoglobin in the first 24–72 h is more likely due to bleeding from raw tissue surfaces or the tracking of blood into the retroperitoneal spaces, and will usually settle with conservative management and the use of pro-thrombotic agents, such as tranexamic acid, and blood replacement. Bleeding after this time, is most likely due to infection and should be managed accordingly.

Unreplaced fluid loss is most commonly seen when surgery is both prolonged and extensive, and is the result of poor fluid replacement, loss of fluid from exposed tissue, third spacing of fluid and unrecognised or underestimation of blood loss. Patients who receive pre-op bowel prep can suffer from dehydration and electrolyte disturbance through gastrointestinal fluid loss exacerbated by pre-op fasting.

Other factors that require close monitoring of fluid balance and fluid replacement include loss of gastrointestinal fluid due to vomiting, diarrhoea, fistulae, high output stomas (especially ileostomies) or bowel oedema secondary to bowel obstruction. Pyrexia, infection and sepsis can also cause increased insensible fluid loss, local sequestration of fluid and tissue oedema, and although more difficult to measure, must be replaced.

Women with advanced ovarian cancer, will often have poor nutrition and increased capillary permeability with associated hypoalbuminaemia, exacerbating the problem of local sequestration of fluid which can manifest as peripheral and sacral oedema, abdominal oedema and ascites. These women are often intra-vascularly depleted and therefore more likely to require intra-operative inotropic support and in the immediate post-op period.

19.3.3 Colloids and Crystalloids

The most common crystalloids used are normal saline and Ringer's lactate solution. Ringer's lactate is generally preferred because it can buffer metabolic acidosis and avoids the hyperchloraemic acidosis associated with large volume normal saline infusions. There is a risk, however, of hyperkalaemia when using Ringer's lactate in patients with an acute kidney injury or chronic kidney disease.

Colloid solutions are theoretically retained in the intravascular space more than crystalloids. The use of colloids in patients with sepsis have been shown to be associated with poorer outcomes leading to safety concerns being raised in this group of patients. Colloid solutions also carry risks of anaphylaxis, coagulopathy and acute kidney injury.

The important points to remember are the need for early recognition and the rapid treatment of hypovolaemic states, the prompt use of blood and blood products in haemorrhage, and most importantly, the surgical treatment of any underlying cause.

19.3.4 Inotropic Agents

Cardiac output is the volume of blood pumped by each ventricle per minute, and is determined by preload, afterload, heart rate, rhythm, contractility and the balance of oxygen demand and supply (Cardiac output = heart rate × stroke volume). If the cardiac output remains low after correcting any hypovolaemia with a fluid challenge, inotropic or other vasoactive drugs are used to optimise myocardial contractility by balancing myocardial oxygen supply and demand, and increase the stroke volume.

The most commonly used inotropes are epinephrine (adrenaline) and dobutamine. Norepinephrine (noradrenaline) is a vasopressor and is used to increase and maintain systemic vascular resistance (SVR) within the normal range (Mean arterial pressure = Cardiac output × Total peripheral resistance).

Inotropes and vasodilators can only be used safely where a full range of cardiac monitoring is available. These patients are most typically looked after in critical care, and never on an ordinary surgical ward.

The following table show the drugs most commonly used for haemodynamic support, the choice of which will depend on the likely cause of shock (Table 19.1).

19.4 Respiratory Complications

Respiratory failure occurs when there is inadequate pulmonary gas exchange such that blood oxygen and carbon dioxide cannot be maintained at normal levels.

Common causes of respiratory failure in the post-op patient can be broadly classified into three groups:

1. <u>A fall in functional residual capacity (FRC) without pulmonary vascular dysfunction</u>—most commonly seen in atelectasis, sputum retention, pneumonia or respiratory depression caused by drugs such as opiates.
2. <u>A fall in functional residual capacity (FRC) with pulmonary vascular dysfunction</u>—includes left ventricular failure, fluid overload, pulmonary hypertension, pulmonary embolism and adult respiratory distress syndrome (ARDS).
3. <u>Airflow obstruction</u>—asthma and chronic obstructive pulmonary disease (COPD).

Factors that increase the risk of respiratory problems post-op include age, obesity, pre-existing respiratory disease such as asthma, COPD, obstructive sleep apnoea, musculoskeletal problems that restrict the ability to deep breathe such as kyphosis and scoliosis (especially after midline laparotomies), smoking and upper abdominal surgery (especially diaphragmatic stripping).

Hypoxia should be treated with humidified high flow oxygen (10–15 L/min) through a non-rebreather mask. Dry, cold gas may contribute towards thickening of airway secretions and promote sputum retention.

It is not within the scope of this chapter to go into the detail of each method of respiratory sup-

Table 19.1 Table of drugs used to provide haemodynamic support

Drug	Receptor	Effect	Clinical use
Norepinephrine	α- and β- adrenoceptor agonists, predominantly α agonist	Peripheral vasoconstriction	Acute hypotension Sepsis and septic shock
Phenylephrine	α-adrenoceptor agonists	Peripheral vasoconstriction	Hypotension secondary to peripheral vasodilation
Epinephrine	α- and β- adrenoceptor agonists, predominantly β- adrenoceptor agonist at low doses	Positive inotropic and chronotropic effects. Vasoconstricts at high doses	Hypotension Septic shock Anaphylaxis Cardiac arrest
Dopamine	α- and β- adrenoceptors. Dopamine (DA) 1 and 2 receptors	Low dose: splanchnic vasodilatation, increased renal and hepatic blood flow (DA1). High dose: vasoconstriction	Hypotension Septic shock
Dopexamine	DA1, DA2 and β- adrenoceptor agonist	Increases splanchnic blood flow	Cardiogenic shock
Dobutamine	β- adrenoceptor agonist	Increases cardiac output and vasodilation	Cardiogenic shock

port, but important for the Gynaecological Oncologist to be aware of the step-wise escalation of the support that may be required as respiratory function worsens.

- Oxygen delivery via conventional nasal cannula and face masks
- High flow oxygen via non-rebreather mask
- Continuous positive airway pressure (CPAP)
- Non-invasive ventilation by mask (NIV)
- Intubation and ventilation

Adequate analgesia and early chest physiotherapy are important preventors of respiratory compromise in the post-op patient.

19.4.1 Understanding of ABGs and Acid-Base Balance

Arterial blood gases (ABGs) are useful in the assessment and management of sick patients and can provide a guide to acid-base status (pH), ventilation (PaO_2 and $PaCO_2$) and tissue perfusion (lactate and base excess). Abnormalities in ABGs may arise before a patient becomes obviously unwell and provides clinicians with the opportunity for early intervention, by providing useful additional information such as haemoglobin, sodium and calcium and glucose levels.

The arterial partial pressure of oxygen (PaO_2) is a reflection of the amount of oxygen dissolved in the blood. A normal level does not necessarily ensure effective oxygen utilisation by the tissues, but it does reflect adequate oxygen delivery by the respiratory and cardiovascular systems. It is important to remember, however, that a normal PaO_2 in a patient on high flow oxygen can be falsely reassuring and may in fact represent a severely compromised patient.

19.4.2 Common Surgical Respiratory Problems

Atelectasis This is an absence of gas from all or part of the lung. It is commonly seen following abdominal procedures, especially midline laparotomies and is exacerbated in the elderly, smokers, the overweight and those with underlying lung disease. Reduced lung expansion from pain and splinting leads to retention of secretions and distal airway collapse. The symptoms and signs are cough, chest pain or breathing difficulty, low oxygen saturations, pleural effusion, cyanosis and tachycardia and is diagnosed on chest x-ray (CXR). Proactive management such as pre-operative deep breathing exercises, early mobilisation, adequate analgesia and chest physiotherapy will help reduce the risk.

Pneumonia This is most commonly bacterial or chemical secondary to aspiration. Symptoms of pneumonia include a productive cough, chest pain, pyrexia and difficulty breathing. The diagnosis is made by a raised white cell count and C-reactive protein (CRP), CXR and sputum culture. Treatment is with appropriate antibiotics and chest physiotherapy.

Pulmonary Embolism This is an obstruction of a vascular branch beyond the right ventricular outflow tract, usually from an associated deep vein thrombosis. PEs are relatively common in post-op Gynae Oncology patients, with risk factors including age, female sex, major abdominal surgery and thrombocythaemia. Common symptoms include dyspnoea, pleuritic chest pain, cough, haemoptysis, tachypnoea, tachycardia and hypoxia. Although It can also be found incidentally on a pre-op computerised tomography (CT) scan, the diagnosis is made most commonly by CT pulmonary angiography (CTPA) and less commonly, by a ventilation-perfusion (VQ) scan.

Treatment is with anticoagulation therapy, most commonly low molecular weight heparin (LMWH) initially. Depending on the need for adjuvant treatment, patients undergoing chemotherapy or radiotherapy are usually kept on LMWH until the completion of oncological treatment. This is to reduce the risk of drug interactions more commonly associated with oral anticoagulant therapy. Conversion to oral anticoagulants such as warfarin, or other novel oral anticoagulants (NOACs) can then be made, and treatment is usually continued for a further 3–6 months. Women who develop PEs severe enough to cause haemodynamic and respiratory instability should be considered for thrombolytic treatment or embolectomy, but this has to be balanced against the risk of bleeding especially in the post-op period.

If a PE is diagnosed pre-op, consideration should be given to the insertion of an IVC filter if surgery is within 4 weeks of the commencement of anticoagulation treatment. However, IVC filters are in themselves thrombogenic, so a balance of risks and benefits must be considered. Monitoring of anti-Xa levels may be warranted in special circumstances such as extremes of body weight, in patients with large thrombi and those with renal dysfunction.

19.5 Renal Failure, Prevention and Management

Acute kidney injury (AKI) in the post-op patient is not uncommon and is often preventable. Management includes careful fluid balance in the peri-operative period and early intervention to prevent worsening renal function and the need for renal replacement therapy.

Although reversible in the short term, repeated and sustained insults can result in tubular necrosis and irreversible renal damage. Reasons for abnormal renal function in women with gynaecological malignancies are summarized in Table 19.2.

Common causes of AKI are classified as:

A. Pre-renal—hypovolemia, sepsis, low cardiac output
B. Renal—acute tubular necrosis, ischaemic injury (hypoxia, hypoperfusion), nephrotoxic injury (drugs, contrast), abdominal compartment syndrome
C. Post-renal—bladder outflow obstruction, bilateral ureteric obstruction

Key points to consider in the development of AKI in the surgical patient:

- Normal renal function requires adequate renal perfusion which is dependent on adequate blood pressure
- A surgical patient with poor urine output usually requires more fluid. However, caution should be used when administering fluid, especially in the elderly, those with significant co-morbidities and patients with hypoalbuminaemia and sequestration of fluid
- Absolute anuria is usually due to urinary tract obstruction
- Poor urine output in a surgical patient is not initially treated with diuretics

Established AKI will require renal replacement therapy (haemodialysis, haemofiltration), and is not within the scope of this chapter.

19.5.1 Management of Life-Threatening Complications

Hyperkalaemia Acute hyperkalaemia (K^+ above 6.5 mmol/L) or a rapid rate of rise requires immediate treatment to prevent life-threatening cardiac dysrhythmias and VF/asystolic arrest.

Table 19.2 Causes of abnormal renal function in women with gynaecological malignancies

- Age
- Underlying co-morbidities such as hypertension and diabetes
- Sequestration of fluid due in increased vascular permeability, reduced intravascular oncotic pressure and reduced intravascular circulating volume
- Poor post-op fluid balance and fluid replacement
- Underestimation of blood loss and replacement
- Disease process—hydronephrosis and hydroureters due to compression of the renal tract by tumour
- Use of pre-op bowel preparations and prolonged fasting
- Unrecognised intra-operative urinary tract injury
- Post-operative urinary tract complications (ureteric fistulas, breakdown of tissue following ureteric reimplantation/bladder reconstruction and repair)
- Use of nephrotoxic drugs—especially if chronic e.g. ACE inhibitors, diuretics, NSAIDS

Table 19.3 Drugs commonly used to treat life-threatening hyperkalaemia

Drug	Route	Dose	Mechanism of action	Pros and Cons
Calcium gluconate	IV	10–30 mL of 10% solution	Membrane stabiliser	Rapid effect but transient action
Insulin/dextrose	IV	IV, 10–20 μ Actrapid in 100 mL of 20% dextrose over 30 min	Drives potassium into cells	Rapid effect, intermediate action but may cause hypoglycaemia
Sodium bicarbonate	IV	50 mmol over 5–10 min followed by infusion of 1.36% or 1.4% solution at 100 mL/h	Transfer of potassium into cells by exchange of hydrogen across membrane	Rapid effect—intermediate action, best with metabolic acidosis; beware sodium overload
Salbutamol	IV infusion or nebulised	5–10 μg/min	Transfer of potassium into cells	Rapid effect, short action; risk of tachycardia, vasodilator effect, frequent use can raise serum lactate

Management includes identifying and stopping the underlying cause such as blood transfusions, drugs that reduce renal potassium excretion (e.g. potassium-sparing diuretics and ACE inhibitors), intravenous fluids containing potassium and potassium supplements. Drugs commonly used to treat acute life-threatening hyperkalaemia are shown in Table 19.3.

Pulmonary Oedema Presents with shortness of breath, tachycardia and tachypnoea. Crepitations and wheeze may be heard on auscultation, and the diagnosis confirmed on CXR. Management includes sitting the patient upright, stopping all IV infusions and administering high flow oxygen (10–15 L/min) aiming for saturations of greater than 94%. Treatment with diuretics is key to offload fluid in the lungs, and furosemide is most commonly used (250 mg in 50 mL saline over 1 h). Escalation to critical care should be considered in the presence of oligo/anuria, continued tachypnoea (>30/min), signs of fatigue, respiratory failure (PaO_2 < 8 kPa, $PaCO_2$ > 7 kPa) and acidosis (pH < 7.2).

19.6 Sepsis and Multiple Organ Failure

Sepsis and hospital-acquired infections are the most common complications seen in post-op patients. Failure to adequately treat infection can lead to sepsis, organ dysfunction and, eventually, multi-organ failure and death. Patients undergoing treatment for gynaecological cancers are particularly at risk, with contributory factors including age, indwelling devices such as catheters and drains (chest and pelvic), central lines and epidurals, immunosuppression secondary to disease, chemotherapy or steroids, and midline abdominal incisions that increase the risk of chest infections due to atelectasis.

Management of suspected sepsis involves prompt recognition, identification of infection and prompt and accurate treatment. Blood should be sent for haematological and biochemical indices, with particular attention to white cell count, CRP and lactate. Cultures should be obtained from blood, urine, drain fluid, wounds and lines. Antibiotics should be targeted and administered urgently. Hypotensive patients or those with a lactate level ≥ 4 mmol/L should be given 30 mL/kg crystalloid with reassessment of volume responsiveness and tissue perfusion. Fluid balance with measurement of hourly urine. Escalation to critical care for inotropic support should be considered in patients with persistent hypotension (MAP ≤ 65 mmHg) or increased lactate levels [3]. Table 19.4 shows the antibiotic regimen used in suspected sepsis in the UK (Table 19.4) [4]. Table 19.5 shows examples of the common causes of sepsis in patients undergoing surgery for gynaecological cancer (Table 19.5).

It is definitely worth mentioning neutropenic sepsis within this section (although it is not

Table 19.4 The antibiotic regimen used in suspected sepsis

Suspected source of sepsis	Antimicrobial regimen	Antimicrobial regimen—penicillin allergy	
		Age <70 years	Age >70 years
If no source apparent, haemodynamically unstable	Piperacillin-Tazobactam 4.5 g IV TDS	[b]Ciprofloxacin 400 mg IV BD Plus Teicoplanin 400 mg IV BD for 3 doses then 400 mg IV OD thereafter Plus Metronidazole 500 mg IV TDS	Tigecycline 100 mg IV stat then 50 mg IV BD Plus [a]Gentamicin 3 mg/kg (ideal body weight) IV as a stat does pending culture results Plus Metronidazole 500 mg IV TDS
Hospital Acquired pneumonia (Non-severe)	Doxycycline 200 mg oral loading dose then 100 mg PO OD or Co-Trimoxazole 960 mg PO BD		
Hospital Acquired pneumonia (Severe)	Teicoplanin 400 mg IV 12 hourly for 3 doses then 400 mg daily Plus [a]Gentamicin 3 mg/kg (ideal body weight) IV as a stat does pending culture results; or Amoxicillin 1 g IV TDS Plus Temocillin 2 g IV BD; or Piperacillin-Tazobactam 4.5 g IV TDS If aspiration pneumonia add Metronidazole 500 mg IV TDS	Teicoplanin 400 mg IV 12 hourly for 3 doses then 400 mg IV OD Plus [b]Ciprofloxacin 500 mg PO BD	Teicoplanin 400 mg IV 12 hourly for 3 doses then 400 mg IV OD; or Linezolid 600 mg IV BD
Mild surgical wound cellulitis	Co-amoxiclav 625 mg TDS PO	[b]Ciprofloxacin 500 mg BD PO Plus Metronidazole 400 mg TDS PO	Co-trimoxazole 960 mg BD Plus Metronidazole 400 mg TDS PO
Severe/deep incisional cellulitis (including pelvic cellulitis)	Piperacillin-Tazobactam 4.5 g IV TDS	[a]Gentamicin 3 mg/kg (ideal body weight) IV as a stat does pending culture results Plus Tigecycline 100 mg IV stat then 50 mg IV BD	
Complicated (upper) Urinary Tract Infection	Co-amoxiclav 1.2 g IV TDS; or Cefuroxime 1.5 g IV TDS	[b]Ciprofloxacin 500 mg PO BD; or [a]Gentamicin 5 mg/kg IV as a stat dose	[a]Gentamicin 3 mg/kg (ideal body weight) IV as a stat does pending culture results Plus Trimethoprim 200 mg PO BD
Catheter associated Urinary Tract Infection	[a]Gentamicin 5 mg/kg (ideal body weight) IV as a stat dose pending cultures		

[a]Use Gentamicin with caution in the elderly, those with impaired renal function and if prescribed other nephrotoxic medication (e.g. diuretics, ACE inhibitors, NSAIDs). **DO NOT use Gentamicin if allergic, Myasthenia Gravis or if CrCl < 30 mL/min: in such cases discuss with a Consultant Microbiologist.** If Gentamicin needs to be continued beyond one dose, take a trough level 23 h post dose and refer to the Adult Once Daily Gentamicin Guidelines regarding subsequent dosing

[b]Do not use in patients with a history of Clostridium difficile infection, and use with caution in patients with risk factors for Clostridium difficile infection e.g. frail and elderly. Discuss an alternative agent with a Medical Microbiologist

strictly a post-op complication), as it is not uncommon for the Gynaecological Oncologist to be faced with a neutropenic septic patient. Classically seen 7–10 days following carboplatin and paclitaxel chemotherapy, these patients present with sepsis and a neutrophil count <1 × 10^9/L. Treatment must be immediate, aggressive and targeted to prevent death. Management of the sepsis is as above, however, in addition, the patient must be barrier nursed, and consideration given to the administration of Granulocyte Colony Stimulating Factor (GCSF) to stimulate the bone marrow to produce granulocytes and stem cells.

19.7 Surgical Site Management

The ability to anticipate problems is an important skill to acquire, allowing earlier and targeted intervention and decreasing the chance of deterioration. Operative mortality can be in excess of 50% among patients who develop organ failure. Some examples of anticipated postoperative complications associated with tumour site are shown in Table 19.6.

The risk of complications can be reduced by clear documentation of operation notes, any intra-operative difficulties, and clear post-operative instructions, especially with regards to antibiotic administration, anticoagulation, drains, nutrition and mobilisation.

The warning signs of significant pathology include:

- Neutropenia (neutrophil count $<1 \times 10^9$/L)—can be seen in overwhelming sepsis or significant immunosuppression
- Grossly elevated White cell count (>20–25 $\times 10^9$/L)—sign of infection, infarction, collection, post-splenectomy
- Metabolic acidosis and elevated lactate—tissue hypoperfusion secondary to ischaemia or sepsis

Any delay in performing definitive investigations, decision making or implementing correct and appropriate treatment invariably leads to a worse outcome.

19.7.1 Specific Surgical Site Complications

Abdominal Compartment Syndrome The presence of an elevated intra-abdominal pressure that causes a disruption of regional blood flow eventually leading to organ failure and should be recognised early. This should be considered in women with intra-abdominal bleeding, large volume ascites and acute kidney injury, and in those with sepsis and aggressive fluid resuscitation

Table 19.5 Common causes of sepsis in Gynaecological Oncology

Surgical	Non-surgical
Anastomotic leak	Respiratory
Surgical site	Urinary, nephrostomy and catheter related
Urinary secondary to obstruction	Intravenous lines, especially CVP
Collection/abscess	Soft tissue infection e.g. cellulitis
Necrotic tissue/tumour	

Table 19.6 Post-operative problems associated with tumour site

Tumour site	Type of surgery	Potential post-operative complication
Ovary	Radical surgery including upper abdominal (diaphragmatic stripping, splenectomy, resection of tail of pancreas) and gastrointestinal procedures	Haemorrhage, ileus, wound breakdown, abscess/collection, anastomotic leak, stoma complications (prolapse, hernia, retraction, bleeding, necrosis), infection (chest, urine, wound), pleural effusion, pancreatic fistula/leak, thromboembolism, pain
Endometrium	Hysterectomy, pelvic and para-aortic lymphadenectomy	Urinary fistula, vascular injury, lymphocyst, abscess/collection, infection (chest, urine, wound), thromboembolism, pain
Cervix (Vagina)	Radical hysterectomy, pelvic and para-aortic lymphadenectomy	Urinary fistula, vascular injury, lymphocyst, anastomotic leak (bowel or urinary if post exenteration), abscess/collection, infection (chest, urine, wound), thromboembolism, pain
Vulval	Vulvectomy and groin node dissection	Wound breakdown, infection (wound, urine), recurrent cellulitis, lymphoedema, lymphocyst, neuralgia, urinary retention

causing extra-vascular sequestration or 'third-spacing'. Treatment is decompression of the abdomen. Patients undergoing laparotomy and have very oedematous bowel and tissue, and where primary closure is not possible, or deemed to be high risk for compartment syndrome, the abdomen can be left open and covered with various temporary abdominal closure devices and bowel bags. It is also important to remember that leaving the abdomen open can result in bowel damage and fistula formation. Re-look laparotomies are carried out every 24–48 h and some patients require a staged closure if the abdomen cannot be closed completely.

Burst Abdomen Wound dehiscence can be superficial involving the skin or deep where the rectus sheath is no longer intact (sheath dehiscence). Risk factors include obesity, diabetes, poor nutritional status (hypoalbuminaemia), long-term use of steroids, would infection and poor surgical technique. While a superficial wound dehiscence is visible and therefore easy to diagnose, a sheath dehiscence should be considered in the presence of serosanguinous fluid discharging from the wound, with or without symptoms of bowel obstruction. Management of a superficial wound dehiscence will include keeping the would clean and dry, treating infection and allowing the wound to heal by secondary intention. Immediate management of a sheath dehiscence would be to keep the exposed viscera warm and moist using sterile saline soaked swabs, minimise fluid loss and maintain body temperature. The patient should be kept nil by mouth and preparations made for a return to theatre. Administration of prophylactic broad spectrum antibiotics should be administered to reduce the risk of infection.

Dehiscence of Groin Wounds More common than abdominal wound dehiscence is the dehiscence of the groin wounds following groin node dissection for vulval cancer. This is because of the location of the wound and the difficulty in keeping the wounds clean, dry and immobile. This is exacerbated by with the drainage of lymph fluid often associated with this type of surgery. The risk of infection is high, and this complication is management by regular dressings and wound packing using alginate and hydrogel dressings. In these cases, the wounds heal by secondary intention and recover is often protracted. Any signs of infection should be treated promptly with targeted antibiotics.

Postoperative Bleeding Despite anticipating bleeding problems, postoperative haemorrhage can be covert, with the only sign being progressive haemodynamic deterioration. Primary haemorrhage occurs at the time of surgery. If difficult to control—particularly if from the liver, pelvis or other inaccessible sites -consideration should be given to packing the affected area, with a view to returning the patient to theatre at 48 h for removal of packs and reinspection of the operative site. Reactive haemorrhage occurs in the immediate post-operative period. This requires prompt detection and a return to theatre. Examining the abdomen for signs of distention and peritonism, as well as any drains may give an indication of intra-abdominal bleeding. Assessing the haematocrit in the drain fluid can sometimes be helpful in establishing if the patient is bleeding, especially if the fluid draining appears to be heavily blood stained. It is imperative that when assessing adequate haemostasis at the end of surgery, this is done when the patient is normotensive, so that you are not reassured of haemostasis in the hypotensive patient, as a return to theatre to secure any bleeding will be more likely.

Anastomotic Leak The signs of anastomotic leakage are of systemic instability with abdominal pain and/or peritonism, tachycardia and pyrexia. However, there may be a far more insidious presentation with low grade pyrexia, a prolonged ileus or failure to recover. It should be recognised that a defunctioning stoma does not exclude the possibility of an anastomotic leak. Risk factors for a leak include conditions that cause vascular dysfunction and impair wound healing such as diabetes, hypertension, immunosuppression, age and malnutrition; intra-operative factors such as surgical technique (poor anatomical blood supply, unrecognised mesenteric vessel damage, poor anastomotic technique), bleeding and excessive blood loss, poor tissue quality, infection/contamination, and the use of inotropic agents; post-operative complications such as intra-abdominal collection and infection, obstruction, constipation and ischaemia.

Necrotising Fasciitis Most gynaecological oncologists may only see two or three cases of necrotising fasciitis in their career lifetime, but should always be suspected in patients with influenza-type symptoms and localised pain or discomfort, especially in the presence of painful swelling and a purplish rash. The skin marking will then blister with blackish fluid, and patients undergo systemic collapse due to sepsis. Mortality is high in up to 75% of cases. The treatment is prompt, aggressive surgical debridement, with wide excision of all tissue back to healthy bleeding edges, broad-spectrum antibiotics and admission to critical care.

Stoma Complications Stomas may be loop or end, defunctioning or permanent, and involve the small or large bowel. They may be faecal or urinary stomas, such as ileal conduits. Small bowel stomas are most commonly ileostomies, and it is important to remember that the contents from an ileostomy are irritant on the skin, and therefore, when fashioning an ileostomy, a spout or 'rose bud' is formed. A bridge is sometimes used when forming a loop ileostomy, and if so tends to be left for 7 days. The use of a bridge delays stoma education, so consideration should be given to performing a 'bridgeless' ileostomy wherever possible. A colostomy will be more flushed to the skin, as the bowel contents are more solid and less irritant. A bluish or non-bleeding stoma should raise concerns of poor vascularity and should be refashioned as they are likely to become necrotic. Other stoma complications include prolapse, retraction, stenosis, and may require surgical intervention if problematic.

Urinary Tract Injury/Fistula Consider this as a possibility in women complaining of watery vaginal discharge or copious amount of urine-like fluid in the drain. Injuries may be immediate if they have occurred at the time of surgery, and are likely to be detected while the patient is still in hospital. Ureteric and urinary fistulae present more commonly on day 10–14, once the patient has been discharged, and are more likely to be due to devascularisation or thermal injury. Definitive diagnosis is best made with a CT Intravenous Urogram (CT IVU), but it is important to remember that a negative CT IVU does not exclude a fistula and should be repeated if the index of suspicion continues to remain high. Other less invasive tests include testing the fluid for urea and creatinine, and comparing this to serum and urinary levels. A level compatible with serum, does not however, exclude a urinary tract injury and a CT IVU should still be performed if the index of suspicion is high.

Cellulitis A common post-op complication, usually caused by *Staph aureus*. Prompt treatment with antibiotics is the mainstay of treatment. Marking the cellulitic area with a stoma marking pen will help assess the response to treatment.

Pancreatic Leak/Pancreatic Fistula Seen most commonly in patients undergoing upper abdominal cytoreductive surgery for ovarian cancer. This can occur following either inadvertent damage to the pancreatic tail during splenectomy or secondary to resection of tumour involving the pancreatic tail. A non-vacuum silastic drain should be inserted into the splenic bed, and day 3 and 5 blood and drain fluid should be measured for amylase levels. Any concerns regarding a leak or a fistula should be discussed an Hepato-Pancreato-Biliary (HPB) or upper GI surgeon. Most pancreatic leaks or fistulas are managed conservatively, although endoscopic intervention may be necessary in severe cases.

Pleural Effusion Post-op pleural effusions can occur secondary to congestive cardiac failure, pneumonia and pulmonary embolism, but can also occur following diaphragmatic stripping. Small effusions can be managed conservatively, with treatment of the underlying cause. Larger effusions may require drainage but should most certainly be tapped for cytology as a positive result will upstage the disease and may affect the need for or the type of adjuvant treatment.

Lymphocysts and Lymphoedema Most commonly seen after groin node dissection. The incidence has been reduced with the introduction of sentinel node detection and the avoidance of a full groin lymphadenectomy. While most lymphocysts are self-limiting, lymphoedema should be actively managed especially if severe. Prompt treatment with antibiotics in the presence of cellulitis, regular massaging and moisturising will help reduce the complications in chronic cases.

19.8 Peri-operative Enteral and Parenteral Nutrition

Malnutrition represents a deficiency or imbalance in nutrient supplies to the body, resulting in adverse effects on body composition and function. The National Institute for Health and Care Excellence (NICE) defines malnutrition using the following criteria [5]:

- Body Mass Index (BMI) < 18 kg/m^2
- Unintentional weight loss >10% within the last 3–6 months
- BMI <20kg/m^2 and Unintentional weight loss >10% within the last 3–6 months

Patients should be considered at risk if they have:

- Poor oral intake for more than 5 days and/or are likely to have on-going poor intake for 5 days or longer
- Poor absorptive capacity and/or high nutrient losses and/or increased nutritional needs from catabolic causes

Most surgical patients will have a nutrient deficiency, and metabolic changes are seen patients with cancer, in the stress response to surgery, and in sepsis. Cancer itself is a catabolic state, and along with symptoms of anorexia, early satiety, nausea and vomiting make maintaining adequate nutrition difficult, and exacerbate the problem of malnutrition.

Some patients who are admitted in a good nutritional state may go on to develop malnutrition as an in-patient. This is seen most commonly in women undergoing extensive surgery who then develop post-op complications such pneumonia, high output stoma, oral thrush, nausea and vomiting, which prevent them from eating adequately.

It is crucial to consider nutritional support for those with established malnourishment and to identify and treat those at risk. If left untreated, malnutrition is associated with increased post-operative complications, infection, increased length of hospital stay and greater mortality.

Potential or established malnutrition can be easily missed, and as a result, numerous screening tools have been developed to help with the identification of 'at risk' individuals. All hospitalised patients should undergo nutritional screening on admission, and at least weekly thereafter during their inpatient stay. The most commonly used, and validated, nutritional screening tool in the UK is MUST (Malnutrition Universal Screening Tool), which uses similar indicators to those described by NICE (Fig. 19.2) [6]. Other forms of assessment which can be done in clinic include asking the patient's family/friend accompanying them to clinic whether they have lost weight especially around their face and arms. This is obviously subjective and may not be apparent until a significant amount of weight has been lost. The use of food charts and low serum albumin levels should also be considered when assessing nutritional status. Other tools may include measurement of skin fold thickness.

The typical daily nutritional requirements are markedly altered in critical illness, where the response to stress and injury results in a significant rise in basal metabolic rate (BMR), and hence nutrient demand.

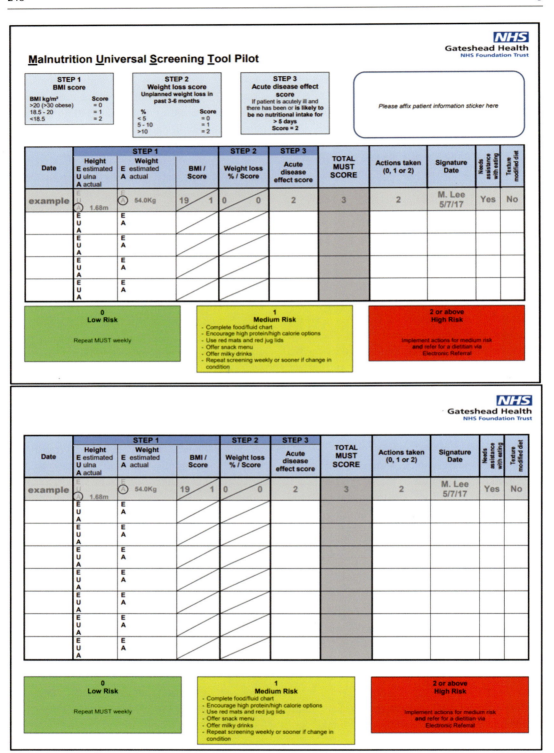

Fig. 19.2 Malnutrition universal screening tool

19.8.1 Treatment and Methods of Nutritional Support

The types of nutrition available are either via the **enteral or the parenteral route**.

19.8.1.1 Enteral Feeding

Wherever possible, feeding by the enteral route should be maintained. Sustained failure to feed using this route may lead to gut atrophy. In the Gynaecological Oncology setting, the use of enteral or parenteral feeding should have a definitive end point in sight. This can either be in the post-operative period to support recovery, or in the pre-treatment optimisation setting. In the latter situation, a period of a week is usually sufficient to assess response to treatment. In this group of patients, where the aim is to salvage and optimise so that they are fit enough to receive treatment, there must be a conversation with the patient and her family before the commencement of feeding to ensure that a clear understanding is reached and that feeding may be stopped if she continues to deteriorate despite active and aggressive medical intervention. This is to avoid the difficulty of having to stop nutritional support should the patient continue to deteriorate and be palliated.

Women receiving nutritional support should also be given 5 days of Pabrinex, which contains the water-soluble vitamins B1 (thiamine), B2 (riboflavin), B3 (nicotinamide) and B6 (pyridoxine) and C (ascorbic acid), preferably by the intravenous rather than the intramuscular route.

Types of Enteral Feeding
- Oral supplements. These can be protein or carbohydrate supplements, and should be used in conjunction with, and not as a substitute for, an oral diet. It is also important to remember that patients with cancer often suffer from altered taste and so adjustments to accommodate this should be made.
- Nasogastric (NG) feeding- This is commonly used when oral intake is deemed insufficient or unsafe, such as in patients with swallowing difficulties or impaired consciousness. In the Gynaecological Oncology patient, this is most often used in women with advanced ovarian cancer requiring optimisation prior to treatment with surgery or neoadjuvant chemotherapy, or following extensive upper abdominal and bowel surgery. These patients are often nutritionally deplete prior to admission, and may not be able to tolerate an oral diet in the immediate post-operative period. Successful feeding by this route requires access to a functioning gastrointestinal tract. Contraindications to nasogastric feeding include bowel obstruction, ischaemic bowel, massive gastrointestinal haemorrhage, severe diarrhoea/vomiting, small bowel fistula, and patient refusal. When there is a failure to absorb NG feed due to ileus, starting patients on a low volume of 10 mL/h elemental feed will reduce the risk of gut atrophy while maintaining a small degree of nutrition until the ileus resolves. Nasogastric feed may be delivered as a bolus or continuously over 16–24 h. The use of prokinetics helps to increase luminal transport and smooth muscle contraction in the gut, and the following drugs are commonly used—metoclopramide 10 mg IV tds, erythromycin 250 mg IV bd, domperidone 10 mg IV tds.
- Nasojejunal or nasoduodenal feeding—The use of a nasogastric/nasoduodenal tube should be considered in patients requiring enteral feeding who have high gastric aspirates. This allows the feed to be administered through the nasojejunal tube, while gastric fluid can be aspirated through the nasogastric component.
- Tube enterostomy—Tube enterostomy (gastrostomy, jejunostomy or duodenostomy) should be considered in patients who require prolonged nutritional support (>4 weeks), or if access via the oral/nasal route is not possible. The use of tube enterostomy feeding is not common in the gynaecological oncology patient.

Complications of Enteral Feeding
- Tube displacement—This is a common complication that can have serious consequences.

The position of the tube must be checked following its insertion and prior to administration of each feed.
- Pressure necrosis/fistulation—Pressure necrosis of the nasal passage can occur when the tube remains in place for long periods, and can lead to fistula formation.
- Tube blockage—Feeding tubes are finer than the NG tubes used for drainage, and therefore more susceptible to blockage. Most blockages can be resolved by flushing the tube with sterile water.
- Pulmonary aspiration—The risk of aspiration is increased in patients who have high aspirates, are vomiting, who have reduced levels of consciousness, or may be the result of tube misplacement. Large volume aspiration leading to pneumonia is associated with a high mortality rate.
- Diarrhoea—The cause is usually multifactorial and is most commonly due to antibiotic use and gut atrophy.

19.8.1.2 Parenteral Feeding

Parenteral nutrition should be considered in malnourished patients who are unable to tolerate enteral feeding, such as those with a non-functional gastrointestinal tract (e.g. bowel obstruction, small bowel fistulae) or who are unconscious (e.g. ventilated patients).

Total parenteral nutrition (TPN) must be administered into a central vein because of its high osmolality, and can precipitate thrombophlebitis if not. Peripheral parenteral nutrition (PPN) can be administered as a temporary alternative until central access is obtained. It is important to be aware that PPN does not provide equivalent nutrient replacement to TPN. Insertion of a long line will be required in patients receiving TPN for a prolonged period.

Complications of Parenteral Feeding
- Infection—Most of these arise from central lines, and the risk can be reduced by ensuring that lines are kept for no more than 7 days, adopting strict aseptic techniques during the insertion and handling of central line, and by allocating a dedicated lumen for the administration of TPN. In cases of suspected line sepsis, the line should be removed, the tip sent for culture and sensitivity, and appropriate antibiotics commenced.
- Line occlusion—Line blockage can be due to blockage within the lumen of the line, compression of the line, or malpositioning.
- Central venous thrombosis—The risk is increased in patients with long-term central lines, those with recurrent line infections, and those in whom multiple line changes are required. Treatment is with anticoagulation, therapy, and the duration of treatment will depend upon the extent of the thrombus and whether or not the central line is still required.
- Fluid and biochemical abnormalities—Patients on TPN can suffer from fluid overload, hyperglycaemia, hypertriglyceridaemia and electrolyte disturbances, so regular monitoring of these is essential with adjustment of the TPN as necessary.
- Refeeding syndrome—Refeeding syndrome occurs following the rapid reintroduction of carbohydrates (enterally or parenterally) in malnourished patients and may be fatal if unrecognised. It is characterised by marked hypophosphataemia, and the clinical effects vary greatly in type and severity. There is no diagnostic test for refeeding syndrome, and treatment should be started based upon a suggestive history or clinical picture.

19.9 Post-op Analgesia

Pain is inevitable following surgery, and pain control is important in ensuring as rapid a recovery as possible. Uncontrolled pain increases the risk of atelectasis by impairing the ability to cough and clear secretions, limits mobility and increases the risk of venous thromboembolism.

19.9.1 Principles of Acute Pain Management

The most important principle in surgical pain control is prevention. Simple measures such as taking regular analgesia, avoiding tension in the surgical wound and preventing drains or other tubes pulling on tissues or sutures is important. The aim is to keep the patient pain free and she should be encouraged to take her analgesia regularly in the immediate post-operative period (even if she is not in pain).

The choice of pain relief depends on many different factors including the site, nature and type of surgery, intensity of pain, co-morbidities and the ongoing clinical condition of the patient. The management options include:

- Oral preparations such as paracetamol, non-steroidal anti-inflammatory drugs and opioids.
- Regional anaesthetic techniques including epidural and spinal anaesthesia, rectus sheath catheters.
- Patient controlled analgesic system (PCAS)
- Local anaesthetic infiltrations along the wound

A combination of medication and regional anaesthetic techniques is desirable for many patients in the immediate post-operative period.

19.10 Summary and Conclusion

To conclude, surgery is a significant physiological insult, exacerbated when this is performed in a patient who is significantly unwell either due to the direct effects of the tumour (e.g. tumour necrosis or acute kidney injury) or because of systemic effects (anorexia, weight loss, biochemical and haematological abnormalities). For the best outcome, a combination of careful assessment, risk identification and pre-treatment optimisation, individualised treatment plans, and good post-operative care need to be ensured. The common complications are cardiovascular, respiratory, surgical site infections and complications, acute kidney injury, sepsis and multi organ failure. Steps should be taken to recognise them early and manage effectively. Ensuring right post operative feeding and pain management are other important aspects.

> **Key Points**
> 1. Identify the patient at risk and the types of complications they are at risk of.
> 2. Optimise the patient as much as possible prior to any form of treatment.
> 3. Act in a targeted and timely manner when faced with a clinically deteriorating patient.
> 4. Ask for help and escalate level of care promptly.
> 5. Good post-operative care is essential to ensure good patient outcomes.

References

1. American College of Surgeons. ACS national surgical quality improvement program [online]. 2004. Available from https://www.facs.org/quality-programs/acs-nsqip. Accessed 27 June 2021.
2. Royal College of Physicians. National Early Warning Score (NEWS) 2 [online]. 2017. Available from https://www.rcplondon.ac.uk/projects/outputs/national-early-warning-score-news-2. Accessed 27 June 2021.
3. National Institute for Health and Care Excellence (NICE). Sepsis: recognition, diagnosis and early management. NICE Guideline 51. London: NICE; Updated 2017.
4. Adapted from Antimicrobial Clinical Guidelines, Gateshead Health NHS Foundation Trust 2021.
5. National Institute for Health and Care Excellence (NICE). Nutrition support for adults: oral nutrition support, enteral tube feeding and parenteral nutrition. Clinical Guideline 32. London: NICE; Updated 2017.
6. Malnutrition Universal Screening Tool (MUST), Gateshead Health NHS Foundation Trust 2021.

Annexure: Staging of Gynaecological Cancers

Cancer Cervix (FIGO 2019 Staging)

FIGO stage*	Description	TNM staging**
Stage I	The carcinoma is strictly confined to the cervix (extension to the corpus should be disregarded)	T1N0M0
IA	Invasive carcinoma that can be diagnosed only by microscopy with maximum depth of invasion ≤5 mm[a]	T1a N0M0
	IA1 Measured stromal invasion ≤3 mm in depth	T1a1 N0M0
	IA2 Measured stromal invasion >3 mm and ≤5 mm in depth	T1a2N0M0
IB	Invasive carcinoma with measured deepest invasion >5 mm (greater than stage IA); lesion limited to the cervix uteri with size measured by maximum tumor diameter[b]	T1bN0M0
	IB1 Invasive carcinoma >5 mm depth of stromal invasion and ≤2 cm in greatest dimension	T1b1N0M0
	IB2 Invasive carcinoma >2 cm and ≤4 cm in greatest dimension	T1b2N0M0
	IB3 Invasive carcinoma >4 cm in greatest dimension	T1b3N0M0
Stage II	The cervical carcinoma invades beyond the uterus, but has not extended onto the lower third of the vagina or to the pelvic wall	T2N0M0
IIA	Involvement limited to the upper two-thirds of the vagina without parametrial invasion	T2aN0M0
	IIA1 Invasive carcinoma ≤4 cm in greatest dimension	T2a1N0M0
	IIA2 Invasive carcinoma >4 cm in greatest dimension	T2a2N0M0
IIB	With parametrial invasion but not up to the pelvic wall	T2bN0M0
Stage III	The carcinoma involves the lower third of the vagina and/or extends to the pelvic wall and/or causes hydronephrosis or non-functioning kidney and/or involves pelvic and/or paraaortic lymph nodes	T3N0/ N1M0
IIIA	Carcinoma involves lower third of the vagina, with no extension to the pelvic wall	T3aN0M0
IIIB	Extension to the pelvic wall and/or hydronephrosis or non-functioning kidney (unless known to be due to another cause)	T3bN0M0
IIIC	Involvement of pelvic and/or paraaortic lymph nodes (including micrometastases)[c], irrespective of tumor size and extent (with r and p notations)[d]	T3cN1M0
	IIIC1 Pelvic lymph node metastasis only	T3c1N1M0
	IIIC2 Paraaortic lymph node metastasis	T3c2N1M0

© The Editor(s) (if applicable) and The Author(s), under exclusive license to Springer Nature Switzerland AG 2022
K. Singh, B. Gupta (eds.), *Gynecological Oncology*, https://doi.org/10.1007/978-3-030-94110-9

FIGO stage*	Description	TNM staging**
Stage IV	The carcinoma has extended beyond the true pelvis or has involved (biopsy proven) the mucosa of the bladder or rectum. A bullous edema, as such, does not permit a case to be allotted to stage IV	Any T Any N M1
IVA	Spread of the growth to adjacent organs	
IVB	Spread to distant organs	

[a]Imaging and pathology can be used, when available, to supplement clinical findings with respect to tumor size and extent, in all stages. Pathological findings supercede imaging and clinical findings
[b]The involvement of vascular/lymphatic spaces should not change the staging. The lateral extent of the lesion is no longer considered
[c]Isolated tumor cells do not change the stage but their presence should be recorded
[d]Adding notation of r (imaging) and p (pathology), to indicate the findings that are used to allocate the case to stage IIIC. For example, if imaging indicates pelvic lymph node metastasis, the stage allocation would be Stage IIIC1r; if confirmed by pathological findings, it would be Stage IIIC1p. The type of imaging modality or pathology technique used should always be documented. When in doubt, the lower staging should be assigned
*FIGO staging
**TNM staging

Ovarian Cancer (FIGO Staging 2014)

FIGO stage	Description	TNM staging[a]
Stage I	**Tumor confined to ovaries or fallopian tube(s)**	T1-N0-M0
IA	Tumor limited to one ovary (capsule intact) or fallopian tube; no tumor on ovarian or fallopian tube surface; no malignant cells in the ascites or peritoneal washings	T1a-N0-M0
IB	Tumor limited to both ovaries (capsules intact) or fallopian tubes; no tumor on ovarian or fallopian tube surface; no malignant cells in the ascites or peritoneal washings	T1b-N0-M0
IC	Tumor limited to one or both ovaries or fallopian tubes, with any of the following:	T1C-N0-M0
	IC1: Surgical spill	T1C1-N0-M0
	IC2: Capsule ruptured before surgery or tumor on ovarian or fallopian tube surface	T1C2-N0-M0

FIGO stage	Description	TNM staging[a]
	IC3: Malignant cells in the ascites or peritoneal washings	T1C3-N0-M0
Stage II	**Tumor involves one or both ovaries or fallopian tubes with pelvic extension (below pelvic brim) or primary peritoneal cancer**	T2-N0-M0
IIA	Extension and/or implants on uterus and/or fallopian tubes and/or ovaries	T2a-N0-M0
IIB	Extension to other pelvic intraperitoneal tissues	T2b-N0-M0
Stage III	**Tumor involves one or both ovaries or fallopian tubes, or primary peritoneal cancer, with cytologically or histologically confirmed spread to the peritoneum outside the pelvis and/or metastasis to the retroperitoneal lymph nodes**	
IIIA	IIIA1: Positive retroperitoneal lymph nodes only (cytologically or histologically proven)	T1/T2-N1-M0
	IIIA1(i) Metastasis up to 10 mm in greatest dimension	
	IIIA1(ii) Metastasis more than 10 mm in greatest dimension	
	IIIA2: Microscopic extrapelvic (above the pelvic brim) peritoneal involvement with or without positive retroperitoneal lymph nodes	T3a2-N0/N1-M0
IIIB	Macroscopic peritoneal metastasis beyond the pelvis up to 2 cm in greatest dimension, with or without metastasis to the retroperitoneal lymph nodes	T3b-N0/N1-M0
IIIC	Macroscopic peritoneal metastasis beyond the pelvis more than 2 cm in greatest dimension, with or without metastasis to the retroperitoneal lymph nodes (includes extension of tumor to capsule of liver and spleen without parenchymal involvement of either organ)	T3c-N0/N1-M0
Stage IV	**Distant metastasis excluding peritoneal metastases**	Any T, any N, M1
Stage IVA	Pleural effusion with positive cytology	
Stage IVB	Parenchymal metastases and metastases to extra-abdominal organs (including inguinal lymph nodes and lymph nodes outside of the abdominal cavity)	

[a]T tumor, N lymph nodes, M metastasis

Annexure: Staging of Gynaecological Cancers

Cancer of Corpus Uteri (FIGO Staging 2009 and American Joint Committee on Cancer (AJCC))

FIGO stage	Description[c]	TNM staging[a]
Stage I	Tumor confined to the corpus uteri	T1 N0 M0
IA	No or less than half myometrial invasion	T1a N0 M0
IB	Invasion equal to or more than half of the myometrium	T1b N0 M0
II	Tumor invades cervical stroma, but does not extend beyond the uterus[b,d]	T2 N0 M0
III	Local and/or regional spread of the tumor	T3 N0–N1 M0
III A	Tumor invades the serosa of the corpus uteri and/or adnexae[b]	T3a N0 M0
III B	Vaginal involvement and/or parametrial involvement[b]	T3b N0 M0
IIIC	Metastases to pelvic and/or para-aortic lymph nodes[b] IIIC1 Positive pelvic nodes T1–T3 N1 M0 IIIC2 Positive para-aortic nodes with or without positive pelvic lymph nodes	T1–T3 N1 M0
IV	Tumor invades bladder and/or bowel mucosa, and/or distant metastases	
IVA	Tumor invasion of bladder and/or bowel mucosa	T4 Any N M0
IVB	Distant metastasis, including intra-abdominal metastases and/or inguinal nodes	Any T Any N M1

[a]T tumor, N lymph nodes, M metastasis
[b]Positive cytology has to be reported separately without changing the stage
[c]For all but stage IVB, grade (G) indicates percentage of tumor with a nonsquamous or nonmorular solid growth pattern:
- G1: ≤ 5%
- G2: 6–50%
- G3: >50%

Nuclear atypia excessive for the grade raises the grade of a G1 or G2 tumor by 1. In serous adenocarcinomas, clear cell adenocarcinomas, and squamous cell carcinomas, nuclear grading takes precedence. Adenocarcinomas with squamous differentiation are graded according to the nuclear grade of the glandular component
Carcinosarcomas should be staged as carcinoma
[d]Endocervical glandular involvement only should be considered as Stage I and no longer as Stage II

Cancer Vulva (FIGO 2021 Staging)

FIGO stage	Description	
I	Tumor confined to the vulva	
IA		Tumor size ≤2 cm and stromal invasion ≤1 mm[a]
IB		Tumor size >2 cm or stromal invasion >1 mm[a]
II	Tumor of any size with extension to lower one-third of the urethra, lower one-third of the vagina, lower one-third of the anus with negative nodes	
III	Tumor of any size with extension to upper part of adjacent perineal structures, or with any number of nonfixed, nonulcerated lymph node	
IIIA		Tumor of any size with disease extension to upper two-thirds of the urethra, upper two-thirds of the vagina, bladder mucosa, rectal mucosa, or regional lymph node metastases ≤5 mm
IIIB		Regional[b] lymph node metastases >5 mm
IIIC		Regional[b] lymph node metastases with extracapsular spread
IV	Tumor of any size fixed to bone, or fixed, ulcerated lymph node metastases, or distant metastases	
IVA		Disease fixed to pelvic bone, or fixed or ulcerated regional[b] lymph node metastases
IVB		Distant metastases

[a]Depth of invasion is measured from the basement membrane of the deepest, adjacent, dysplastic, tumor-free rete ridge (or nearest dysplastic rete peg) to the deepest point of invasion
[b]Regional refers to inguinal and femoral lymph nodes

Cancer Vagina (FIGO 2009 Staging)

Stage	Description
Stage I	Tumor should be confined to the vaginal wall
Stage II	The carcinoma has involved the subvaginal tissue but has not extended to pelvic wall
Stage III	The carcinoma has extended to the pelvic side wall, with involvement of the obturator internus, levator ani, or piriformis, external or internal iliac vessels, or bony structures

Stage	Description
Stage IVA	Tumor invades adjacent organs, involving the mucosal layer of the bladder, rectum, or urethra, or extension beyond the true pelvis. Bullous oedema of bladder does not permit a case to be allotted to stage IV
Stage IVB	Presence of distant metastases, including disease in the lungs or liver

TNM and Corresponding FIGO 2009 Staging for Vaginal Cancer

Stage	TNM
0[a]	Tis N0 M0
I	T1N0 M0
II	T2N0M0
III	T1–T3N1M0 T3 N0M0
IVA	T4 Any N M0
IVB	Any T Any N M1

[a]FIGO no longer includes stage 0 (Tis)

FIGO Staging System for Uterine Leiomyosarcomas and Endometrial Stromal Sarcomas (2009)

Stage	Definition
I	Tumor limited to uterus
IA	Tumor size less than or equal to 5 cm
IB	Tumor size more than 5 cm
II	Tumor extends beyond the uterus, within the pelvis
IIA	Adnexal involvement
IIB	Involvement of other pelvic tissues
III	Tumor involves abdominal tissues
IIIA	One site
IIIB	More than one site
IIIC	Metastasis to pelvic and/or para-aortic lymph nodes
IV	
IVA	Tumor invades bladder and/or rectum
IVB	Distant metastasis

FIGO Staging System for Adenosarcomas (2009)

Stage	Definition
I	Tumor limited to uterus
IA	Tumor limited to endometrium/endocervix with no myometrial invasion
IB	Less than or equal to half myometrial invasion
IC	More than half myometrial invasion
II	Tumor extends beyond the uterus, within the pelvis
IIA	Adnexal involvement
IIB	Involvement of other pelvic tissues
III	Tumor invades abdominal tissues
IIIA	One site
IIIB	More than one site
IIIC	Metastasis to pelvic and/or para-aortic lymph nodes
IV	
IVA	Tumor invades bladder and/or rectum
IVB	Distant metastasis

References

1. Bhatla N, Berek JS, Cuello Fredes M, Denny LA, Grenman S, Karunaratne K, Kehoe ST, Konishi I, Olawaiye AB, Prat J, Sankaranarayanan R, Brierley J, Mutch D, Querleu D, Cibula D, Quinn M, Botha H, Sigurd L, Rice L, Ryu HS, Ngan H, Mäenpää J, Andrijono A, Purwoto G, Maheshwari A, Bafna UD, Plante M, Natarajan J. Revised FIGO staging for carcinoma of the cervix uteri. Int J Gynaecol Obstet. 2019;145(1):129–35. https://doi.org/10.1002/ijgo.12749. Erratum in: Int J Gynaecol Obstet. 2019 Nov;147(2):279–80.
2. Corrigendum to Revised FIGO staging for carcinoma of the cervix uteri [Int J Gynecol Obstet 145(2019) 129–35]. Int J Gynecol Obstet. 2019;147(2):279–80. https://doi.org/10.1002/ijgo.12969. Erratum for: Int J Gynaecol Obstet. 2019;145(1):129–35.
3. Prat J, FIGO Committee on Gynecologic Oncology. Staging classification for cancer of the ovary, fallopian tube, and peritoneum: abridged republication of guidelines from the International Federation of Gynecology and Obstetrics (FIGO). Obstet Gynecol. 2015;126(1):171–4.

4. Based on staging established by the International Federation of Gynecology and Obstetrics (FIGO) and American Joint Committee on Cancer (AJCC), AJCC Cancer Staging Manual. 8th ed. New York: Springer. 2017.
5. Olawaiye AB, Cotler J, Cuello MA, Bhatla N, Okamoto A, Wilailak S, Purandare CN, Lindeque G, Berek JS, Kehoe S. FIGO staging for carcinoma of the vulva: 2021 revision. Int J Gynaecol Obstet. 2021;155(1):43–7.
6. American Joint Committee on Cancer. Vagina. In: Amin MB, Edge S, Greene F, Byrd DR, Brookland RK, et al, editors. AJCC cancer staging manual. 8th ed. New York: Springer; 2017. 649–656.

Index

A
Abdominal adhesiolysis, 112
Abdominal compartment syndrome, 244
Ablative methods, 89
    advantages and disadvantages of, 92
    cryotherapy, 89, 90
    prerequisites for, 89
    thermal ablation, 90, 91
Acid-base balance, 240
Acute bowel obstruction, 111
    alternative treatment, 112, 113
    conservative management, 111
    surgical management, 112
Acute kidney injury (AKI), 241
    causes of, 241
    development of AKI in surgical patient, 241
Acute pain management, 250–251
Adenocarcinoma in situ, AIN, 185
Adequate exposure, 56
Adhesiolysis, 56
Adjuvant chemotherapy by histology, 128
Adjuvant EBRT, 156
Adjuvant radiotherapy, 157
ADNEX model, 223
Adult granulosa cell tumour (AGCT), 196
Airflow obstruction, 238
Alpha fetoprotein, 6
Alvimopan, 67
American Joint Committee on Cancer (AJCC) staging, 232
Anaemia, 108
Analgesic ladder, 118, 170
Anastomotic leak, 245
Anti-angiogenic agents, 127
Anticoagulation therapy, 240
Antimicrobial prophylaxis, 64
Anti-neoplastic therapy, 113, 114
Arterial and central venous pressure measurements, 237
Arterial blood gases (ABGs), 240
Arterial injuries, 76
Arterial partial pressure of oxygen (PaO_2), 240
Artificial intelligence techniques, 232
Ascites, 113
    anti-neoplastic therapy, 113
    chylous ascites, 119, 120
    definition of, 113
    diuretic therapy, 113
    drainage of, 113
    indwelling catheters, 113
    malignant, 165
Atelectasis, 240
Avascular necrosis, 82

B
Bad news, 23
Benign/malignant ovarian tumors, 6
Benzodiazepines, 166
Bevacizumab, 128, 132, 165
Biochemical response assessment, 126
Bladder injury, 83
Bleeding in advanced gynaecological cancers, 163–165
Body mass index, 4
Bowel injury, 83
Bowel obstruction (BO), 111
Brachytherapy, 147, 149, 152–154
Breathlessness, 165, 166
Burst abdomen, 245

C
CA125, 5
Calvert formula, 126
Cancer Care Review, 28
Cancer incidence and mortality, 1
Cancer pain, 117
    analgesic ladder for, 118
    interventions for, 118
    management of, 118
    mechanism of, 117
    opioids for, 118
    physical modalities for, 118, 119

Cancer surgery
  before operation
    consenting, 52, 53
    decision-making, 56
    exploration, 55, 56
    multidisciplinary approach, 52
    noise level, 54
    operation, 55
    patient selection, 52
    prehabilitation, 53
    resection, 57
    surgeon, 54, 55
    team, 53, 54
    theatre environment, 53, 54
  postoperative period, 57, 58
Cancer susceptibility genes (CSGs), 207
Cancer syndromes, 209
Cannabidiol (CBD) oil, 33
Carbohydrate antigen 19-9 (CA19-9), 6
Cardiac output, 238
Cardiac toxicities, 110
Cardiopulmonary exercise testing (CPEX), 235
Cardiovascular complications, 236
Carvedilol, 110
Catumaxomab, 165
Cell cycle, 126
Cellulitis, 246
Central venous pressure (CVP), 237
Central venous thrombosis, 250
Cervical biopsy, 88
Cervical cancer, 75, 157
Cervical epithelial neoplasia, 203
Cervical glandular neoplasia, 185, 186
Cervical intraepithelial neoplasia (CIN), 89, 183
Cervical squamous neoplasia, 183–185
Cervical tumours, 203
Cervix
  cervical glandular neoplasia, 185, 186
  cervical squamous neoplasia, 183–185
  HPV in situ hybridisation, 186
Chemotherapy, 126
Chemotherapy agents, 124
Chemotherapy drugs, 126
Chemotherapy-related side-effects, 107, 108
  cardiac toxicities, 110
  gastrointestinal toxicities, 108, 110
  haematologic toxicities, 108
  neurologic toxicities, 110
Chest tube drainage, 102–104
Choriocarcinoma, 197
Chylous ascites, 119, 120
CLASS protocol, 20, 21
  acknowledge emotions, 21
  body language, 21
  context (setting), 21
  family members/friends, 21
  listening skills, 21
  strategy, 22
  summary, 22
  touch, 21
Clavien-Dindo classification, 74
Clear cell carcinomas of endometrium, 202
Clinical practice, 35
Cognitive Behaviour Therapy (CBT), 29
Cold coagulation, *see* Thermal ablation
Cold knife conisation, 93–95
Colloids, 238
Colposcopy, 87–89
Communication
  best practices for, 20, 21
  CLASS protocol, 21
    acknowledge emotions, 21
    body language, 21
    context (setting), 21
    family members/friends, 21
    listening skills, 21
    strategy, 22
    summary, 22
    touch, 21
  definition of, 19
  flows of, 19, 20
  informed consent, 23
    express consent, 24
    implied consent, 23
    model for, 24, 25
  Montgomery ruling, 24
  reviewing decisions, 24
  with other specialities, 22, 23
  with vulnerable patients, 22
Complete transection of the ureter, 82
Computed tomography (CT), 223–226, 231
Concurrent chemoradiation (CCRT), 147, 157, 158
Concurrent chemotherapy, 157
Conservative management, 111, 167
Contrast enhanced CT (CECT) study, 224
Contrast induced nephropathy (CIN), 224
Coordinator, 14
Cowden's syndrome, 209
C-reactive protein (CRP), 81
Crushing injury, 82
Cryotherapy, 89, 90
Crystalloids, 238
Cystoscopy, 101, 102
Cytokeratins, 175

D

D-dimmers, 115
Deep vein thrombosis (DVT), 115, 116
Dehiscence of groin wounds, 245
Dexrazoxane, 110
Diagnostic test accuracy (DTA) studies, 41, 43
Diarrhoea, 108, 110, 250
Differentiated VIN, 182
Diuretic therapy, 113

Dostarlimab, 134
Drains, 64

E
Eastern Cooperative Oncology Group (ECOG), 3
Eastern Cooperative Oncology Group performance status (ECOG PS), 37
Education and Support Elements, 28
Effective communication, 19, 20
Embolism, 77, 80
Emotional support, 32
Endometrial biopsy, 95
Endometrial cancer (EC)
    diagnosis, genetic testing at, 213, 214
    hormonal therapy in, 139–142
    immunotherapy in, 134, 135
    radiotherapy in, 156, 157
    SACT in, 132–134
    types of, 178
Endometrial carcinomas, 197, 198
Endometrial stromal nodules, 182
Endometrial stromal sarcomas, 203
Endometrioid carcinomas of endometrium, 197–201
Endoscopic procedures, 164
Enhanced Recovery After Surgery (ERAS), 61
    benefits of, 69
    cancer prehabilitation
        definition of, 61
        medical optimization, 62
        nutritional interventions, 62
        physical interventions, 62
        psychological and social interventions, 62, 63
    discharge, 67
    early ambulation, 67
    minimizing surgical insult, 64
    pain management, 65, 66
    perioperative fluid management, 65
    peri-operative normoglycemia maintenance, 63
    perioperative nutrition, 66
    preoperative bowel preparation, 63
    prevention of post-operative ileus, 67
    standard anaesthetic protocol, 65
    surgical site infection reduction bundle, 64
    VTE and prophylaxis, 63, 64
Enhancing the QUAlity and Transparency Of health Research (EQUATOR) Network, 43
Enteral feeding, 249
    complications, 249, 250
    types of, 249
Enteral/parenteral route, 249
Epithelial ovarian cancer (EOC), 5, 143, 144
Estimated glomerular filtration rate (eGFR, 224
European Society of Medical Oncology, 200
Evidence-based medicine (EBM), 35
    critical appraisal (appraise), 44
        GRADE framework, 45
        support critical appraisal, 44, 46
    in gynaeoncology, 45, 46
    searching for evidence (acquire)
        guidelines and synthesised summaries, 44
        hierarchy of evidence, 36
        primary research studies, 36–43
        systematic reviews, scoping reviews and meta-analysis, 43, 44
    structured question, 35, 36
Excisional biopsy, 91–95
Express consent, 24
External beam radiotherapy (EBRT), 147, 151, 158
External iliac venous injury repair, 76
Extramammary Paget's disease (EMPD), 182, 183

F
Fallopian tube, 178
Family survivorship, 33
FDG PET CT, 231
Fine needle aspiration biopsy of superficial groin lymph, 98
Fluid and biochemical abnormalities, 250
Fluorine 18 fluoro-2-deoxy-D-glucose (^{18}F-FDG), 229
Full-thickness wound dehiscence, 99–101
Functional residual capacity (FRC) with pulmonary vascular dysfunction, 238

G
Gastrointestinal toxicities, 108, 110
General Medical Council (GMC), 15, 16, 20
Generic working, 55
Genetics, 207, 208
    advantages of, 210, 211
    cancer syndromes, 209
    disadvantages of, 211
    endometrial cancer diagnosis, genetic testing at, 213, 214
    ovarian cancer diagnosis, genetic testing at, 212, 213
    population testing, 214
    traditional family history (FH), 211, 212
    variants, classes of, 210
Germ cell tumour, 176, 197
Grading of Recommendations Assessment, Development and Evaluation (GRADE) framework, 44
Granulocyte Colony Stimulating Factor (GCSF), 244
Granulosa cell tumours (GCT), 144
Gross Tumour Volume (GTV), 151
Gynaecological malignancy, 19, 27
Gynae Oncology
    diagnostic pathway, 1, 2
    hematological Investigations, 5, 6
    hereditary and genetic factors, assessment of, 4
    histopathology and cytology, 8
    history and physical assessment, 2, 3
    hub and spoke model, 2
    imaging, 6, 7
    nutritional assessment, 4
    psychological and social assessment of, 5
Gynandroblastoma, 196

H

Haematologic toxicities, 108
Haemorrhage
    management of, 76
    primary, 76
    reactionary, 76, 77
    secondary, 76, 77
    vascular injury, 76–79
Hallmarks of cancer, 124
Health and Social Care Act 2012 (HSCA), 16
Hematuria, 164
Heparin-induced thrombocytopenia (HIT), 116
Hepato-Pancreato-Biliary (HPB), 246
Hereditary breast and ovarian cancer (HBOC), 209
Hereditary cancer, 5
High-dose-rate (HDR) brachytherapy, 149
High-grade cervical glandular intraepithelial neoplasia (HGCGIN), 185
High grade serous carcinoma (HGS), 193–195
High grade serous ovarian cancer, 129
High-resolution CT (HRCT), 224
Holistic approach
    cancer journey
        palliation and end of life, 31, 32
        recurrence, 31
        remission, 31
        support at diagnosis, 28
        support during treatment, 28–31
    coping mechanisms, 32
    families and carers, support for, 33
    holistic needs, 27
    recovery package, 28
Holistic Needs Assessment (HNA), 28
Homologous recombination deficiency (HRD), 131, 194–195
Hormonal therapy (HT) in gynaecological malignancies, 139
    endometrial cancer (EC), 139–142
    ovarian cancer, 143, 144
    uterine sarcomas, 142, 143
Hormone replacement therapy (HRT), 29
Hospital-acquired infections, 242
HPV-independent VIN, 182
HPV in situ hybridisation (ISH), 186
Hub and spoke model, 1, 2
Hyperkalaemia, 241
Hypofractionated radiotherapy, 151
Hypovolaemia, 237
Hypoxia, 238
Hysteroscopy, 95, 96

I

Idea, Development, Exploration, Assessment, Long-term follow-up (IDEAL) network, 35
Image guided brachytherapy (IGBT), 154
Image guided interventions, 230, 231
Image Guided Radiotherapy (IGRT), 147, 151
Immunohistochemistry (IHC)
    cervix
        cervical glandular neoplasia, 185, 186
        cervical squamous neoplasia, 183–185
        HPV in situ hybridisation, 186
    definition of, 173
    for diagnosis, 173, 174
    fallopian tube, 178
    MMR immunohistochemistry, 180
    for ovary, 174
        carcinoma, 174
        germ cell tumour, 176
        metastatic carcinomas, 176, 178
        neuroendocrine neoplasms, 176
        p53, 174, 175
        pseudomyxoma peritonei, 178
        sex cord-stromal tumours, 175
        WT1, 175
    predictive information, 174
    prognostic information, 174
    serous fluid cytology, 188
    undifferentiated malignancies, 186, 188
    uterine corpus, 178, 180
    uterine mesenchymal neoplasms, 180, 182
    vulva
        EMPD, 182, 183
        vulval squamous neoplasia, 182, 183
Implied consent, 23
Incisional hernias, 84
Indwelling catheters, 113
Infections, 80, 81, 250
Inferior vena cava (IVC) filters, 117
Informed consent, 23
    express consent, 24
    implied consent, 23
    model for, 24, 25
Inotropic agents, 238
Intensity-Modulated Radiotherapy (IMRT), 147, 151
Intermittent pneumatic compression (IPC) devices, 116
International Ovarian Tumor Analysis (IOTA), 6
Interstitial brachytherapy (ISBT), 147, 154
Intra-cavity brachytherapy (ICBT), 147, 153
Intrapleural application of fibrinolytic, 114
Invasive squamous cell carcinoma, 185
Iodinated water-soluble contrast agents, 224

J

Juvenile granulosa cell tumour, 196

L

Large loop excision of the transformation zone (LLETZ), 92, 93
Lead, 14
Leiomyosarcomas, 203
Life-prolonging surgery, 52
Life-threatening complications, management of, 241
Li-Fraumeni syndrome (LFS), 210
Ligation/acute angulation, 82
Line occlusion, 250
Lloyd-Davies position, 55
Loop electrosurgical excision procedure (LEEP), *see* Large loop excision of the transformation zone (LLETZ)

Loperamide, 108
Low grade endometrial stromal sarcomas (LG-ESS), 142, 143
Low grade serous carcinoma (LGSC), 195
Low grade serous ovarian cancer (LGSOC), 132
Low molecular weight heparin (LMWH), 116
Lymphadenectomy, 81
Lymphadenectomy in Ovarian Neoplasms (LION) trial, 35
Lymphatic complication, 81
Lymph nodes evaluation, 230
Lymphocysts, 247
Lymphoedema, 247
Lymphovascular space invasion (LVSI), 132
Lynch syndrome (LS), 174, 197, 209

M
Magnetic resonance imaging (MRI), 226, 228, 229, 232
Malignancy index, 6
Malignant ascites, 165
Malignant bowel obstruction (MBO), 166–168
Malignant melanoma, 204
Malignant pleural effusion (MPE), 114
Malnutrition, 4, 247
MEK inhibitors, 132
Memorial Sloan Kettering Cancer Surgical Secondary Events (SSE) Database, 74
Mesenchymal tumours, 204
Metastatic carcinomas, 176, 178
Methotrexate, 135
Meticulous haemostasis, 57
Microcystic stromal tumour, 196
Microsatellite instability (MSI), 209
Minimally invasive surgery (MIS), 64
Mini Nutritional Assessment tools, 4
Minor surgical procedures
    ablative methods, 89
        advantages and disadvantages of, 92
        cryotherapy, 89, 90
        prerequisites for, 89
        thermal ablation, 90, 91
    chest tube drainage, 102–104
    colposcopy, 87–89
    cystoscopy, 101, 102
    definition of, 87
    endometrial biopsy, 95
    excisional biopsy, 91–95
    fine needle aspiration biopsy of superficial groin lymph, 98
    hysteroscopy, 95, 96
    paracentesis, 98, 99
    pyometra drainage, 96
    Tru cut biopsy, 97, 98
    vulval biopsy, 96, 97
    wound dehiscence, management of, 99–101
Mismatch repair (MMR) immunohistochemistry, 180
Mitogen-activated protein kinase (MAPK) pathway, 124
Modern energy devices, 57
Monsel's paste, 164
Montgomery ruling, 24

mTOR inhibitors, 139
Mucinous carcinoma (MC), 196
Multidisciplinary approach, 52
Multi-disciplinary team (MDT), 11, 12, 22
    characteristics of, 12, 13
    environment, 14, 15
    governance and responsibilities, 15
    legal position of, recommendations, 15, 16
    limitations, 16, 17
    people and processes, 13, 14
Multiple organ failure, 242, 244
Multiplex Ligation-dependent Probe Amplification (MLPA), 195

N
Nasoduodenal feeding, 249
Nasogastric (NG) feeding, 249
Nasogastric tube (NGT), 111
Nasojejunal feeding, 249
National Health Services (NHS) cancer plan, 12
National Institute for Clinical Excellence (NICE), 200
Nausea/vomiting, 108
Necrotising enterocolitis, 110
Necrotising fasciitis, 246
Neo(adjuvant) treatment, 128
Nerve injury, 83
Neuroendocrine neoplasms, 176
Neurologic toxicities, 110
Neutropenia, 108
Neutropenic sepsis, 242
Non-aspiration capillary-action technique, 98
Non-steroidal anti-inflammatory drugs (NSAIDs), 118
Normothermia, 64

O
Observational studies, 37, 39, 40
Olaparib, 132
Oncology practitioner, 1
Opioids, 118, 166
Oral supplements, 249
Organs at risk (OAR), 147
Ovarian cancer diagnosis, genetic testing at, 212, 213
Ovarian cancer, hormonal therapy (HT) in
    epithelial ovarian cancer (EOC), 143, 144
    granulosa cell tumours (GCT), 144
Ovarian carcinomas, 193–196
Ovarian clear cell carcinoma (OCCC), 196
Ovarian endometrioid carcinoma (OEC), 195–196
Ovarian high grade serous carcinomas, 178
Ovarian tumors
    germ cell tumours, 197
    high grade serous carcinoma, 193–195
    low grade serous carcinoma, 195
    mucinous carcinoma, 196
    ovarian clear cell carcinoma, 196
    ovarian endometrioid carcinoma, 195–196
    sex cord stromal tumours, 196–197
    undifferentiated/de-differentiated carcinoma, 196

Ovary, IHC for, 174
   carcinoma, 174
   germ cell tumour, 176
   metastatic carcinomas, 176, 178
   neuroendocrine neoplasms, 176
   p53, 174, 175
   pseudomyxoma peritonei, 178
   sex cord-stromal tumours, 175
   WT1, 175

P
p16, 183, 184, 186
p53, 174, 175
Packing, 56
Pain assessment, 31, 168
Pain management, 31, 65, 66
Palliation, 31, 32, 158
Palliative care, 161
   bleeding in advanced gynaecological cancers, 163–165
   breathlessness, 165, 166
   current status of, 161, 162
   definition of, 161
   end-of-life care, 169
   malignant ascites, 165
   malignant bowel obstruction, 166–168
   management of other symptoms, 168, 169
   pain, 168
   services, 162
   symptom management, 163
   timing of, 162, 163
Palliative gastrostomy tubes, 112
Palliative radiotherapy, 151
Pancreatic leak/pancreatic fistula, 246
Paracentesis, 98, 99, 165
Paralytic ileus, 84
Parenteral feeding, 250
Partial transection of the ureter, 82
Patient Generated Global Assessment Tool (PG-SGA), 4
PEComas, 182
Pelvic brim, 81
Peri-operative enteral and parenteral nutrition, 247, 249, 250
Personalised medicine, 127
Person centred coordinated care, 20
Peutz-Jeghers syndrome (PJS), 196, 209
Platinum based chemotherapy in early-stage disease (FIGO I-II), 128
Platinum free interval, 129
Pleural effusion, 114, 166, 247
Pleural space, 114
Pleurectomy, 114
Pleurodesis, 114, 166
PleurX drain, 102–104, 114
Pneumonia, 240
Polyadenosine diphosphate ribose polymerase (PARP) inhibitors, 41, 42, 108, 129–132
Population, intervention, comparison, outcome and design (PICOD), 35–36

Population testing, 214
Post-operative analgesia, 250, 251
Postoperative bleeding, 245
Post-operative care, 235
   arterial and central venous pressure measurements, 237
   cardiovascular complications, 236
   colloids and crystalloids, 238
   factors influencing need for haemodynamic support, 237
   inotropic agents, 238
   patient at risk identification, 235, 236
   renal failure (*see* Acute kidney injury (AKI))
   respiratory complications, 238, 240
      ABGs and acid-base balance, 240
      atelectasis, 240
      pneumonia, 240
      pulmonary embolism, 240, 241
   surgical site management, 244–247
Preferred Reporting Items for Systematic Reviews and Meta-Analyses (PRISMA) guidelines, 43
Prehabilitation, 53
   definition of, 61
   medical optimization, 62
   nutritional interventions, 62
   physical interventions, 62
   psychological and social interventions, 62, 63
Presacral haemorrhage/bleeding, 76
Primary antibody, 173
Primary debulking surgery, 128
Primary palliative care, 162
Primary research studies, 36
Primary tubo-ovarian carcinomas, 175
Primary vulval and vaginal malignancies, 232
Progesterone, 139
Progestins, 142
Proton beam therapy (PBT), 147
Pseudomyxoma peritonei, 178
Psychotherapy, 118, 119
Pulmonary aspiration, 250
Pulmonary embolism (PE), 115, 240, 241
Pulmonary oedema, 242
Pyometra drainage, 96

R
Radiation therapy, 164
Radiobiology, 149
Radiogenomics, 232
Radiological response, 127
Radiology investigations
   computed tomography, 223–226
   ^{18}F-FDG PET CT, 229, 230
   image guided interventions, 230, 231
   lymph nodes evaluation, 230
   MRI, 226, 228, 229
   recommended imaging pathways, 231
   ultrasound, 221
      cervical, 223
      endometrial, 223

Index

ovarian, 221–223
Radiomics, 232
Radiotherapy, 147
  in cervical cancer, 157
  in endometrial cancer, 156, 157
  in palliation, 158
  planning and delivery, 151, 152
  radiation physics, 147, 149
  toxicity, 150, 151
  in vaginal cancer, 158
  in vulval cancer, 158
Randomised control trials (RCT), 36–38
RAS-MAPK signalling pathway, 133
Reactionary haemorrhage, management of, 77
Reducing early salpingectomy and delayed oophorectomy (RRESDO), 211
Refeeding syndrome, 250
Renal failure, *see* Acute kidney injury (AKI)
Renal replacement therapy, 241
Respiratory complications, 238, 240
  arterial blood gases and acid-base balance, 240
  atelectasis, 240
  pneumonia, 240
  pulmonary embolism, 240, 241
Response assessment, 126
Royal College of Obstetricians and Gynaecologist (RCOG), 20

S

Secondary antibody, 173
Secondary haemorrhage, management of, 77
Selective oestrogen receptor modulators (SERM), 139
Sepsis, 242, 244
Serous carcinomas of endometrium, 200, 202
Serous fluid cytology, 188
Serous intraepithelial carcinoma (STIC), 178
Sertoli Leydig cell tumour (SLCT), 196
Serum albumin ascitic gradient (SAAG), 113
Sex cord stromal tumours (SCST), 175, 196–197
Sex cord tumour with annular tubules (SCTAT), 196–197
Shift in fluid balance, 84
Small cell carcinoma of hypercalcaemic type, 197
Specialty palliative care, 162
Stents, 112
Stoma complications, 246
Suction aspiration technique, 98
Superficial dehiscence, 99
Superficial groin lymph, fine needle aspiration biopsy of, 98
Surgical complications, 75
  vs. adverse effect/sequelae of surgery, 73, 74
  defined, 73
  factors affecting rates, 74, 75
  intra-operative, 75
    haemorrhage, 76–79
    infections, 80, 81
    lymphatic complication, 81
    nerve injuries, 83
    paralytic ileus, 84
    shift in fluid balance, 84
    thrombosis and embolism, 77, 80
    visceral injuries, 81–84
  late postoperative complications, 84
  prevention of, 84
  professional duty of candour, 73
  terminology for incidence of, 75
Surgical site infection reduction bundles, 64
Surgical site management, 244–247
Systemic anti-cancer treatment (SACT), 123
  advanced disease (FIGO III-IV), 128
  cervical, vulval and rare gynaecological cancers, 135
  early stage disease (FIGO I-II), 128
  in endometrial cancer, 132–134
  immunotherapy in endometrial cancer, 134, 135
  LGSOC, target treatment in, 132
  PARP inhibitors in ovarian cancer, 129–132
  principles, 123–128
  relapsed disease, 129
Systemic therapy, 164

T

Table-mounted surgical retractors, 56
Targeted agents used in gynaecological cancer, 127
Therapeutic thoracentesis, 114
Thermal ablation, 90, 91
Thrombocytopenia, 108
Thrombosis, 77, 80
Total pain, 168, 169
Total parenteral nutrition (TPN), 250
TP53 mutations (*TP53*muts), 180, 193
Traction-countertraction, 57
Traditional family history (FH), 211, 212
Transabdominal ultrasound, 221
Transcutaneous arterial embolization, 164
Transcutaneous electrical nerve stimulation (TENS) therapy, 118–119
Translational research, 39, 41, 42
Transvaginal sonography (TVS), 6, 221
Treatment Summary, 28
Tru cut biopsy, 97, 98
Tube enterostomy, 249
Tumor markers, 5, 6
Tumour boards, 12
Tumour necrosis factor (TNF), 113
Tunneled Pleural Catheter (TPC), 114
T2-weighted imaging (T2 WI), 226

U

Ultrasound, 221, 231
  cervical, 223
  endometrial, 223
  ovarian, 221–223
Ultrasound guided fine needle aspiration (US-FNAC), 98
Undifferentiated/de-differentiated carcinoma, 196
Undifferentiated malignancies, 186, 188
Unfractionated heparin, 116
Ureter crossing the uterine vessels, 81

Ureteric injuries, 81–83
Urinary catheters, 64
Urinary tract injury/fistula, 246
Uterine corpus, 178, 180
Uterine leiomyosarcomas (u-LMS), 142
Uterine mesenchymal neoplasms, 180, 182
Uterine sarcomas, 231
Uterine sarcomas, hormonal therapy (HT) in
    low grade endometrial stromal sarcomas (LG-ESS), 142, 143
    uterine leiomyosarcomas (u-LMS), 142
Uterine tumours
    carcinosarcomas, 202
    clear cell carcinomas, 202
    endometrial carcinomas, 197, 198
    endometrial stromal sarcomas, 203
    endometrioid carcinomas, 197–201
    leiomyosarcomas, 203
    molecular stratification, 197
    serous carcinomas of endometrium, 200, 202
Uterine tumours resembling ovarian sex cord tumour (UTROSCT), 182

V
Vaginal brachytherapy (VBT), 147, 154
Vaginal cancer, 158
Vaginal packing, 164
Variants, classes of, 210
Variants of Uncertain Significance (VUS), 210
Vascular injuries, management of, 76–79
Venous injuries, 76

Venous thromboembolism (VTE), 63, 64, 107
    clinical presentation and diagnosis, 115, 116
    epidemiology and aetiology, 115
    mechanical prophylaxis, 116
    pharmacological prophylaxis, 116, 117
    treatment, 117
Vesicoureteric junction, 81
Visceral injuries
    bladder injuries, 83
    bowel injuries, 83
    nerve injuries, 83
    ureteric injuries, 81–83
Volumetric Modulated Arc Therapy (VMAT), 147, 151
Vulva
    EMPD, 182, 183
    vulval squamous neoplasia, 182, 183
Vulval and vaginal tumours, 203–204
Vulval biopsy, 96, 97
Vulval cancer, 158
Vulval intraepithelial neoplasia (VIN), 182
Vulval squamous neoplasia, 182, 183, 203–204

W
Warfarin, 241
Wound dehiscence, management of, 99–101
WT1 nuclear expression, 175

Z
Zero-sum fluid balance, 65

Printed in the United States
by Baker & Taylor Publisher Services